INTRODUCTION TO HOSPITAL ACCOUNTING

Second Edition

INTRODUCTION TO HOSPITAL ACCOUNTING

L. Vann Seawell, DBA, CPA
Professor of Accounting
Indiana University

HFMA
Healthcare Financial Management Association
Oak Brook, Illinois

Kendall/Hunt Publishing Company
Dubuque, Iowa

Library of Congress Catalog Card Number: 86–80043

ISBN 0–8403–3905–4

Fourth Printing, 1986

Printed in the United States of America

B 403905 01

To Stanley A. Pressler,
who got me started—
which I appreciate—
and gave me his friendship
—*that* I treasure.

Foreword to the 1977 Revised Edition

Hospitals are becoming increasingly aware of the financial resources necessary for continued delivery of the institutional health care required by local communities. This need is expressed in accounting terms with figures derived from a sound bookkeeping system.

In the short time span since the Hospital Financial Management Association entered the field of textbook publishing with the 1971 edition of Dr. Seawell's *Introduction to Hospital Accounting*, a number of significant publications have been added to accounting literature—notably the American Institute of CPAs' *Hospital Audit Guide*, the American Hospital Association's *Chart of Accounts for Hospitals* and Dr. Seawell's *Hospital Financial Accounting: Theory and Practice*. Reflecting the sophistication in hospital accounting evidenced by these publications, Dr. Seawell has expanded the present text from its 1971 predecessor.

The Hospital Financial Management Association represents many thousands of individuals whose responsibility is the practical application of accounting knowledge in hospitals. Dr. Seawell, with over 20 years of experience in the hospital accounting environment, epitomizes the growing number of academicians currently interested in health care economics and financial management.

It is an honor to publish this volume authored by Dr. Seawell.

Robert M. Shelton, FHFMA, CAE
Hospital Financial Management Association

Preface

The origins of this book may be traced back more than twenty years to when Professor Stanley A. Pressler of the Indiana University Graduate School of Business urged one of his students to take a serious interest in the accounting and financial practices of hospitals. With his guidance and encouragement, I prepared a mimeographed booklet for use in connection with a correspondence study course in hospital accounting. That course, the first of its kind, was cosponsored by Indiana University and the American Association of Hospital Accountants (later to become the Hospital Financial Management Association). Its success led me to write *Principles of Hospital Accounting* (Physicians' Record Company, 1960), which subsequently was revised and retitled *Introduction to Hospital Accounting* for publication by HFMA in 1971.

Historically, then, the present volume is a fourth edition of an effort extended over two decades; yet this book bears little resemblance to its predecessors. I have attempted not a limited revision but an almost completely *new* introduction to hospital accounting. The number of chapters, pages, illustrations, and assignment exercises in this edition is more than double that of the 1971 edition. While still introductory in nature, much of the discussion within these pages is aimed at a level of sophistication appropriate to the considerable progress which hospital accounting has made in recent years. In addition, a glossary of accounting and financial terms has been added, and an entirely new practice set has been developed. An instructor's manual is available to adopters. A number of other changes were made largely in response to helpful comments received from users of the previous edition. I am most grateful for their interest and assistance, and I welcome criticisms and suggestions from readers of this edition.

The publication of this book is but another reflection of the dedication of the HFMA board of directors, committees, officers, and staff to an ongoing educational program in the health care field. I deeply appreciate this opportunity to contribute again to that program, hoping that my writing may prove worthy of their trust and support. While I dare not attempt to list the names of all who have assisted me in this undertaking, I must single out the following persons to whom I owe a special debt of gratitude: Robert M. Shelton, HFMA executive director; William L. Fill, HFMA administrative assistant; Patricia Rummer, HFMA director of publications; James T. Whitman, HFMA treasurer; Arthur Schmidt, AHA Hospital Administrative Services associate director; Juanita A. Raman, HFMA book editor; and Marcy Schuering, HFMA secretary specialist. None of these individuals, however, has any responsibility for whatever errors of commission or omission may appear in this text. Such responsibility is entirely mine.

Last, but most important, I wish to express my deepest appreciation to my wife, Emma, whose love and understanding sustained me over the long and lonely hours demanded by this work.

L. Vann Seawell

Bloomington, Indiana
May 18, 1977

Contents

1
Nature and Function of Hospital Accounting

Accounting is an essential service activity found in all economic entities and organizations, regardless of type or size. The primary purpose of accounting is to provide useful financial information about an organization's activities and affairs. This information is intended to be used for purposes of intelligent decision making by the organization's management and by interested external groups such as investors, creditors, governmental agencies, and the public at large. Because these decisions directly affect the manner in which a limited amount of resources is allocated and employed in our economy, accounting information plays a significant role in determining the types and quantities of products and services that are produced and consumed. With this in mind, the recording and reporting of adequate and reliable financial information relevant to users' needs clearly must be viewed as a function of extreme importance in our economic system.

In this book, the economic entity with which we are specifically concerned is the hospital enterprise organized and operated either on a not-for-profit or profit-seeking basis. This emphasis on accounting as related to the hospital organization in particular seems warranted because, while the basic principles of accounting are substantially the same for all types of organizations, hospital enterprises have many unique characteristics which require specialized applications of accounting principles and procedures. In addition, the health care business has grown to massive economic and social significance, demanding an increasingly higher order of accounting and financial reporting practices. It seems reasonable to assume that this requirement will be realized most effectively and quickly through educational materials and programs dealing specifically with the hospital industry and its particular accounting problems. There is no doubt, however, that hospitals benefit greatly from the use of time-proven accounting techniques and business methods that have been developed by commercial enterprises.

In seeking solutions to the serious problems being encountered currently in the provision of health care at reasonable costs, hospital managements are more heavily dependent than ever before upon the information generated by a highly sophisticated accounting system. The effectiveness of hospital managers at all levels is directly related to the quality of the information provided by hospital accountants, including business office personnel engaged in the least glamorous bookkeeping tasks. A similar dependency upon, and need for, more and better financial information about hospitals also exists with respect to third-party payers, planning agencies, and other external groups.

Your interest in hospital accounting may arise from a desire to become a hospital accountant or auditor, or in order to increase your capabilities in these areas. On the other hand, you may be preparing yourself for a career in hospital administration as a nonaccounting executive, recognizing that this preparation would not be adequate or complete without a study of accounting principles. In either event, this book is intended to serve as an introductory course emphasizing the methodology of hospital accounting but also providing an understanding of the meaning and managerial uses of accounting information. The broad coverage of subjects allows this book to be used as a complete course for those having no interest in an accounting career. The depth of coverage, however, is sufficient to permit others to continue their accounting education at an intermediate level.

In this chapter we shall examine some of the characteristics of the hospital enterprise, the economic environment in which it pursues its objectives, and the role of accounting in its management. You will see that there is a critical and continuous need for financial information about hospital activities and affairs, that this information is required for internal management purposes and also by external users, and that the accounting process provides that information. Then, in introductory fashion, we will explore the nature and content of financial statements developed by the accounting process. Your concern will be to obtain a general knowledge of the hospital business and a basic understanding of the end product of accounting—the financial statements—before getting involved in the details of accounting methodology, beginning with the next chapter.

Hospital Environment

The importance of the health care industry in this country is indicated by its size and rate of growth. Health care is the second largest American industry (after construction) with annual expenditures in excess of $85 billion. No other nation spends so much of its gross national product for health care as does the United States. In addition, with these expenditures increasing by about 14% annually, health care is the nation's fastest growing industry. It is generally agreed that this trend is not likely to change significantly in the near future. A greater emphasis, however, will be placed upon efforts to assure maximum returns from this huge investment in terms of the quality and quantity of health care services provided to the American public.

1 *Nature and Function*

The single largest component of the health care industry by far is the network of over 7,100 hospitals with a total of about 1.6 million beds and some $35 billion in assets. Over the last 25 years, spending on hospital care has risen from about $4 billion to nearly $40 billion per year. In recent years, hospital costs have increased an average of approximately 14% annually, and hospitals have been subjected to price controls and other regulations established by the federal government.

Aside from inflation, the rather dramatic rise in spending on hospital care since 1950 is attributable to a vastly greater demand for, and utilization of, an increasingly wide range of hospital services. This expanded demand has required an increase in hospital personnel of from about 800 thousand employees in 1946 to about 3 million in 1976. The average earnings of hospital employees also have risen substantially because of the application of minimum wage laws to hospitals, greater competition for the available labor force, and unionization. In addition, the last quarter century has produced technological changes that have required the use of sophisticated and expensive equipment operated by skilled and highly paid technicians. We also should recognize the advent of Medicare and other governmental programs as yet another factor contributing to the increase in hospital costs.

One of the most important environmental influences on hospital operations is, of course, the third-party reimbursement system. Whereas most commercial businesses are paid directly by their customers for services and products sold to them, hospitals receive payment for a large majority of their revenues through reimbursement from third-party payers, including governmental agencies, Blue Cross plans, and commercial insurers. (It should be clearly understood that, although a third party is billed on behalf of the patient, the patient is still the debtor.) Many reimbursements are made on a retrospective cost basis, although some are based on hospital charges or on negotiated rates. The full financial needs of hospitals, however, generally are not recognized under existing reimbursement systems. As a result, hospital managers often are engaged in a desperate struggle, attempting to maintain the financial integrity of their institutions. Individual philanthropy and community fund-raising drives have declined in importance as sources of supplementary funds, and hospitals are now financing their long-term capital needs through bond issues and other forms of debt.

HOSPITAL ORGANIZATION

The largest category of American hospitals is comprised of short-term, general hospitals usually referred to as community hospitals. Most of these are voluntary, not-for-profit enterprises operated under corporate charters granted by the various states. Other hospitals are either government institutions or privately owned businesses conducted on a profit-seeking basis. Although major emphasis in this book is given to community hospitals, much of the discussion is relevant to all types of hospitals and other health care organizations.

Regardless of the type of ownership, the essential function and primary mission of all hospitals is patient care. This is the basic objective and purpose of the hospital: the provision of quality service at reasonable costs to persons in need of medical attention and hospital care. In addition, hospitals also perform vital roles in the areas of medical research and education.

In carrying out these tasks, hospitals employ many different types of physical, financial, and human resources. These resources, if they are to be utilized in an economical and effective way, must be segregated into manageable organizational units in which authority is centralized and responsibility is clearly assigned for each function. The duties of each employee should be carefully defined, and interrelationships among individuals and organizational segments should be soundly structured so that all personnel may work together in a coordinated, cooperative effort. It is only through a well-conceived plan of organization that the hospital achieves its service and financial objectives.

A hospital's organizational pattern generally is expressed in a formal organization chart such as the one shown in figure 1. You should understand that this chart is illustrative only; there is no single plan of organization applicable to all hospitals. Different organizational structures arise because of differences in hospital size, range of services, personnel capabilities, and other characteristics.

At the top of the organizational structure is the hospital's governing board which often is called the board of directors or board of trustees. The ultimate authority and responsibility for the proper and prudent management of the hospital's affairs rests with this group. Typically the board will carry out its function through a number of standing committees, such as finance, medical affairs, and public relations. The board members, however, do not directly manage the day-to-day operations of the hospital; this authority is delegated to the hospital's chief executive, who has the title of administrator, director, or president. Similarly, authority and responsibility for the medical aspects of hospital activity are assigned to a physician known as the medical director or chief of staff. The administrator and medical director, since their responsibilities are interdependent, must work always in close cooperation.

It is not possible, even in small hospitals, for the administrator to exercise continuous and direct personal supervision of all hospital activities. As indicated in figure 1, the work of the hospital necessarily must be organized into major divisional units such as nursing services, other professional services, general services, and fiscal and administrative services. Each of the divisional units is headed by a manager or director having authority and clearly assigned responsibility for its operations. Each division head is responsible to the administrator who, in turn, is responsible to the governing board.

The nursing services division, headed by the director of nursing, has the responsibility for daily patient-care activities. Employees of the division include nurses, nurses' aides, surgical technicians, ward clerks, and orderlies. The division is comprised of many departments, including nursing units generally organized by medical-service classifications, operating rooms, delivery rooms, emergency rooms, and central supply.

Figure 1
Hospital Organization Chart

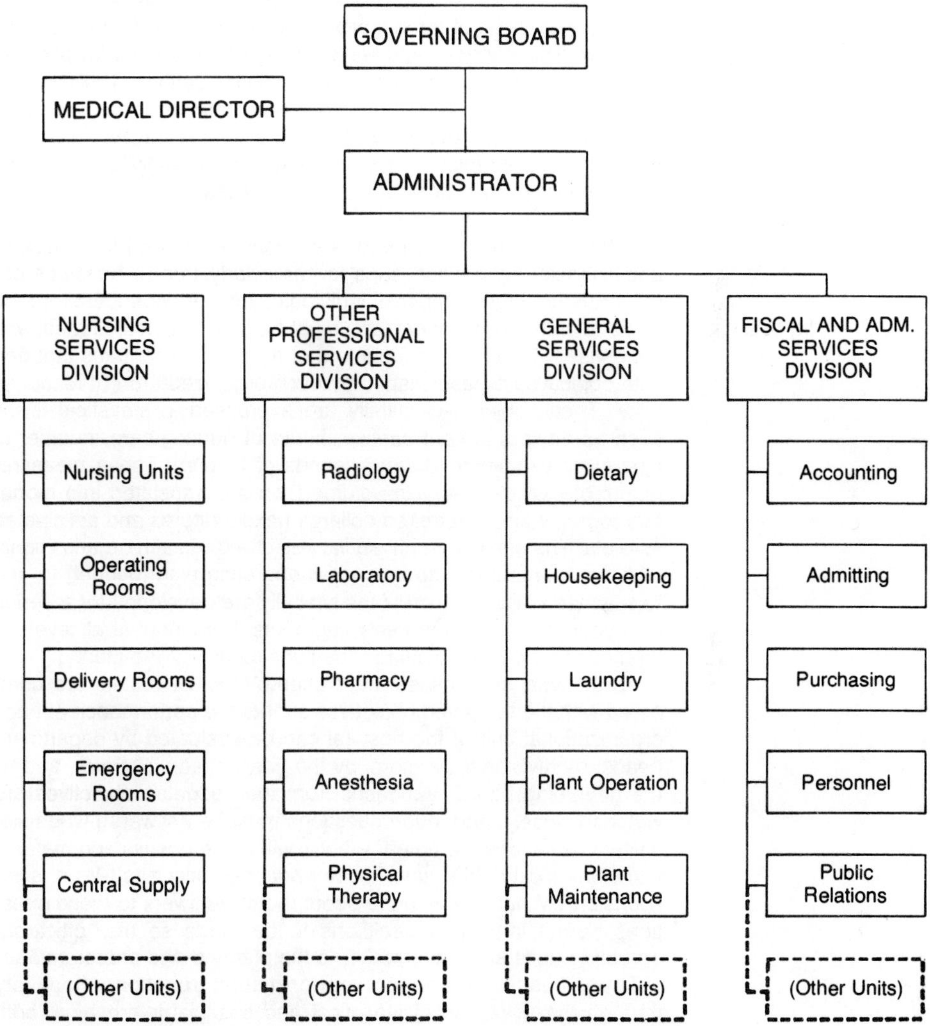

The other professional services division offers ancillary services to the hospital's patients. This division is subdivided into major professional departments such as laboratory, radiology, pharmacy,

EEG, EKG, and physical therapy. These departments, some of which are headed by physicians, provide essential diagnostic and therapeutic services.

The general services division is responsible for various support services necessary to patient care and to the operation of other departments of the hospital. Departments organized within this division include dietary, laundry and linen, housekeeping, and plant operation and maintenance. Some hospitals have contracted with outside firms to perform certain of these support functions.

A fourth division of the hospital is that of fiscal and administrative services. This division includes such departments as admitting, accounting, purchasing, personnel, and public relations. The accounting department itself is divided into subordinate organizational units, including payroll, accounts receivable, accounts payable, budgets, and general accounting. The division is headed either by the hospital controller or by a director of fiscal services.

Need for Statistical and Financial Information

Within any enterprise, there is an imperative need for statistical and financial information. This is particularly true of hospitals because of the large number of individual, yet interdependent, organizational units whose operations must be planned, coordinated, and supervised. Effective management of the hospital requires that definite objectives be established by each organized area of responsibility. These objectives initially are expressed in statistical terms such as days of patient service, hours of nursing care, number of laboratory examinations, and pounds of laundry. These measurements of expected service volume then are translated into monetary terms, such as required dollars of expenditures and anticipated receipts. The service and financial objectives of each organizational unit are coordinated into an overall operating plan (budget) for the hospital as a whole. Such plans typically are developed for a period of a year, broken into monthly segments. Personnel at all levels in the hospital may participate in the construction of the plan.

As the year progresses, each month's actual results are compared with the budgeted objectives so that the performance of each organizational unit of the hospital can be evaluated by department heads, by divisional directors, by the hospital administrator, and by the governing board. Variances from the budgeted objectives are watched closely, and tough questions must be answered when significant deviations are noted. Where, within the hospital, do material variations exist? Why have these variances occurred? Who is responsible? What can be done about them? Answers to these questions permit intelligent decisions to be made so that off-target operating units are redirected onto the planned and proper course.

Thus, hospital managers perform their function effectively through the utilization of statistical and financial information, both historical and projected. This information is essential to the manager in *planning* the hospital's operations, in *evaluating* the actual performance of hospital personnel, and in *taking corrective action* to overcome unfavorable conditions and trends. Of course, the information must be timely, adequate, relevant, and reliable, or the manager's decisions are likely to be ill advised and unsound.

In addition to the internal use of statistical and financial data by management, groups external to the hospital also make important use of much of the same information. These external groups include third-party payers, banks, suppliers, planning agencies, and hospital associations. Hard decisions are made by all these groups, and they have a crucial impact on the ability of the hospital to pay its expenses, borrow money, obtain credit, acquire new plant and equipment, add new services, and pursue research and educational programs. You can be sure that these decisions will not favor the hospital that is unable or unwilling to supply the kinds of statistical and financial information that necessarily must be required by these external groups.

Accounting Function

The hospital accounting function, simply stated, is to provide useful information about the hospital's activities and affairs. This information is of a statistical and financial character; it is both historical and projected in nature. As you have seen, this information has vitally important uses in the internal management of the hospital and equally important uses in the decisions made by parties external to the hospital. In short, accounting is an information system; it is the source of information absolutely essential to the management of the individual hospital and to the functioning of the hospital industry.

Hospital accounting can be defined as the accumulation, communication, and interpretation of historical and projected economic data relating to the financial position and operating results of a hospital enterprise, for purposes of decision making by its management and other interested parties. Let us examine the several parts of this definition.

The term *accumulation* refers to the process of recording and classifying the business transactions and financial events that occur in the economic life of the hospital. This, if you wish, is the "bookkeeping" aspect of the accounting function. It involves several mechanical operations which you will discover at a later point.

By *communication* is meant the reporting of recorded information to those who utilize it. There are many types of accounting reports, and they contain different kinds of information. While the content of these reports generally depends upon the particular needs of users, there is a substantial body of information that is believed to serve certain common interests of all users. So this general-purpose information is routinely reported in financial statements called *balance sheets* and *income statements.* There are other basic required reports, but you will not need to concern yourself with them at this time.

The word *interpretation* refers to the effort made by accountants to analyze and evaluate reported information so that it may be better understood and more easily utilized by decision makers. It is not enough for the accountant merely to record and report; the accountant's responsibility extends to the function of assisting users in the interpretation of reported data. This is necessary if users are to comprehend fully the significance of the information and utilize it to the fullest extent. More will be said about this matter in subsequent chapters.

Much of the information recorded and reported through the accounting process, of course, is historical in nature. Historical economic data are required for many purposes, including reimbursement and payroll tax reports. At least an equal share of the accountant's time, however, is spent in the development of annual budgets, long-range plans, and other projections of data into the future. Financial forecasting is a major part of the accounting task.

The information generated by the accounting process is of 2 basic types. Balance sheets report *financial-position* information; income statements report information relating to *operating results.* The financial position of a hospital at a particular point in time is measured in terms of the hospital's resources (assets), obligations (liabilities), and equity. The operating results of a hospital for a given period of time are measured in terms of revenues earned and expenses incurred during that period. These terms—*assets, liabilities, equity, revenues,* and *expenses*—will be defined and described fully later in this chapter.

Finally, the definition of accounting indicates that the financial statements developed in the accounting process are intended to be useful for decision-making purposes. If accounting information were not useful, there would be no need for accounting and no demand for accountants.

Financial Statements

As you have learned, hospital accounting is a service activity whose primary function is the provision of useful quantitative information about the financial position and operating results of the hospital enterprise. Financial statements are the end product of the accounting process. They are the means by which the information developed by the accounting process is communicated to hospital managements, creditors, third-party payers, and others who use the information as a basis for making economic decisions. Your understanding of the accounting process will be considerably enhanced if we briefly examine here two of the basic financial statements before dealing with the procedures through which financial information is accumulated by accountants.

The several different types of financial statements usually prepared by accountants are illustrated and described at appropriate points in this book. For the present, however, you will be concerned only with 2 of these: (1) the balance sheet and (2) the income statement. These statements are illustrated in figures 2 and 3 for a hypothetical Happy Valley Hospital. A number of simplifications and condensations of the data have been made to facilitate an introductory discussion of the essential elements and features involved. More specific attention to practical application will be given in subsequent chapters.

To be useful, accounting information must be not only relevant but accurate and reliable, as well. The accuracy and reliability of the monetary and statistical data provided in accounting reports is dependent upon an effective system of *internal control.* This system has been defined as follows:

> Internal control comprises the plan of organization and all of the coordinate methods and measures adopted within a business to safeguard its assets, check the accuracy and reliability of its accounting data, promote operational efficiency, and encourage adherence to prescribed managerial policies.[1]

Such a system greatly reduces the possibility of serious errors in the accumulation and communication processes of accounting, thereby giving hospital managers more confidence in accounting information and in decisions based upon such information. The hospital accountant is responsible for the development and operation of the internal control system as an integral part of the accounting process. We will describe specific internal-control methods and procedures at various points throughout this book.

BALANCE SHEET

A balance sheet is a presentation of the financial position of a hospital at a particular point in time. It also may be referred to as a statement of financial condition (or position). Financial position is measured in terms of resources (assets) owned and obligations (liabilities) owed by the hospital at a given date. The difference between these resources and obligations is the hospital's *net assets*, variously called "equity," "capital," or "net worth." Thus, in the simplest terms, a balance sheet indicates how "well off" a hospital is at a particular date by listing the things of value which the hospital owns in relation to its debts to suppliers, employees, and other creditors. The excess of things owned over things owed is the hospital's equity at that date.

The balance sheet gets its name from the fact that it depicts a balance (an equality) between total assets, on one side, and the total of liabilities and equity, on the other side. This equality is known as the *accounting equation*:

$$\text{ASSETS} = \text{LIABILITIES} + \text{EQUITY}$$

or

$$\text{ASSETS} - \text{LIABILITIES} = \text{EQUITY}$$

To put it in personal terms, let us say that today you have $25,000 of assets (cash and other property) and $10,000 of liabilities (unpaid bills and other debts). By subtracting your liabilities from your assets, we can determine that your equity (net worth) is $15,000. You could, of course, prepare a personal balance sheet for yourself, listing $25,000 of assets on the left and reporting $25,000 of liabilities and equity on the right side. This relationship of total assets to total liabilities and equity is fundamental to the debit-and-credit methodology employed in accounting operations, as you shall see in the next chapter.

---

[1]Committee on Auditing Procedure, *Internal Control* (New York: American Institute of Certified Public Accountants, 1949), p. 6.

Figure 2
Happy Valley Hospital
Balance Sheet
December 31, 1976
(000's Omitted)

Assets			*Liabilities and Equity*	
Cash		$ 540	Accounts payable	$ 300
Accounts receivable		2,500	Notes payable	275
Inventory		200	Accrued expenses payable	795
Prepaid expenses		60	Deferred income	30
Total current assets		3,300	Total current liabilities	1,400
Long-term investments		400	Long-term liabilities	3,200
Land, buildings, and equipment	$7,200		Total liabilities	4,600
Less accumulated depreciation	2,100	5,100	Hospital equity	4,200
Total assets		$8,800	Total liabilities and equity	$8,800

• ***Statement Heading***. Figure 2 presents the balance sheet of Happy Valley Hospital at December 31, 1976. Notice that the heading of the statement contains (1) the name of the accounting entity, (2) the name of the statement, and (3) the date of the statement. These 3 elements should always be included in the heading provided for this statement.

The *accounting entity* in this case is Happy Valley Hospital. This is one of the most important and basic accounting concepts. Under this concept, the hospital itself is personified as an entity (or being) separate and distinct from its governing board, management, and other employees. The hospital is regarded as a person capable of owning property, incurring debts, buying and selling, rendering services, and taking other economic actions. Thus, we say that "the hospital purchased equipment," that "the hospital borrowed $100,000 from the local bank," or that "the hospital paid $160,000 of salaries and wages to its employees last month." The accountant thinks of the hospital as an entity for whose economic activity a financial record must be kept. The object of the accountant's attention and effort is the hospital itself, not the personal affairs of board members, administrators, and employees. Activity recorded in the accounting records of the hospital is limited to the financial affairs and business transactions of the hospital as an economic person.

As noted earlier, the name of this financial statement is *balance sheet*, but you should be aware of alternate titles such as "statement of financial position." The name most widely used, however, is *balance sheet*, and this term will be used throughout this book.

The *date* of the Happy Valley Hospital balance sheet is December 31, 1976, a specific point in time. A balance sheet is analagous to a snapshot which portrays a situation existing at a given moment. It is a picture of the financial position of Happy Valley Hospital on December 31, 1976, only. The picture likely was somewhat different on December 30 and probably will be different again on January 1, 1977. This is true because business transactions will occur every day, and consequently the dollar amounts of assets and liabilities also change daily.

The particular assets and liabilities to be included in balance sheets, and the dollar amounts at which they are stated, are determined by the application of a body of rules, procedures, methods, and standards known as *generally accepted accounting principles*. Special attention is given to this very important matter in the author's *Hospital Accounting—Theory and Practice.* For our present purposes, it is enough that you understand that there are prescribed and generally accepted accounting principles which accountants employ in recording and reporting financial information.

• ***Assets***. *Assets* may be defined as the economic resources of the hospital that are recognized and measured in conformity with generally accepted accounting principles. As indicated in figure 2, the assets of Happy Valley Hospital total $8,800 at December 31, 1976. The following is a brief explanation of each of the assets included in that balance sheet:

1. *Cash* is the amount of money on hand and in bank checking accounts maintained by the hospital.
2. *Accounts receivable* represent the amount of money due the hospital from patients and their third-party payers for services provided to them but for which the hospital has not yet been paid.
3. *Inventory* is the cost of foodstuffs, fuel, drugs, and other medical supplies purchased by the hospital but not yet used or consumed.
4. *Prepaid expenses* include expense items such as insurance, interest, and rent which have been paid in advance. These items are assets in the sense that their prepayment will provide future benefits (insurance protection, use of borrowed money, and use of space or leased equipment) to the hospital.
5. *Long-term investments* represent the cost of corporate and governmental securities which the hospital owns and intends to hold for a period of time in excess of one year.
6. *Land, buildings, and equipment* consist of the original acquisition cost of tangible plant assets used in hospital operations.
7. *Accumulated depreciation* reflects the amount of plant-asset costs consumed by the use of the assets and treated as an operating expense of the hospital during the time that has elapsed since the assets were acquired. Notice that accumulated depreciation is deducted from the cost of the plant assets and that only the remaining "undepreciated" balance of cost is included in the total assets reported in the balance sheet.

Items 1–4 above are totaled and presented in the balance sheet as *total current assets*. For the present, we consider *current assets* as consisting of cash plus other assets which will be converted into cash, or consumed by operations, within one year from the balance sheet date. All other assets (items 5–7) can be referred to as *noncurrent* (long-term) *assets*.

You have noticed that most assets are reported in the balance sheet at acquisition cost rather than current market value. The valuation of assets at historical cost is a basic accounting principle. This basis of valuation is employed in accounting because it is a permanent and objective measurement, and because we assume that the monetary unit is reasonably stable; that is, that the purchasing power of money does not change materially over time. This assumption, because of recent inflationary trends, naturally has been challenged by various groups who argue that assets should be presented in balance sheets at either "fair values" or estimated replacement costs. Other authorities advocate, instead, adjusting the historical costs to reflect changes in the purchasing power of the dollar. One of these proposals may well become a generally accepted practice in the future, but it is a topic beyond the scope of this book.

Another point worth noting at this time concerns the *sequence* in which the assets are listed in the balance sheet. Observe that the sequence generally is an order of liquidity. The most-liquid asset (cash) is listed first; the least-liquid assets (land, buildings, and equipment) are last in sequence. This is a standard practice in financial reporting.

Finally, you should understand that certain economic resources of the hospital are not included as assets in the balance sheet. A hospital may enjoy good public relations and high employee morale, but, while these things may be regarded as resources of great value to the hospital, they are not formally recognized as assets in accounting. They are excluded from recorded assets because of the great difficulty involved in making an objective measurement of them in monetary terms. This problem is being studied, and perhaps someday a satisfactory solution will be forthcoming.

• ***Liabilities***. *Liabilities* may be defined as the economic obligations of the hospital that are recognized and measured in conformity with generally accepted accounting principles. The following is a brief description of the liabilities presented in the Happy Valley Hospital balance sheet:

1. *Accounts payable* are amounts owed by the hospital to suppliers and other trade creditors for merchandise and services purchased from them but for which the hospital has not yet paid.
2. *Notes payable* generally consist of short-term borrowings by the hospital from banks and other financial institutions. These debts usually are in the form of promissory notes issued by the hospital to the lender.
3. *Accrued expenses payable* are liabilities for expenses (employee salaries and wages, for example) that have been incurred by the hospital but for which the hospital has not yet paid.
4. *Deferred income* represents income (nursing school tuition, for example) that has been received in cash by the hospital but which the hospital has not yet earned and for which it is obligated to provide some specific service in the future.
5. *Long-term liabilities* typically are mortgage loans or hospital bond issues which will not be paid off by the hospital in the near future (usually well beyond one year from the date of the balance sheet).

As you can see in figure 2, items 1–4 above are totaled and reported as *total current liabilities*; that is, obligations that will be paid by the use of current assets within one year from the balance sheet date. The long-term liabilities of the hospital therefore may be referred to as *noncurrent liabilities*.

Liabilities, generally speaking, are measured in terms of the dollar amounts that will be required to discharge them. Long-term liabilities, however, sometimes may be reported in the balance sheet at the present value of the future payments required for their liquidation; but again, we must postpone a discussion of this matter.

As was true of assets, recognition problems also exist with respect to liabilities. When is an obligation a liability in the accounting sense? As you pursue your study of this book, you will discover items which you may consider liabilities but which are not so treated in accounting. Similarly, you may encounter accounting liabilities which you have not previously regarded as such. This is but another example of the patience you must have in beginning your study of hospital accounting. Full explanations cannot be given of all matters in the early stages; your complete comprehension of the various points will eventually be achieved but only through a gradual process.

Liabilities are presented in the balance sheet more or less in the order in which they will be paid. The proper sequence, however, is not always easy to determine, and compromises often must be made. It is essential, however, that the balance sheet show a figure of total current liabilities and a figure for total liabilities (current and noncurrent) as indicated in figure 2. Readers of the balance sheet of the hospital are entitled to have this information.

• ***Equity***. *Hospital equity* may be defined simply as the excess of hospital assets over hospital liabilities. It is the hospital's residual ownership interest in its own assets after the claims of creditors against these assets have been satisfied. Hospital equity is increased by profits earned by the hospital; it is decreased by operating losses.

Much further on in this book, the subject of fund accounting will be introduced. Fund accounting is employed by a majority of hospitals and consists basically of segregating assets, liabilities, and equity into self-balancing groups or "funds." When this accounting procedure is used, a separate balance sheet can be prepared for each fund; or a single balance sheet may be prepared in which assets, liabilities, and equity are classified and reported according to the particular fund with which they are associated.

INCOME STATEMENT

An income statement is a presentation of the operating results of a hospital for a specified period of time. It also may be referred to as the "statement of revenues and expenses," the "profit-and-loss statement," or simply the "operating statement." In any event, this statement reports the revenues earned and the expenses incurred by the hospital during a given period of time, such as a month, a quarter, or one year. The difference between the revenues and expenses of the period is reported as *net income* (or *net loss*, if total expenses exceed total revenues). This "bottom-line" figure also may be called "net profit."

• ***Statement Heading***. Figure 3 presents the income statement of Happy Valley Hospital for the year ended December 31, 1977 (the year following the hospital's balance sheet illustrated in figure 2). The heading of the statement includes (1) the name of the accounting entity, (2) the name of the statement, and (3) the period of time encompassed by the statement. These elements should always appear in the heading provided on income statements.

Figure 3
Happy Valley Hospital
Income Statement
Year Ended December 31, 1977
(000's Omitted)

Patient service revenues:		
Daily patient services	$ 6,000	
Other professional services	4,000	
Total	10,000	
Less deductions from patient service revenues	1,000	
Net patient service revenues		$9,000
Other operating revenues		500
Total operating revenues		9,500
Less operating expenses:		
Nursing services	$ 3,400	
Other professional services	2,700	
General services	1,800	
Fiscal and administrative services	1,400	
Total operating expenses		9,300
Operating income		200
Add nonoperating revenues		130
Net income for the year		$ 330

The *accounting entity* is identified here, as in the balance sheet previously discussed, as Happy Valley Hospital. It is the economic unit or organization whose activities are reported in the financial statement. A careful identification of the entity is required so that it is distinguished from all other similar or related entities, such as the Happy Valley college, church, nursing home, or manufacturing company. As pointed out before, under the entity concept the hospital is personified as an economic unit separate and distinct from its governing board, management, and employees.

The name, *income statement,* identifies and explains its function.

Observe that the illustrative income statement is dated "*year ended* December 31, 1977." This specifies the *accounting period* to which the income statement items are related (i.e., the 12 calendar months of 1977). It would be improper and misleading to date the statement simply "December 31, 1977," as this would imply that the information relates to a single day or, at best, to an unspecified period of time ending on that day. Income statements often are prepared for periods of a month or a quarter as well as for annual periods, and it is essential that the particular time period covered be clearly disclosed in the statement heading. Balance sheets also are prepared on a monthly or quarterly basis as well as annually. Financial statements prepared during the course of a year (monthly income statements and balance sheets, for example) are referred to as *interim* statements. For the present, however, you will be concerned only with annual financial statements.

The previously discussed balance sheet presented the assets, liabilities, and capital of Happy Valley Hospital at December 31, 1976. These resources and obligations, of course, became the opening balances for the 1977 year; in other words, the closing cash balance on December 31, 1976, becomes the opening cash balance on January 1, 1977. As the 1977 year unfolds day by day, Happy Valley Hospital will complete thousands of individual business transactions. Services will be provided to patients, supplies will be purchased and used, employees will be paid salaries and wages, cash receipts will arise from billings to patients and third parties, and various other operating activities will take place.

Figure 4
Happy Valley Hospital
Balance Sheet
December 31, 1977

Assets		
Cash		$ 575
Accounts receivable		2,600
Inventory		420
Prepaid expenses		80
Total current assets		3,675
Long-term investments		380
Land, buildings, and equipment	$7,500	
Less accumulated depreciation	2,210	5,290
Total assets		$9,345
Liabilities and Equity		
Accounts payable		$ 360
Notes payable		200
Accrued expenses payable		831
Deferred income		24
Total current liabilities		1,415
Long-term liabilities		3,400
Total liabilities		4,815
Hospital equity		4,530
Total liabilities and equity		$9,345

At the end of the 1977 year, another balance sheet can be prepared as shown in figure 4. This statement presents the financial position of the hospital at December 31, 1977. (A vertical, or report, format is employed here simply to illustrate an alternative form of presentation for balance sheets.) This balance sheet, however, does *not* reveal the details of *operating results* for the 1977 year; so an income statement is needed to disclose what happened during the 12-month interval between December 31, 1976, and December 31, 1977. Income statements, in this way, are connecting links between successive balance sheets.

• ***Revenues***. Hospital revenues consist primarily of economic values earned by the hospital through the provision of services, and sale of products, to patients. They also include receipts of unrestricted gifts and contributions from donors. Revenues typically are evidenced by an increase in hospital assets, either cash or accounts receivable in most instances.

The revenues of a hospital are determined by the application of generally accepted accounting principles. In conformity with these principles, certain increases in assets are recognized as revenues; other asset increases are not. Cash received from an outpatient for a laboratory examination, for example, is revenue. A billing made to an inpatient for a day's room and board is recorded as an increase in accounts receivable and is recognized as revenue too. In each case, the revenue is recorded when it is *earned* (that is, at the time the related service is rendered and the hospital has either received cash or has a legal claim against the patient for the value of the service provided). On the other hand, the receipt of cash arising from the borrowing of money from a bank is *not* revenue.

Hospital revenues arising from patient-care services are measured in terms of the value of those services as evidenced by the hospital's full, established rates (prices) for those services. This is true whether the hospital actually collects its full charges, less than full charges, or nothing for the services provided. Many third-party payers of hospital services, for example, pay less than the hospital's established rates. Hospitals also provide a very considerable amount of service to indigent patients at nominal rates or on a free (charity) basis. Also on occasion, certain financially sufficient patients simply fail to pay the hospital for services they have received, and so bad debts are incurred by the hospital.

Nevertheless, *all* patient-care services rendered by the hospital must be recorded as revenues measured in terms of the hospital's full rates. Figure 3 reports $10,000 of gross patient service revenues, for example, of which $1,000 is estimated to be uncollectible for the reasons indicated in the above paragraph. This produces $9,000 of net patient service revenues or, if you prefer, "collectible" patient service revenues. You should understand, however, that much of this $9,000 has not yet been collected in cash: the December 31, 1977, balance sheet (figure 4) reports $2,600 of accounts receivable!

There are 2 other categories of revenue in the illustrative income statement. "Other operating revenues" may be comprised of cafeteria sales, parking-lot fees, rentals received, tuition from educational programs, research grants, and similar operating items. "Nonoperating revenues," shown at the foot of the income statement, consist mainly of unrestricted gifts, contributions from donors, and income from investments.

The illustrative income statement presents the revenues

of the hospital in condensed form. In actual practice, of course, much more detail would be required. Necessary details often are provided in supplementary schedules to accompany the summary income statement. Such schedules would supply detailed information about the amounts of revenues earned by each organizational unit (revenue derived from each nursing unit, revenue from operating rooms, revenue from laboratory, and so on). In addition, the revenues would be classified into outpatient and inpatient categories. Detailed classifications of revenue deductions, other operating revenues, and nonoperating revenues also would be provided in supplementary schedules.

• ***Expenses***. *Hospital expenses* may be defined roughly as the costs of services, supplies, and other items purchased and consumed by the hospital in the provision of patient-care services during a given period of time. In accordance with generally accepted accounting principles, expenses are recognized and measured in the time period in which they are incurred or consumed in providing hospital services. This may or may not be the same time period in which they are paid. When supply items are purchased for cash, for example, their costs are considered to be assets (inventory). Only when supply items are consumed in hospital operations are their costs recognized and reported as expenses. Like most assets, expenses are measured in terms of historical costs.

The operating expenses in figure 3 are reported in a *functional* classification; that is, according to the divisional organizational units of the hospital. In actual practice, these divisional expense totals would be supported by supplementary schedules in which details, classified by individual department and type of expense, would be provided. The general services expense of $1,800, for example, would be broken down by department (dietary, housekeeping, plant operation) and by type of expense (salaries and wages, supplies, purchased services). Illustrations of such schedules appear at a subsequent point in this book.

Rather than report expenses in a functional classification as seen in figure 3, Happy Valley Hospital might report its expenses in an *object of expenditure*, or *natural, classification* in the manner shown as follows:

Operating expenses:	
Salaries and wages	$6,080
Supplies	1,753
Utilities	1,020
Depreciation	110
Interest	206
Other	131
Total operating expenses	$9,300

This natural classification of expense typically appears in the published financial statements of hospitals. In internal management reports, hospital expenses are primarily classified functionally so as to associate the expenses with organizational units and individuals who are responsible for them. This procedure, known as *responsibility reporting*, is especially useful for managerial control purposes.

The net income of Happy Valley Hospital for 1977 is $330 as indicated in figure 3. As noted earlier, a net income (profit) increases the equity of the hospital. So, if we add the 1977 net income to the equity balance at December 31, 1976, we should obtain the hospital equity figure appearing in the balance sheet at December 31, 1977:

Hospital equity, December 31, 1976 (figure 2)	$4,200
Add net income for 1977 (figure 3)	330
Hospital equity, December 31, 1977 (figure 4)	$4,530

Had there been an operating loss in 1977, the loss would have been subtracted in this computation. Recognize, however, that this is something of a simplification in that factors other than net income (or loss) affect the hospital equity balance. But this point too is a matter for subsequent discussion.

You should now have a general understanding of 2 of the basic financial statements comprising the end product of accounting. With this accomplished, we can move on to a study of the accounting operations which produce the financial information contained in these statements.

QUESTIONS

1. What are the basic objective and purpose of the hospital enterprise?

2. Draw up a simple organization chart for a hypothetical hospital to indicate your understanding of the basic organizational structure generally found in hospitals.

3. State briefly the function of a hospital's (a) governing board, (b) medical director, and (c) administrator.

4. Why is there a need for information about a hospital's financial position and operating results?

5. Describe briefly some of the major characteristics of the economic environment in which today's hospitals are operated.

6. What is the primary function of hospital accounting?

7. State briefly the purpose of a balance sheet.

8. Define *assets*. List 5 examples of assets which appear in hospital balance sheets.

9. Distinguish between current and noncurrent assets. Give an example of each.

10. Define *liabilities*. List 5 examples of liabilities which appear in hospital balance sheets.

11. Distinguish between current and noncurrent liabilities. Give an example of each.

12. State the accounting equation in 2 alternative forms.

13. Valley Hospital's balance sheet at April 30 includes $4,750,000 of assets and $2,500,000 of hospital equity. What is the amount of Valley Hospital's liabilities at April 30?

14. What information should be provided in the heading of a balance sheet?

15. State briefly the purpose of an income statement.

16. Define *revenues*. List 4 examples of revenues which appear in hospital income statements.

17. Define *expenses*. List 4 examples of expenses which appear in hospital income statements.

18. Distinguish between (a) a functional classification of expenses and (b) a natural classification of expenses.

19. What information should be provided in the heading of an income statement?

20. "In a hospital balance sheet, assets are reported at their fair market values." Do you agree? Explain.

21. "In a hospital income statement, revenues represent cash receipts, and expenses represent cash disbursements of the period." Do you agree? Explain.

22. What are interim financial statements?

23. In hospital accounting, when should revenues and expenses be recognized and recorded?

24. What is the *accounting entity* concept?

25. What are 2 of the major objectives of an effective system of internal control in hospitals?

PROBLEMS

A. Fillbill Hospital provides you with the following information which relates to its financial position at September 30, 1977:

Accrued expenses payable	$ 780
Inventory	510
Accumulated depreciation	2,600
Accounts payable	420
Prepaid expenses	90
Cash	600
Deferred income	15
Land, buildings, and equipment	8,200
Accounts receivable	2,450
Notes payable	150
Long-term investments	400
Bonds payable (due 1987)	3,500

Required. Prepare in good form a balance sheet at September 30, 1977, for Fillbill Hospital.

B. Patricia Hospital provides you with the following information which relates to its operating results for the year ended December 31, 1977:

Nursing service expenses	$4,100
Deductions from patient service revenues	900
Other professional service revenues	4,600
General service expenses	1,900
Nonoperating revenues	140
Fiscal and administrative service expenses	1,200
Daily patient service revenues	6,320
Other professional service expenses	2,610
Other operating revenues	450

Required. Prepare in good form an income statement for Patricia Hospital for the year ended December 31, 1977.

C. Bobshell Hospital provides you with the following information which relates to its financial position at August 31, 1977, and its operating results for the year then ended:

Accounts payable	$ 310
Nonoperating revenues	90
Accounts receivable	2,850
Deferred income	60
Long-term investments	590
Nursing service expenses	4,300
Bonds payable (due 1990)	4,100
Daily patient service revenues	6,830
Fiscal and administrative service expenses	1,600
Cash	340
Notes payable	180
Land, buildings, and equipment	8,600
Deductions from patient service revenues	970
Prepaid expenses	70
Other professional service expenses	2,900
Other professional service revenues	4,560
Accrued expenses payable	820
Accumulated depreciation	3,200
Inventory	240
Hospital equity, August 31, 1976	3,780
Other operating revenues	630
General service expenses	2,100

Required. Prepare in good form (1) an income statement for Bobshell Hospital for the year ended August 31, 1977, and (2) a balance sheet for Bobshell Hospital at August 31, 1977.

D. Gayner Hospital provides you with the following information which relates to its financial position at October 31, 1977, and its operating results for the month then ended:

Bonds payable (due 1985)	$2,100
Salaries and wages expense	5,180
Prepaid expenses	40
Hospital equity, September 30, 1977	3,060
Daily patient service revenues	4,630
Interest expense	120
Nonoperating revenues	110
Cash	170

Deferred income	20
Deductions from patient service revenues	420
Accounts payable	170
Land	250
Utilities expense	980
Other operating revenues	380
Notes payable	200
Accounts receivable	1,930
Accumulated depreciation	1,580
Accrued expenses payable	490
Other professional service revenues	3,060
Supplies expense	1,210
Building and equipment	5,000
Inventory	190
Depreciation expense	240
Other operating expenses	70

Required. Prepare in good form for Gayner Hospital (1) an income statement for the month ended October 31, 1977, and (2) a balance sheet at October 31, 1977.

I

Basic Record-Keeping Procedures

2 Analysis of Business Transactions

The economic life of a hospital consists of a continuous stream of business transactions. At frequent intervals, for example, a hospital will purchase medical and surgical supplies for its inventory. An invoice will be received in due course from the supplier, and a check will be written in payment of the billing. As required, the supplies are issued from inventory for use in the provision of patient-care services. Certain of the supplies may not be itemized on the patient's bill separately; other supplies are directly chargeable. Eventually patients' accounts will be collected, and the cash receipts are deposited in the hospital's bank accounts. The cycle then begins anew.

Transactions of many different types occur daily in large numbers. Over a period of a few months, a hospital may complete thousands of individual transactions. Certainly, there must be a system by which this mass of activity can be efficiently processed and recorded so that the desired information about the hospital's business transactions can be produced on a timely and accurate basis. That system, of course, is the *accounting system*. This chapter, and several of the chapters immediately following, will be directed to a description of basic elements and operations found in all accounting systems.

In addition to making certain simplifying assumptions, we also will assume that the accounting records involved are manually maintained in handwritten and typewritten form. It is true, of course, that virtually all hospitals today necessarily employ various types of accounting equipment ranging from a simple bookkeeping machine to sophisticated electronic data processing devices. Nevertheless, an exposition of the accounting process is greatly facilitated, and the procedural operations are more easily learned, when a manual system is assumed. You also should understand that accounting principles are not altered by the employment of accounting equipment; the principles are the same for manual systems as for mechanized and electronic systems. You can better understand what various types of accounting equipment do, if you learn how manual records are maintained. How to program, instruct, and otherwise operate such equipment, however, is beyond the scope of this book.

Documentary Evidence

In making records of business transactions, accountants must first be made aware that transactions have occurred. A system must be devised to document *all* business transactions as they occur or at the earliest practicable point after their occurrence. It is of critical importance that no transaction be overlooked and go unrecorded. A failure to recognize and record all transactions results in lost revenues and incomplete financial information.

Documentary evidences of transactions include purchase requisitions, purchase orders, receiving reports, invoices, checks written and checks received, patient service requisitions, charge tickets, cash register tapes, cash receipt slips, deeds and contracts, bank deposit slips, correspondence with patients and creditors, intrahospital memoranda, and all other forms and business papers. This is the "red tape" for which accountants often are blamed. While these documents are vital to the accounting process, they often have primary purposes and supplemental uses that are not directly related to accounting.

The documentation should provide all essential facts involved in the transaction. Accountants are particularly interested in dates, authorizations, an accurate identification of the services, supplies and other items involved, quantities, and dollar amounts. Without this information, the integrity of the accounting records would be subject to question.

Thus, accountants require, to the extent possible, verifiable and objective evidence of the occurrence of bona fide transactions and of all essential facts involved. Not everything recorded in the accounting records, however, can be documented, or documented to the same degree. A certain amount of the information recorded and reported by accountants is in the nature of approximations and estimates based upon professional judgment and experienced opinion. This is one aspect of accounting which makes it interesting and challenging.

Accounting Equation

The accounting equation, or model, was introduced briefly in the preceding chapter. This equation, you may remember, was expressed as follows:

ASSETS = LIABILITIES + EQUITY

The left side of the equation represents assets, the things of value owned by the hospital (i.e., cash, receivables, inventory, plant assets, and so on). The right side of the equation consists of liabilities and equity, claims against the assets of the hospital. These claims consist of the amount of assets owed to creditors (accounts payable, wages payable to employees, loans payable to banks, and other obligations) and the residual ownership interest in assets accruing to the hospital entity itself (equity). The equation must always balance; it expresses an equality that exists throughout the accounting process.

When a business transaction occurs, the accountant must analyze the transaction in terms of its effect on the equation. A determination is made of the increase and/or decrease effects of each transaction on each element of the equation. Each transaction is analyzed to determine the amounts by which it increased and/or decreased assets, liabilities, or equity. The amounts are measured in terms of dollars. Documentary evidences provide the information needed to make the analysis.

Let us assume, as a starting point, that a hospital has $5,000 of assets, $2,000 of liabilities, and $3,000 of equity. The equation is

ASSETS	=	LIABILITIES	+	EQUITY
$5,000	=	$2,000	+	$3,000

Now assume that the hospital borrows $600 from a bank. What are the effects of this transaction upon the accounting equation? Which of the elements of the equation were increased or decreased? The answer is seen below:

ASSETS	=	LIABILITIES	+	EQUITY	
$5,000	=	$2,000	+	$3,000	(previous balances)
+600		+600			(effect of transaction)
$5,600	=	$2,600	+	$3,000	(resulting balances)

As a result of the bank loan, the hospital has $600 more assets (cash received from the bank) and $600 more liabilities (the debt owed to the bank which must be paid in the future). The receipt of a cash loan has no effect on the hospital's equity. Nor is the cash receipt regarded as revenue.

Assume that the hospital repays $100 (disregarding interest) of the principal amount of the bank loan. The analysis is

ASSETS	=	LIABILITIES	+	EQUITY	
$5,600	=	$2,600	+	$3,000	(previous balances)
−100		−100			(effect of transaction)
$5,500	=	$2,500	+	$3,000	(resulting balances)

The hospital disbursed $100 cash, thereby reducing its assets *and* its liability to the bank (from $600 to only $500). Repayment of the bank loan (disregarding interest) has no effect on the hospital's equity. Nor does this expenditure constitute expense.

Assume that the hospital purchases $300 of supplies on account (on credit). In this transaction the hospital obtains a new asset (inventory) and incurs a liability (accounts payable) to pay the supplier at an agreed future date. The analysis is

ASSETS	=	LIABILITIES	+	EQUITY	
$5,500	=	$2,500	+	$3,000	(previous balances)
+300		+300			(effect of transaction)
$5,800	=	$2,800	+	$3,000	(resulting balances)

This transaction has no effect on the hospital's equity; and neither is it a transaction that requires the recognition of revenue or expense.

Assume that the hospital purchases a new item of equipment for $400 cash. The analysis is shown below:

ASSETS	=	LIABILITIES	+	EQUITY	
$5,800	=	$2,800	+	$3,000	(previous balances)
+400					(effect of transaction)
−400					
$5,800	=	$2,800	+	$3,000	(resulting balances)

The effect of this transaction is to increase one asset (equipment) and decrease another asset (cash). There is no effect on the liabilities or equity. Nor is there any revenue or expense to recognize.

Now let us consider a transaction that affects the hospital's revenue and therefore its equity. Assume that the supplies previously purchased in one of the transactions above are sold to patients for $350 and charged to their accounts (no cash is yet received from them). The analysis is

ASSETS	=	LIABILITIES	+	EQUITY	
$5,800	=	$2,800	+	$3,000	(previous balances)
+350				+350	(effect of transaction)
$6,150	=	$2,800	+	$3,350	(resulting balances)

This transaction produces an increase in the hospital's assets (patients' accounts receivable). Every transaction, however, has at least 2 effects. What is the other effect? Since liabilities are unaffected by the transaction, the other effect must be an increase in the hospital's equity. The principle: Revenues, evidenced by increases in assets, are recognized as increases in the hospital's equity.

But you are probably wondering about the *cost* of the supplies which were sold and are no longer in the hospital's inventory! Yes, in addition to the revenue, we must recognize the related *expense*:

ASSETS	=	LIABILITIES	+	EQUITY	
$6,150	=	$2,800	+	$3,350	(previous balances)
−300				−300	(effect of transaction)
$5,850	=	$2,800	+	$3,050	(resulting balances)

Here, assets (inventory) are decreased by the cost of the supplies removed from inventory and sold to patients. The cost of supplies sold (or used) is treated as a reduction of the hospital's equity. The principle is that expenses are recognized as decreases in hospital equity.

If you prefer, we could have recorded the revenue transaction and the expense transaction simultaneously. The analysis would have been

ASSETS	=	LIABILITIES	+	EQUITY	
$5,800	=	$2,800	+	$3,000	(previous balances)
+350				+350	(effect of transactions)
−300				−300	
$5,850	=	$2,800	+	$3,050	(resulting balances)

A point made in the preceding chapter was that net income (profit) increases hospital equity. This is true because revenues increase equity and expenses decrease equity, and net income is the excess of revenues over expenses. As you can see immediately above, hospital equity increased by $50, the profit made on the sale of supplies ($350 − $300 = $50).

Hospitals, however, have so many revenue and expense transactions that it is not feasible to attempt to record them as *direct* additions to, and deductions from, hospital equity. Instead, we expand the accounting equation to include 2 additional elements: revenues and expenses. The expanded equation is

ASSETS = LIABILITIES + EQUITY* + REVENUES − EXPENSES

*Equity balance at beginning of period.

This extension of the equation simply expresses the principle that the equity balance at the beginning of the period is increased by revenues earned and is decreased by expenses incurred during the period. It also allows revenues and expenses to be treated as separate elements of the equation rather than as direct changes in the equity balance.

The expanded equation will be easier to work with if we will add expenses to each side to produce

ASSETS + EXPENSES = LIABILITIES + EQUITY* + REVENUES

*Equity balance at beginning of period.

This avoids having positive and negative elements on the right-hand side of the equation. In subsequent expressions of the equation, the asterisk (*) will be deleted, but keep in mind that *equity* means the equity balance at the beginning of the period (year).

Now, using the expanded equation, let us analyze a new set of transactions for a different hospital with assumed opening balances including $300,000 of assets, $100,000 of liabilities, and $200,000 of equity. The assumed transactions are as follows:

1. The hospital borrowed $25,000 from a bank.
2. The hospital purchased supplies on account for $12,000.
3. Half of the supplies were issued from inventory and used in patient care. Patients were billed for $7,500.
4. The hospital paid $14,000 of salaries and wages to its employees.
5. Patients were billed (charged) for $15,300 of other services.
6. The bank loan was paid off with a disbursement of $26,000 (this includes interest of $1,000).
7. The hospital paid $9,000 on its accounts payable.
8. The hospital collected $18,400 on patients' accounts receivable.

An analysis of the effects of these transactions on the expanded equation is presented in figure 5. Observe that each transaction has at least 2 effects and that the equation balances (left equals right) after each transaction is recorded.

Figure 5
Transaction Analysis

	ASSETS	+	EXPENSES	=	LIABILITIES	+	EQUITY	+	REVENUES
Opening balances	$300,000	+	$ −0−	=	$100,000	+	$200,000	+	$ −0−
Transaction 1	+25,000				+25,000				
Resulting balances	$325,000	+	$ −0−	=	$125,000	+	$200,000	+	$ −0−
Transaction 2	+12,000				+12,000				
Resulting balances	$337,000	+	$ −0−	=	$137,000	+	$200,000	+	$ −0−
	− 6,000		+ 6,000						
Transaction 3	+ 7,500							+	+7,500
Resulting balances	$338,500	+	$ 6,000	=	$137,000	+	$200,000	+	$ 7,500
Transaction 4	−14,000		+14,000						
Resulting balances	$324,500	+	$ 20,000	=	$137,000	+	$200,000	+	$ 7,500
Transaction 5	+15,300								+15,300
Resulting balances	$339,800	+	$ 20,000	=	$137,000	+	$200,000	+	$ 22,800
Transaction 6	−26,000		+ 1,000		−25,000				
Resulting balances	$313,800	+	$ 21,000	=	$112,000	+	$200,000	+	$ 22,800
Transaction 7	− 9,000				− 9,000				
Resulting balances	$304,800	+	$ 21,000	=	$103,000	+	$200,000	+	$ 22,800
	+18,400								
Transaction 8	−18,400								
Resulting balances	$304,800	+	$ 21,000	=	$103,000	+	$200,000	+	$ 22,800
Closing entry (profit)			−21,000				+ 1,800		−22,800
Closing balances	$304,800	+	$ −0−	=	$103,000	+	$201,800	+	$ −0−

At the bottom of figure 5, you see that a closing entry has been made to eliminate the accumulated totals of revenues and expenses from the equation, and to add the excess of revenues over expenses (the net income, or profit) to the opening equity balance. This produces the closing equity balance:

Equity, beginning of period		$200,000
Revenues of the period	$ 22,800	
Less expenses of the period	21,000	
Net income (profit) for the period		+1,800
Equity, end of period		$201,800

In actual practice, closing entries are made at the end of each annual period as a part of the procedure known as "closing the books." Considerable attention is given to this matter in chapter 4.

After the closing entry has been made, the accounting equation consists only of the closing balances for assets, liabilities, and equity. These balances are carried forward into the next accounting period and become the opening balances of that period. A new accounting cycle then begins.

Debit-and-Credit Methodology

In analyzing and recording the effects of business transactions, accountants employ a special method involving debits and credits. This method was first described in writing in a book published in 1494 by an Italian monk named Paciolo. Today, nearly 500 years later, the system described by Paciolo is still being used by accountants throughout the world.

Let us assume, for the moment, that only 5 types of accounts are employed in accounting: (1) assets, (2) expenses, (3) liabilities, (4) equity, and (5) revenues. The relationship among these accounts can be expressed by the basic accounting equation previously discussed:

ASSETS + EXPENSES = LIABILITIES + EQUITY + REVENUES

Paciolo suggested that we refer to the left-hand side of the equation as the *debit* side. The elements of the left-hand side—assets and expenses—are therefore debit items (or debit balances). So, if you make an *addition* to the *left-hand* side of the equation, you are making a debit: in other words, increases in assets and expenses are recorded by making debits to those accounts.

Similarly, Paciolo indicated that the right-hand side of the equation is called the *credit* side. The elements of this side—liabilities, equity, and revenues—are therefore credit items (or credit balances). So, if you are making an *addition* to the *right-hand* side of the equation, you are making a credit: in other words, increases in liabilities, equity, and revenues are recorded by making credits to those accounts.

Thus, increases in assets and expenses are debits; increases in liabilities, equity, and revenues are credits. It logically follows that decreases in assets and expenses are credits, and that decreases in liabilities, equity, and revenues are debits. In summary, the rules of debit and credit are as follows:

1. With respect to asset and expense accounts
   a. Debit to increase
   b. Credit to decrease.
2. With respect to liability, equity, and revenue accounts
   a. Credit to increase
   b. Debit to decrease.

Like all other introductory accounting students, you probably will memorize the rules at first. As you gain experience in the application of the rules to business transactions, however, debit-and-credit analysis will become almost second nature to you.

Many persons begin a study of accounting with certain preconceived (and incorrect) notions about debits and credits. It is widely believed, for example, that a debit is something "bad" and that a credit is something "good." There also exists an erroneous idea that the term *debit* always means "decrease," and that credits are always increases. If you have formed these impressions, try to clear them from your mind. These notions are incorrect and, if not discarded, will impair your understanding of accounting.

Remember that the word *debit*, standing alone, simply means an entry or balance on the left-hand side of an accounting record. A debit means increase only with respect to assets and expenses; a debit to any other type of account is a decrease. Similarly, the word *credit* means nothing more than an entry or balance on the right-hand side of an accounting record. Whether a debit or a credit is an increase or a decrease, then, depends upon the type of account to which it is related.

USE OF ACCOUNTS

Let us now illustrate the recording of debits and credits in accounts. An account form is basically a T shape:

(Account Name)	
(left) Debit side	(right) Credit side

The name of the account appears at the top of the form above the horizontal ruling. (For present purposes, we will use the terms *assets, expenses, liabilities, equity,* and *revenues* as the account names. More-specific account titles will be introduced in the next chapter.) A vertical ruling divides the account into a left side and a right side.

No matter what the account name, however, the left-hand side of an account is the debit side; the right-hand side is the credit side. With respect to assets and expenses, entries made on the left (debit) side are increases (+), and entries made on the right (credit) side are decreases (−). The opposite is true in accounts for liabilities, equity, and revenues. These debit and credit rules are presented here in account form:

ASSETS		+	EXPENSES		=	LIABILITIES		+	EQUITY		+	EXPENSES	
Dr.	*Cr.*		*Dr.*	*Cr.*		*Dr.*	*Cr.*		*Dr.*	*Cr.*		*Dr.*	*Cr.*
(+)	(−)		(+)	(−)		(−)	(+)		(−)	(+)		(−)	(+)

Note that the word *debit* is abbreviated *dr.* and that the word *credit* is abbreviated *cr.* These abbreviations are derived from equivalent words of the Latin language in which Paciolo wrote. They are not English abbreviations.

In figure 5, we analyzed 8 transactions in terms of the accounting equation. These same 8 transactions now will be illustrated in account form, using debits and credits. You will recall the assumed balances at the beginning of the period:

Assets	
Bal. 300,000	

Expenses	

Liabilities	
	Bal. 100,000

Equity	
	Bal. 200,000

Revenues	

The 5 accounts, as a group, will be referred to as the *ledger*. As you can see, the ledger is "in balance"; that is, total debits equal total credits.

The first transaction to be analyzed and entered in this ledger is one in which the hospital borrows $25,000 from a bank. This transaction creates $25,000 of additional assets (cash) and $25,000 of additional liabilities (the amount now owed to the bank). The entry, numbered *1*, is shown below:

Assets	
Bal. 300,000	
(1) 25,000	

Expenses	

Liabilities	
	Bal. 100,000
	(1) 25,000

Equity	
	Bal. 200,000

Revenues	

Thus, the required entry is a $25,000 debit to assets and a $25,000 credit to liabilities. The entry increases assets to a balance of $325,000 and increases the liabilities to a balance of $125,000, and the ledger remains in balance.

The second transaction is the purchase of supplies (inventory) on account for $12,000. The entry, numbered *2*, will appear in the following form:

Assets (Debit)	Assets (Credit)	Expenses (Debit)	Expenses (Credit)	Liabilities (Debit)	Liabilities (Credit)
Bal. 300,000					Bal. 100,000
(1) 25,000					(1) 25,000
(2) 12,000					(2) 12,000

Equity (Debit)	Equity (Credit)	Revenues (Debit)	Revenues (Credit)
	Bal. 200,000		

This transaction, which produces a new asset and a new liability, is recorded as a $12,000 debit to assets and a $12,000 credit to liabilities. Every transaction entry will have at least 2 effects; every entry will include at least one debit and one credit.

Do not fall into the trap of assuming that a transaction entry is always an increase in one account and a decrease in another. Each of the 2 entries made above was an increase in one account and an increase in another. No decreases at all were recorded. Other types of transactions are recorded by a decrease in one account and a decrease in another (or the same) account, with no increase in any account. Still other transactions require an increase in one account and a decrease in another. So, it is possible to have any combination of increases and decreases.

Before continuing, notice that the ledger is still in balance. The debit total of assets, $337,000—or $300,000 + $25,000 + $12,000—equals the credit totals of liabilities, $137,000—or $100,000 + $25,000 + $12,000—and equity, $200,000. This equality of debit and credit balances must be maintained at all times.

The next transaction consists of the sale of half the supplies inventory to patients for $7,500. Since all the supplies purchased in transaction 2 cost $12,000 but only half of them were sold, the cost of the supplies sold is therefore $6,000. This $6,000 must be removed from assets (inventory) and charged to expenses (supplies expense). The $7,500 billing to patients must be charged to patients' accounts receivable (debited to assets) and recorded as revenues earned by the hospital. The entry, numbered *3*, is

Assets (Debit)	Assets (Credit)	Expenses (Debit)	Expenses (Credit)	Liabilities (Debit)	Liabilities (Credit)
Bal. 300,000	(3) 6,000	(3) 6,000			Bal. 100,000
(1) 25,000					(1) 25,000
(2) 12,000					(2) 12,000
(3) 7,500					

Equity (Debit)	Equity (Credit)	Revenues (Debit)	Revenues (Credit)
	Bal. 200,000		(3) 7,500

This entry includes 2 debits and 2 credits. Entries having more than one debit or credit are referred to as *compound entries*. You also will encounter compound entries having 2 or more debits but only one credit, and entries having 2 or more credits but only one debit.

In transaction 4, the hospital pays $14,000 of salaries and wages to its employees. The entry, numbered *4*, is

Assets		Expenses		Liabilities	
Bal. 300,000	(3) 6,000	(3) 6,000			Bal. 100,000
(1) 25,000	(4) 14,000	(4) 14,000			(1) 25,000
(2) 12,000					(2) 12,000
(3) 7,500					

Equity		Revenues	
	Bal. 200,000		(3) 7,500

This entry records a decrease in assets (cash) and an increase in expenses (employees' salaries and wages expense).

The fifth transaction is the billing of hospital patients for $15,300 of services (room and board, laboratory, pharmacy, and so on):

Assets		Expenses		Liabilities	
Bal. 300,000	(3) 6,000	(3) 6,000			Bal. 100,000
(1) 25,000	(4) 14,000	(4) 14,000			(1) 25,000
(2) 12,000					(2) 12,000
(3) 7,500					
(5) 15,300					

Equity		Revenues	
	Bal. 200,000		(3) 7,500
			(5) 15,300

This entry records an increase in hospital assets (accounts receivable) and an increase in hospital revenues (revenues from services to patients). A portion of the accounts receivable established in this entry will be collected in cash in the eighth transaction.

Transaction 6 consists of the repayment of the bank loan of $25,000 plus $1,000 of interest assumed to be due the bank. The required entry, numbered *6*, includes 2 debits and one credit:

Assets		Expenses		Liabilities	
Bal. 300,000	(3) 6,000	(3) 6,000		(6) 25,000	Bal. 100,000
(1) 25,000	(4) 14,000	(4) 14,000			(1) 25,000
(2) 12,000	(6) 26,000	(6) 1,000			(2) 12,000
(3) 7,500					
(5) 15,300					

Equity (Dr.)	Equity (Cr.)
	Bal. 200,000

Revenues (Dr.)	Revenues (Cr.)
	(3) 7,500
	(5) 15,300

Of this $26,000 cash disbursement, $1,000 is interest expense, and the remaining $25,000 is a reduction of liabilities (elimination of the bank loan payable).

The seventh transaction is the payment by the hospital of $9,000 of accounts payable to its suppliers. The required entry, numbered *7*, is

Assets (Dr.)	Assets (Cr.)
Bal. 300,000	(3) 6,000
(1) 25,000	(4) 14,000
(2) 12,000	(6) 26,000
(3) 7,500	(7) 9,000
(5) 15,300	

Expenses (Dr.)	Expenses (Cr.)
(3) 6,000	
(4) 14,000	
(6) 1,000	

Liabilities (Dr.)	Liabilities (Cr.)
(6) 25,000	Bal. 100,000
(7) 9,000	(1) 25,000
	(2) 12,000

Equity (Dr.)	Equity (Cr.)
	Bal. 200,000

Revenues (Dr.)	Revenues (Cr.)
	(3) 7,500
	(5) 15,300

These accounts payable arose in transaction 2 when the liabilities account was credited for $12,000. Now, since $9,000 of the accounts payable are being paid, the liabilities account is debited. The difference of $3,000 remains unpaid as part of the credit balance in the liabilities account.

The last transaction is the receipt of $18,400 in payment of a portion of accounts receivable due from patients for supplies and services provided to them in previous transactions (transactions 3 and 5). The required entry, numbered *8*, is

Assets (Dr.)	Assets (Cr.)
Bal. 300,000	(3) 6,000
(1) 25,000	(4) 14,000
(2) 12,000	(6) 26,000
(3) 7,500	(7) 9,000
(5) 15,300	(8) 18,400
(8) 18,400	

Expenses (Dr.)	Expenses (Cr.)
(3) 6,000	
(4) 14,000	
(6) 1,000	

Liabilities (Dr.)	Liabilities (Cr.)
(6) 25,000	Bal. 100,000
(7) 9,000	(1) 25,000
	(2) 12,000

Equity (Dr.)	Equity (Cr.)
	Bal. 200,000

Revenues (Dr.)	Revenues (Cr.)
	(3) 7,500
	(5) 15,300

This transaction requires entering a debit and a credit to the assets account. The entry, in this case, debits (increases) one type of asset (cash) and credits (decreases) another type of asset (accounts receivable).

Now we should determine the *balance* of each account. Consider, for example, the assets account which consists of an opening balance at the beginning of the period, 5 debits for the increases in assets during the period, and 5 credits for the decreases in assets during the period. The balance of assets at the end of the period may be determined as follows:

Assets			
Bal.	300,000	(3)	6,000
(1)	25,000	(4)	14,000
(2)	12,000	(6)	26,000
(3)	7,500	(7)	9,000
(5)	15,300	(8)	18,400
(8)	18,400		
	378,200		73,400
	73,400		
Bal.	304,800		

Notice that the opening balance of assets plus the debits (increases) during the period total $378,200; the credits (decreases) during the period total $73,400. The difference between the debit and credit totals is the end-of-period balance of assets, that is, a debit balance of $304,800. It is a debit balance because the debit total in the account exceeds the credit total.

A balance for each of the other accounts may be determined in a similar manner. To determine whether or not the ledger is in balance, the individual account balances may be arranged in a *trial balance*, as follows:

	Balances	
	Dr.	Cr.
Assets	$304,800	
Expenses	21,000	
Liabilities		$103,000
Equity		200,000
Revenues		22,800
Totals	$325,800	$325,800

Notice that the accounts for assets and expenses have debit balances, and that the accounts for liabilities, equity, and revenues have credit balances. This is the normal state of affairs. Elements of the left-hand side of the accounting equation are debit items; elements of the right are credit items.

To obtain the end-of-period equity balance (taking into account the net income for the period), a closing entry is required. This entry, labeled *C*, is shown as follows:

Assets

Bal. 300,000	(3) 6,000
(1) 25,000	(4) 14,000
(2) 12,000	(6) 26,000
(3) 7,500	(7) 9,000
(4) 15,300	(8) 18,400
(8) 18,400	

Expenses

(3) 6,000	(C) 21,000
(4) 14,000	
(6) 1,000	
═════	═════

Liabilities

(6) 25,000	Bal. 100,000
(7) 9,000	(1) 25,000
	(2) 12,000

Equity

	Bal. 200,000
	(C) 1,800

Revenues

(C) 22,800	(3) 7,500
	(5) 15,300
═════	═════

The closing entry eliminates the balances of revenues and expenses, and records the $1,800 difference (net income) as an increase in the equity account. The double rules in the accounts for revenues and expenses indicate that these accounts have been closed and have no balance. In the account for expenses, for example, debits equal credits; the account balance is zero.

Need for More-Detailed Information

If financial statements were to be prepared from the accounts developed in the foregoing discussion, the information in those statements would be highly condensed data. The income statement for the period and the balance sheet at the end of the period would contain the following information:

Figure 6

Income Statement

Revenues	$22,800
Less expenses	21,000
Net income for the period	$ 1,800

Balance Sheet

Assets	$304,800
Liabilities	$103,000
Equity	201,800
Total liabilities and equity	$304,800

While these are the kinds of information required by financial statement users, the categories are much too broad to be useful. Considerably more-detailed information must be provided.

From what services and other sources did the hospital earn its revenues, and how much revenue was derived from each source? What is the functional and natural breakdown of the hospital's expenses, and how much expense was incurred in each classification? What specific assets are owned by the hospital, and how much money is invested in each of them? What specific liabilities does the hospital have, and what is the monetary amount of each of them? Which of these assets and liabilities are current, and which are noncurrent?

In the next chapter, we shall begin to develop the detailed information necessary to answer such questions.

QUESTIONS

1. Indicate briefly the need for documentary evidence in accounting. Give 5 examples of documentary evidences used in hospital accounting.
2. Define the term *debit*.
3. Define the term *credit*.
4. "In accounting, debits represent something 'bad' (undesirable), whereas credits represent something 'good' (desirable)." Do you agree? Explain.
5. State the rules of debit and credit with respect to asset and expense accounts.
6. State the rules of debit and credit with respect to liability, equity, and revenue accounts.
7. What are compound entries?
8. What is a trial balance? What is its purpose?
9. Which of the following types of accounts normally have debit balances?
   - a. Assets
   - b. Liabilities
   - c. Equity
   - d. Revenues
   - e. Expenses
10. What is the purpose of a closing entry?

PROBLEMS

A. Assume that General Hospital on May 1 had $29,000 of assets, $12,000 of liabilities, and $17,000 of equity. Subsequently, the following transactions were completed:

1. The sum of $2,500 was borrowed from a bank.
2. The hospital repaid $1,000 (disregard interest) of the bank loan.
3. Supplies costing $1,800 were purchased on account and placed in inventory.
4. A new item of equipment was purchased for $4,600 cash.
5. The amount of $800 was paid on accounts payable.
6. Supplies previously purchased for $700 were sold to patients for $960 cash.
7. Patients' accounts were charged for $1,770 of hospital services rendered to them.
8. Cash collections on patients' accounts amounted to $1,150.

Required. Taking into account the cumulative effects of the 8 transactions and the May 1 balances, what are General Hospital's total assets, total liabilities, and total equity?

B. On October 1 Specific Hospital had $450,000 of assets, $150,000 of liabilities, and $300,000 of equity. Transactions completed during the month of October were as follows:

1. The hospital borrowed $50,000 from a bank.
2. The hospital purchased supplies on account for $20,000.
3. Seventy-five percent of the supplies were issued from inventory and used in patient care. Patients were billed for $21,000.
4. The hospital paid $45,000 of salaries and wages to its employees.
5. Patients were billed for $48,500 of other services.
6. The hospital paid $30,400 (including $400 interest) on the bank loan.
7. The hospital paid $17,000 on its accounts payable.
8. The hospital collected $59,000 on patients' accounts receivable.

Required. Prepare an analysis of the above transactions in the form illustrated in figure 5 at page 30.

C. On December 1 Gibson Hospital had $380,000 of assets, $120,000 of liabilities, and $260,000 of equity. Transactions completed during the month of December were as follows:

1. The hospital borrowed $20,000 from a bank.
2. Supplies purchased on account amounted to $14,000.
3. Supplies issued from inventory and used in patient care amounted to $10,000. Patients were billed for $16,000.
4. Employees were paid $28,000 of salaries and wages.
5. New equipment was purchased for $4,000 cash.
6. Patients were billed for $26,000 of other services.
7. The bank loan was paid off with a disbursement of $20,300 (this includes interest of $300).
8. Payments on accounts payable amounted to $11,000.
9. Collections on accounts receivable were $39,000.

Required. Prepare a debit-and-credit analysis of the above information in T-account form, including a closing entry at December 31. Indicate the balance of each account at December 31.

D. On November 1 Ohio Hospital had $710,000 of assets, $230,000 of liabilities, and $480,000 of equity. Transactions completed during the month of November were as follows:

1. Supplies purchased on account totaled $29,000.
2. Supplies which had cost $26,000 were issued from inventory and used in patient care. Patients were billed $31,000.
3. Employees were paid $84,000 of salaries and wages.
4. Patients were billed for November services.

Daily patient services	$51,500
Other professional services	37,500
Total	$89,000

5. Other operating revenues received in cash came to $2,800.
6. Purchase of new equipment on account was for $12,000.
7. Payments on accounts payable amounted to $24,700.
8. Collections on accounts receivable totaled $102,600.
9. Miscellaneous other expenses paid in cash came to $14,300.

Required (1) Prepare a debit-and-credit analysis of the above information in T-account form, including a closing entry at November 30. (2) Prepare, in as much detail as possible, an income statement for November.

3
Journal, Ledger, and Trial Balance

The preceding chapter was concerned with the analysis of business transactions in terms of their increase and decrease effects on the basic elements of the accounting equation. Only 5 accounts were used in the analysis: assets, expenses, liabilities, equity, and revenues. A much greater number of accounts is needed, however, to provide the detailed information required by hospital management and other financial statement users. Such information is developed by the use of a *chart of accounts*, sometimes called a *classification of accounts*. A relatively simple chart of accounts will be introduced in this chapter.

Also in the previous chapter, transaction entries were recorded directly in the accounts. This procedure is not feasible in actual accounting practice because of the large volume of transactions which must be recorded each day. Instead, the effects of business transactions are recorded initially in an accounting record known as a *journal*. The process of making records of transactions in a journal is called *journalizing*. Subsequently, the journalized information is transferred (by a process called *posting*) into the accounts in the hospital's ledger. The major part of this chapter is devoted to a discussion of these procedures.

ILLUSTRATION DATA

Let us assume that Smalltown is a rapidly growing community but one without a hospital of its own. Since the nearest hospital is located in a city a considerable distance away, the citizens of Smalltown decide to build a hospital for their community. A civic improvement committee is established for the purpose of raising the necessary money for construction, equipment, and initial operating funds (working capital). An extended fund-raising campaign is completed on December 31, 1976, when a goal of $100,000 is achieved. The hospital is incorporated under the laws of the state, and a corporate charter is duly obtained.

Upon receipt of the not-for-profit charter, the Smalltown Hospital begins its corporate existence on January 1, 1977. During the ensuing year, the following transactions are completed by the hospital.

1. On January 1, 1977, the hospital receives its initial equity of $100,000 from the citizens of Smalltown through the Civic Improvement Committee.
2. On January 2, 1977, the hospital issues $50,000 of 8%, 10-year bonds at face value. Interest on these bonds is payable annually on December 31.
3. On January 3, 1977, the hospital purchases plant assets for cash as follows:

Land	$ 25,000
Building	67,000
Equipment	45,000
Total cost	$137,000

   The cost of the building includes the alterations and remodeling of an existing structure previously operated as a hotel.
4. During the year, total purchases of supplies on account by the hospital amount to $28,200. These include dietary supplies, pharmaceuticals, and other medical and surgical supplies.
5. As the year passes, $21,500 of these supplies are issued from inventory for use in hospital operations.
6. Services rendered to patients over the course of the year total $120,300 and are billed to patients as follows:

Routine services	$ 72,180
Ancillary services	48,120
Total revenues	$120,300

   Routine services include room, board, and ordinary nursing care. Ancillary services include those performed by departments such as operating rooms, laboratory, X-ray, and pharmacy.
7. During the year, collections on patients' accounts amount to $94,500. (We will assume no charity service, no bad debts, and no other deductions from revenues.)
8. Payments on accounts payable to suppliers during 1977 are $22,600.
9. During the year, the hospital receives in cash $13,800 of revenues from other sources (including unrestricted contributions and gifts).
10. Over the course of the year, the hospital pays operating expenses as follows:

Salaries and wages	$76,400
Utilities	12,700
Insurance	3,600
Repairs	2,900
Other expenses	1,300
Total	$96,900

11. On October 1, 1977, the hospital obtains a short-term, 10% loan of $12,000 from a local bank.
12. On December 31, 1977, the hospital pays interest expense on the bonds and bank loan as follows:

Interest on bonds	$4,000
Interest on bank loan	300
Total	$4,300

You should understand that the above listing is largely a summary of the perhaps thousands of transactions for 1977. Except in a few cases, individual transactions are not indicated. This also means that, other than where particular dates are specified, the itemization is *not* in the chronological order in which the events occurred. Items 4 through 10, for example, each describe a series of transactions which took place over the entire year at periodic intervals. The hospital rendered patient services daily, cash was received and disbursed every day, supplies may have been purchased weekly, salaries and wages were perhaps paid biweekly or monthly, and so forth.

You now are aware of all the financial activity engaged in by Smalltown Hospital during 1977. Knowing this, what is the hospital's net income for the year? How much cash does Smalltown Hospital have in the bank at the end of the year? At December 31, 1977, what is the amount of accounts receivable due from patients? Inventory? Accounts payable to suppliers? What are the amounts of other hospital assets and liabilities?

Who cares? As you learned in chapter 1, management cares, creditors care, third-party payers care, the banker cares, the bondholders care, governmental agencies care, and the citizens of Smalltown have a considerable interest. All of these groups and others care very much indeed about these questions and the answers to them! Without such information, none of these groups would be able to make intelligent economic decisions.

So, if we can agree that financial information about Smalltown Hospital is important and useful, how do we deal with the problems of accumulating and communicating it? How do we develop and maintain the necessary accounting records, and how do we report the recorded information to those who use it?

CHART OF ACCOUNTS

As noted in the preceding chapter, competent documentary evidence of completed transactions is the first and fundamental requirement of the accounting system. Documentary evidence is essential because the reliability and accuracy of the information produced by the accounting process rests largely upon the extent to which that information is based upon verifiable, objectively determined facts. You realize, of course, that accounting never can become fully objective or completely scientific. Accounting is an art which requires the exercise of judgment and the use of estimates. Wherever possible, however, business transactions are evidenced by objective documentation such as invoices, bank deposit slips, charge tickets, cash receipt slips, and other business papers.

Figure 7
Smalltown Hospital
Chart of Accounts

100 *Assets*

101 Cash
102 Accounts Receivable
103 Inventory

110 Land
111 Building
112 Equipment

200 *Liabilities*

201 Accounts Payable
202 Bank Loan Payable

210 Bonds Payable

300 *Equity*

301 Hospital Equity
302 Revenue and Expense Summary

400 *Revenues*

401 Routine Services Revenue
402 Ancillary Services Revenue
403 Other Revenues

500 *Expenses*

501 Salaries and Wages Expense
502 Supplies Expense
503 Utilities Expense
504 Insurance Expense
505 Repairs Expense
506 Interest Expense
507 Other Expenses

Properly executed documentary evidences make the accountant aware that transactions have occurred. In order to record these transactions in an organized manner, an information-classification system must be used. This system is set forth in a *chart of accounts* such as the one illustrated in figure 7. This chart depicts the manner in which transaction data will be classified and recorded in the accounting records of Smalltown Hospital. It is designed primarily to meet the informational needs of the hospital management, but accounting standards as well as legal, tax, and regulatory agency requirements also influence its design.

The illustrative chart is divided into 5 groups of accounts: assets, liabilities, equity, revenues, and expenses. Each account in the chart is assigned an identifying number. Any account in the "100" series is an asset, any account in the "200" series is a liability, and so on. This numerical coding of the accounts saves clerical time and effort in that it is easier to say, write, or type "501," for example, than it is to say, write, or type "salaries and wages expense." Numerical coding also promotes accuracy and permits one to identify the nature of an account readily. Data processing equipment requires the use of account numbers.

There are 21 accounts in Smalltown Hospital's chart. If the management of Smalltown Hospital required more detailed information about expenditures for, say, utilities, separate accounts could be provided for water, electricity, and heat instead of combining all such expenditures into a single utilities account. Or, rather than a single revenue account for ancillary services, a number of separate accounts could be maintained for individual services such as operating room revenue, laboratory revenue, pharmacy revenue, etc. This, of course, is done in actual practice where charts of accounts generally consist of several hundred individual accounts. Smalltown Hospital's chart of accounts, however, is limited to just 21 accounts for the purposes of this introductory discussion. Notice also that we are not yet ready to introduce accounts for depreciation, prepaid and accrued expenses, bad debts, and various other financial-statement items which you may recall having seen in chapter 1. These complications will be introduced at appropriate points in subsequent chapters.

JOURNAL

Assuming we have documentary evidence supporting Smalltown Hospital's 1977 transactions, and given the hospital's chart of accounts, we can proceed with the task of analyzing and recording the transactions for the year. Each of the 12 transactions previously listed will be analyzed in terms of its effects on the account classifications provided in the chart of accounts. Which account or accounts should be debited, and which should be credited, for each of these transactions? This debit-and-credit analysis will be recorded initially in an accounting record called a *journal*.

As you will see later, there are many types of journals: revenue journals, cash receipt journals, voucher registers, etc. These special journals are illustrated in chapters 11–14. We are concerned at this point, however, only with the *general journal*. This particular form of journal is illustrated in figure 8.

The process of recording transactions in the journal is called *journalizing*. It consists of a formal handwritten or typewritten analysis of the increase and decrease effects of transactions on the

Figure 8
General Journal Form

Date			Accounts and Explanations	Account Numbers	Debit	Credit
Mo.	Day	Yr.	Account(s) to be Debited	No.	Amount	
			Account (s) to be Credited	No.		Amount
			Explanation of the transaction.			
			(EXAMPLE)			
1	1	77	Cash	101	100000	
			Hospital Equity	301		100000
			Receipt of initial equity funds from Civic Improvement Committee.			
1	2	77	Cash	101	50000	
			Bonds Payable	210		50000
			Issue of 8%, 10-year bonds at face value.			

specific account classifications provided in the chart of accounts. You can think of journalizing as maintaining a business diary for the hospital. The journal is a chronological record of financial events in the economic life of the hospital. As each event, or transaction, occurs, it is recorded in the journal. This record, as you can see in figure 8, consists of several elements:

1. The date of the transaction
2. The titles of the accounts affected (increased and/or decreased) by the transaction, i.e., the accounts to be debited and credited
3. A brief explanation of the nature and salient facts of the transaction
4. The account numbers for the accounts being debited and credited
5. The dollar amounts of the debits and credits

These are the essential elements of a *journal entry*. All these elements must be provided for each entry.

Several different kinds of journal entries are made in accounting. Further on in this book, you will learn to make adjusting entries, correcting entries, and closing entries. For the moment, however, we are concerned only with entries to record transactions, that is, *transaction entries*.

All of the transaction entries for Smalltown Hospital for the 1977 year are shown in figure 9. Carefully note the following points:

1. The date on which each transaction occurred ordinarily is written in the column on the far left. For the purposes of this illustration, however, we give each transaction entry a number rather than a specific date.

   Transactions of the same type—purchases of supplies, for example—are summarized for the entire year in this illustration and are recorded by a single journal entry in order to simplify and shorten the presentation. This is why the journal entries are not dated with a specific month and day indication.
2. The titles of the accounts debited and credited, along with a brief explanation of the transaction being recorded, are indicated in the next section of the journal.
   a. The title of the account, or accounts, debited in each entry is written first against the left-hand margin.
   b. The title of the account, or accounts, credited is written underneath the account(s) debited and is indented about an inch or so. This indentation distinguishes the credits from the debits at a mere glance.
   c. The explanation or description of the transaction follows the account titles and is indented about half an inch so that it will not be confused with account titles.

   It is very important that you use the precise account titles indicated by the chart of accounts and that you not "invent" new accounts. Your analysis is limited to the accounts provided in the chart of accounts.

Figure 9
Smalltown Hospital
1977 Journal

Entry No.	Accounts and Explanations	Acct. No.	Debit	Credit
1	Cash	101	100,000	
	Hospital Equity	301		100,000
	Receipt of equity funds from Smalltown Civic Improvement Committee.			
2	Cash	101	50,000	
	Bonds Payable	210		50,000
	Issue of 8%, 10-year bonds at face value.			
3	Land	110	25,000	
	Building	111	67,000	
	Equipment	112	45,000	
	Cash	101		137,000
	Purchase of plant assets.			
4	Inventory	103	28,200	
	Accounts Payable	201		28,200
	Purchase of supplies on account.			
5	Supplies Expense	502	21,500	
	Inventory	103		21,500
	Supplies used.			
6	Accounts Receivable	102	120,300	
	Routine Services Revenue	401		72,180
	Ancillary Services Revenue	402		48,120
	Charges to patients for services rendered.			
7	Cash	101	94,500	
	Accounts Receivable	102		94,500
	Collections on patients' accounts.			
8	Accounts Payable	201	22,600	
	Cash	101		22,600
	Payments on accounts payable to suppliers.			
9	Cash	101	13,800	
	Other Revenues	403		13,800
	Receipt of miscellaneous revenues.			
10	Salaries and Wages Expense	501	76,400	
	Utilities Expense	503	12,700	
	Insurance Expense	504	3,600	
	Repairs Expense	505	2,900	
	Other Expenses	507	1,300	
	Cash	101		96,900
	Payments of operating expenses.			
11	Cash	101	12,000	
	Bank Loan Payable	202		12,000
	Receipt of short-term, 10% loan from local bank.			
12	Interest Expense	506	4,300	
	Cash	101		4,300
	Payment of interest as follows:			
	Interest on bonds $4,000			
	Interest on bank loan 300			
	Total $4,300			

3. The account numbers of the accounts debited and credited in each journal entry are entered in the column provided for them. Do not "invent" new account numbers; use the numerical coding provided by the chart of accounts.
4. The dollar amounts involved in the transaction are written in the debit and credit columns on the right-hand side of the journal. Dollar marks ($) are not necessary.
5. One line is skipped between journal entries so that each entry is set apart from the others on the journal page.

While much accounting is still done manually in this typewritten or handwritten form, most hospitals employ accounting machines and various kinds of electronic data processing equipment. What you see in figure 9 in manual form, however, is the same sort of record made by the use of accounting machines, punched cards, and magnetic tape.

Now let us quickly examine each of the 12 transaction entries appearing in Smalltown Hospital's 1977 journal:

Entry No.

1 The transaction had the effect of increasing the hospital assets (cash) and increasing the hospital's equity. Assets are increased by debits, and equity is increased by credits; so, we record a debit to cash and a credit to hospital equity.

2 The transaction increased the hospital's assets (cash) and its liabilities (bonds payable). Assets are increased by debits, and liabilities are increased by credits; so, we debit cash and credit bonds payable. (This entry is very similar to entry 11.)

3 The transaction increased 3 asset categories (land, building, and equipment) and decreased another (cash). Assets are increased by debits and decreased by credits; so, we debit the accounts for land, building, and equipment, and credit the cash account.

4 The transaction was one in which the hospital acquired an asset (inventory) and incurred a liability (accounts payable); so, we record an addition to the hospital assets and an addition to hospital liabilities.

Further on, you will see that purchased supplies sometimes can be debited directly to supplies expense rather than to inventory. For the present, however, we will debit inventory.

5 The transaction decreased an asset (inventory) and increased the hospital's expenses (supplies expense). Expenses are increased by debits; assets are decreased by credits; so, we record the cost of the supplies used as expense and reduce the inventory.

6 In this summary transaction hospital services were rendered to patients who did not pay for the services at the time they were provided. Revenues earned by the hospital are given accounting recognition, at the time services are rendered.

The transaction, then, increases the hospital's assets and its revenues. Since assets are increased by debits and revenues are increased by credits, we debit accounts receivable and credit the appropriate revenue accounts.

7 Cash collections on patients' accounts increase cash and decrease accounts receivable. No revenue is recognized here; the revenue to which these collections relate has already been recorded in entry 6.

8 When supplies were purchased on account (entry 4), accounts payable were established by a credit. Now, when a portion of these accounts is paid, accounts payable are debited (decreased) and cash is credited (decreased). This entry is a decrease in one account and a decrease in another; this transaction results in no increase in any account.

9 This transaction entry records the receipt of cash representing revenues collected from miscellaneous sources, such as sales receipts from the hospital cafeteria. Certain kinds of revenues may be recorded directly in this manner without using a receivables account.

10 This summary entry records the disbursements made during the year for various operating expenses. The appropriate expense accounts are debited, and cash is credited.

In actual practice, however, all hospital disbursements are run through liability accounts. Salaries and wages, for example, require 2 entries:

Salaries and Wages Expense	$---	
Salaries and Wages Payable		$---
Salaries and Wages Payable	$---	
Cash		$---

This procedure will be introduced later but, for now, we will record expenses directly by debits to expense and credits to cash. We also are disregarding, at this point, matters such as payroll taxes, prepaid expenses, accrued expenses, and depreciation.

11 This entry records the receipt of a short-term (less than one year) loan from a bank. Cash is debited, and the liability to the bank is established by the credit. A similar transaction was recorded in entry 2.

Note carefully that neither in this entry nor in entry 2 was any recognition given to interest, either as a liability or as expense. The point is that, at the time the bank loan was received and at the time the bonds were issued, the hospital owed no interest and therefore had no interest expense. The interest on these obligations is recorded in entry 12.

12 You will recall that the hospital issued $50,000 of 10-year, 8% bonds at the beginning of the year. These bonds have been outstanding all year, so the bond interest expense is $4,000 (i.e., $50,000 × 8%).

The bank loan, on the other hand, was obtained on October 1, 1977. Since the hospital has had the use of the bank's money for only 3 months (October, November, December), the hospital's interest expense is $300 (i.e., $12,000 × 10% × $^3/_{12}$).

We are assuming that interest on the bonds and on the bank loan is paid on December 31, 1977. So, the entry debits interest expense and credits cash for $4,300 or $4,000 + $300. If we assumed, however, that the interest was payable on January 1, 1978, the December 31 entry would be

Interest Expense	$4,300	
Accrued Interest Payable		$4,300

We are not yet ready to take up expense accruals, but this matter will be considered at a later point.

Thus, Smalltown Hospital's 1977 journal provides a chronological record of the effects of the year's transactions on the account classifications set forth in the hospital's chart of accounts. It presents an economic history of the hospital's financial activities for the year.

To assist you in your study of the transaction entries in the 1977 journal of Smalltown Hospital, a classification of routine transaction entries is provided in figure 10. These points should be noted:

1. Transactions completed by a hospital may be classified basically as either cash transactions or noncash transactions. If the transaction produces a cash receipt or requires a cash disbursement, it is a cash transaction. All other transactions, of course, are noncash transactions.
2. If the transaction does not involve a cash receipt or disbursement, it may be (for example) the purchase of supplies on account, a charge to patients for services rendered, or the use of supplies from the hospital's inventory. While there are many other types of noncash transactions, these 3 are the ones with which you are concerned presently.
3. If the transaction is a cash transaction, it is either a cash disbursement or cash receipt transaction. This can be determined simply by reading the description of the transaction as given in the text or in end-of-chapter problems.
   a. If the transaction is a cash disbursement, you will always make a *credit* to cash. Cash disbursements are decreases in cash, an asset. To decrease an asset, you credit the asset.

      Then, you ask; "What do I *debit*?" Simply ask yourself, "For what was the money spent?" Was it spent to acquire an asset? If so, debit the asset. Was it spent to eliminate or reduce a liability? If so, debit the appropriate liability account. Was it spent to pay an expense? If so, debit the appropriate expense account.

      Cash-disbursement transactions may require a debit to equity or to a revenue account, but such transactions are extremely unusual. You need not be concerned with such transactions at this time.

Figure 10
Classification of Routine Transaction Entries

	Dr.	*Cr.*
Noncash-Transaction Entries:		
1. Purchases of supplies on account:		
Inventory	X	
Accounts Payable		X
2. Charges to patients for services rendered:		
Accounts Receivable	X	
Appropriate Revenue Accounts		X
3. Usage of supplies from inventory:		
Supplies Expense	X	
Inventory		X
Cash-Transaction Entries: Cash Disbursements		
1. Acquisition of an asset:		
Appropriate Asset Account	X	
Cash		X
2. Elimination of a liability:		
Appropriate Liability Account	X	
Cash		X
3. Payment of an expense:		
Appropriate Expense Account	X	
Cash		X
Cash Receipts		
1. Collections on patients' accounts:		
Cash	X	
Accounts Receivable		X
2. Incurrence of a liability:		
Cash	X	
Appropriate Liability Account		X
3. Receipt of revenue:		
Cash	X	
Appropriate Revenue Account		X

b. If the transaction is identified as a cash receipt, you will always make a *debit* to cash. To determine the proper *credit*, you simply ask yourself: "What was the source of the cash receipt?" Did the cash arise from collections of patients' accounts? If so, credit accounts receivable. Was the cash obtained through the incurrence of a liability, for example, bank loans or bond issues? If so, credit the appropriate liability account. Does the cash receipt represent revenues provided on a cash basis, that is, cash received at the time the service is rendered? If so, credit the appropriate revenue account.

Cash-receipt transactions rarely require a credit to expense, but a credit to equity sometimes is required (as you have seen in Smalltown Hospital's first journal entry). Also, hospitals will make occasional sales of plant assets which will require a credit to land, buildings, or equipment. Further on, you will deal with some of these transactions.

Remember that figure 10 is a classification of routine, regularly recurring transaction entries only. These routine, regularly recurring, transactions in practice are recorded in specialized journals which are illustrated in subsequent chapters. Until then, we will enter all transactions in a general journal. There also are other kinds of transactions not included in figure 10. And, as mentioned earlier, entries other than transaction entries are made in journals, e.g., adjusting entries and closing entries. You will be introduced to non-transaction entries shortly.

LEDGER

At this point, we have a complete record of the transactions completed by Smalltown Hospital during 1977. This record appears in chronological sequence in the hospital's journal. The journal, however, does not readily or directly provide the information needed for the development of financial statements. It does not provide individual account balances at the end of the year! Nowhere in the journal do we find, for example, the December 31, 1977, cash balance. In an actual situation, the journal may consist of hundreds of pages and include perhaps thousands of transaction entries. Cash receipt and disbursement entries appear in chronological order throughout the pages of the journal, and there is no indication of the year-end cash balance. How, then, do we determine the December 31, 1977, balance of cash or of any other account in Smalltown Hospital's chart of accounts?

To determine year-end account balances, we must transfer the information recorded in the journal to another accounting record called a *ledger*. The process of making this transfer is called *posting*. By posting to the ledger, the journalized information is summarized according to account classification so that all recorded increases and decreases in each account are brought together to permit the determination of individual account balances at the end of the year.

A *ledger account*, as it might appear in actual practice, is illustrated in figure 11. A single page or card ordinarily is used for each account. The title and number of the account appears at the top of the form. Within the form, columns are provided to indicate the various elements of each posting to the account:

1. The date indicated generally is the date as of which the posting is being made. In other words, in posting the 1977 journal entries, the postings to the ledger would be dated December 31, 1977. Sometimes, however, the posting date may be the

Figure 11
Ledger Account

Account Title — Cash				Account No. — 101	
				Balance	
Date		Ref.	Debit	Credit	Debit	Credit
1 1 77		GJ-1	100000		100000	
1 2 77		GJ-1	50000		150000	
1 3 77		GJ-1		137000	13000	

(EXAMPLE)

date the transaction occurred as shown in figure 11, but we will not do this in subsequent illustrations.

2. The next column may be used for memorandum entries or notations of supplemental information of interest to the bookkeeper. You may disregard this column for the time being.
3. The "Ref." column (sometimes shown as "LF," leaf folio) is the posting reference; i.e., the name of the journal and the page number of the journal from which the posting is made. This provides a cross-reference between the ledger and the journal.
4. The next 2 columns are used to show the dollar amounts of debits and credits posted from the various journal entries affecting the account. In this way, all of the increases and decreases in each ledger account (as recorded in the journal) are brought together on a single page so that the balance of each account can be determined.
5. The 2 columns on the far right are used to maintain a running balance (debit or credit, as the case may be) of the account. If debit postings exceed credit postings, the account will have a debit balance, and vice versa.

The example shown in the ledger account assumes that the account is the account for cash, account number 101. What you see in this example are the postings to the cash account of the cash debits and credits from the first 3 entries on page 1 of Smalltown Hospital's general journal.

The ledger account form used in the remainder of this book, however, will be the "T-account" form introduced in the preceding chapter. Figure 12 illustrates how we will make postings to these "T accounts." Notice that no posting dates will be indicated; we will assume that all postings are made on December 31. Instead of using a journal page number as the posting reference, we will simply use the journal entry number, that is, (1), (2), (3), and so on. And, instead of maintaining a running balance in each account, we will wait until all debit and credit postings are made before computing an account balance.

You should recognize that figure 12 illustrates only the postings of the cash debits and credits from the first 3 journal entries. *All* debits and credits in the journal, of course, must be posted to the respective ledger accounts. This will be seen in figure 13.

To summarize, then, the transactions for the period are initially recorded as transaction entries in the hospital's journal (figure 9). While this provides a necessary chronological record of the transactions, it does not accumulate the account balances resulting from those transactions. These end-of-period account balances are needed in order to prepare financial statements. So, the information recorded in the journal must be rearranged and summarized in such a manner that these balances can be determined. This is accomplished by posting (transferring) the journal entries to the ledger accounts.

The ledger contains a separate account for each account listed in the chart of accounts. Since Smalltown Hospital's chart provides for 21 accounts, the hospital's ledger will consist of 21 accounts. This ledger is referred to as the *general ledger*. As there are several different kinds of journals, so are there several different kinds of ledgers. Ledgers other than the general ledger are called *subsidiary ledgers*. Such ledgers include the accounts receivable subsidiary ledger (or "patients' ledger"), the accounts payable ledger, the plant assets subsidiary ledger, and others. Later on,

Figure 12
Illustration of Posting Procedure

(JOURNAL)

Entry No.	Accounts and Explanations	Acct. No.	Debit	Credit
1	Cash	101	100,000	
	Hospital Equity	301		100,000
	Receipt of equity funds from Smalltown Civic Improvement Committee.			
2	Cash	101	50,000	
	Bonds Payable	210		50,000
	Issue of 8%, 10-year bonds at face value.			
3	Land	110	25,000	
	Building	111	67,000	
	Equipment	112	45,000	
	Cash	101		137,000
	Purchase of plant assets.			

(LEDGER)

CASH 101

(1) 100,000	(3) 137,000
(2) 50,000	

Figure 13
Smalltown Hospital
1977 Ledger

Cash 101

(1) 100,000	(3) 137,000
(2) 50,000	(8) 22,600
(7) 94,500	(10) 96,900
(9) 13,800	(12) 4,300
(11) 12,000	
(B) 9,500	

Accounts Receivable 102

(6) 120,300	(7) 94,500
(B) 25,800	

Inventory 103

(4) 28,200	(5) 21,500
(B) 6,700	

Land 110

(3) 25,000	

Building 111

(3) 67,000	

Equipment 112

(3) 45,000	

Accounts Payable 201

(8) 22,600	(4) 28,200
	(B) 5,600

Bank Loan Payable 202

	(11) 12,000

Bonds Payable 210

	(2) 50,000

Hospital Equity 301

	(1) 100,000

Revenue and Expense Summary 302

Routine Services Revenue 401

	(6) 72,180

Ancillary Services Revenue 402

	(6) 48,120

Other Revenues 403

	(9) 13,800

Salaries and Wages Expense 501

(10) 76,400	

Supplies Expense 502	
(5) 21,500	

Utilities Expense 503	
(10) 12,700	

Insurance Expense 504	
(10) 3,600	

Repairs Expense 505	
(10) 2,900	

Interest Expense 506	
(12) 4,300	

Other Expenses 507	
(10) 1,300	

subsidiary ledgers will be discussed, but for now we are concerned only with the general ledger.

While you may have some difficulty at first with the journalizing of transactions in journals, you should have little trouble with postings to the ledger accounts. Posting is simply a matter of copying the journal debits and credits into the ledger accounts. If the journal "says" debit cash, you debit the cash account in the ledger; if the journal entry includes a credit to hospital capital, you post a credit to the ledger account for hospital capital. This procedure is easily learned. Be sure, however, that you post all debits and credits from the journal to the ledger: be careful not to overlook any postings. And, unless you are attentive, you may find yourself posting debits as credits or credits as debits. If you do this, your ledger will not balance.

Figure 13 shows Smalltown Hospital's ledger after all postings of the 12 transactions have been made. It probably would be helpful if you would trace all of these postings from the hospital's journal (figure 9) into the accounts. Notice also in figure 13 that, where an account has more than a single posting and the account balance is not obvious, account balances have been determined. This was done simply by totaling the debits in the account, totaling the credits in the account, and computing the differences between the totals. This difference, either a debit or credit, is shown as the account balance, labeled *B*. If it is a debit balance, it is shown on the left side of the account; credit balances are shown on the right side.

Only one posting appears in many of the ledger accounts because of the fact that the illustration is simplified. In actual practice, of course, most ledger accounts will have multiple postings. If, for example, the hospital pays salaries and wages to its employees on a monthly basis, the salaries and wages expense account will have 12 postings. Too, we have assumed annual postings to the ledger accounts, whereas postings are made monthly in actual practice.

So, do not be misled by the illustration; in an actual hospital, there typically is a considerable amount of activity in each ledger account.

One more point should be made with respect to Smalltown Hospital's ledger. You probably have noticed the revenue and expense summary account (number 302), wondering how and when it is used. The summary account is employed in the process of "closing the books," a procedure that will be discussed in the following chapter. You need not be concerned about this account until then.

TRIAL BALANCE

At this point in Smalltown Hospital's accounting process, it would be interesting to determine whether or not the hospital's ledger is in balance. It should be in balance if we have made equal debits and credits in the journal, if we have posted these debits and credits correctly to the ledger accounts, and if we have made no mathematical errors in computing the balance of each account in the ledger.

Figure 14
Smalltown Hospital
Trial Balance
December 31, 1977

Acct. No.	Account Titles	Dr.	Cr.
101	Cash	$ 9,500	
102	Accounts Receivable	25,800	
103	Inventory	6,700	
110	Land	25,000	
111	Building	67,000	
112	Equipment	45,000	
201	Accounts Payable		$ 5,600
202	Bank Loan Payable		12,000
210	Bonds Payable		50,000
301	Hospital Equity		100,000
302	Revenue and Expense Summary		
401	Routine Services Revenue		72,180
402	Ancillary Services Revenue		48,120
403	Other Revenues		13,800
501	Salaries and Wages Expense	76,400	
502	Supplies Expense	21,500	
503	Utilities Expense	12,700	
504	Insurance Expense	3,600	
505	Repairs Expense	2,900	
506	Interest Expense	4,300	
507	Other Expenses	1,300	
	Totals	$301,700	$301,700

To ascertain whether the ledger is in balance, we can prepare a so-called trial balance.

A December 31, 1977, trial balance for Smalltown Hospital is illustrated in figure 14. It is a listing of all of the accounts in the hospital's ledger, with their debit or credit balances at the end of the year. The sequence in which the accounts are listed is the same as the sequence in which they appear in the ledger (which, incidentally, is the same as the order in which they appear in the hospital's chart of accounts).

Observe that the trial balance indicates that the Smalltown Hospital ledger is in balance. The debit balances total $301,700 as do the credit balances. A warning, however, is in order: the fact that the trial balance shows an equality of debit and credit balances is no guarantee that the figures are accurate. If the documentary evidence is incorrect or misinterpreted, the trial-balance data will be incorrect. If debits and credits were made to the wrong accounts in the journal or ledger, the trial balance will include incorrect figures. Thus, the trial balance is only a partial check on the accuracy of the accounting work of the period. Should the trial balance not balance, however, we *know* that an error has been made someplace in the journal or ledger, or in the trial balance itself.

Smalltown Hospital's December 31, 1977, trial balance will be the taking-off point for the next chapter. In that chapter we will use the trial-balance figures to prepare a set of annual financial statements. Chapter 4 also will illustrate and discuss the use of worksheets, and describe and explain the process known as closing the books.

QUESTIONS

1. Why is documentary evidence essential to the accounting process?

2. What is the purpose of a chart of accounts? What factors influence the design of a hospital's chart of accounts?

3. Distinguish between a chart of accounts and a ledger.

4. How does a chart of accounts differ from a trial balance?

5. Why are numerical codes assigned to the accounts in a chart of accounts? Are these codes identical in all hospitals?

6. Define each of the following terms: (a) *journal,* (b) *journalizing,* and (c) *journal entry*.

7. What are the 5 essential elements of a journal entry?

8. In recording cash receipt transactions in the journal, debits are made to cash. What types of accounts generally would be credited?

9. In recording cash disbursement transactions in the journal, credits are made to cash. What types of accounts generally would be debited?

10. What is the purpose of posting journal entries to ledger accounts?

11. What are the 5 essential elements of a posting to a ledger account?

12. Distinguish between *general* and *subsidiary* ledgers. Give 2 examples of a subsidiary ledger.

13. What is the purpose of a trial balance?

14. "If a trial balance indicates an equality of debit and credit balances, this indicates that the journal and ledger are free of errors." Do you agree? Explain.

15. "The ledger contains a separate account for each account in the hospital's chart of accounts. That is, if the chart of accounts contains 150 accounts, there will be 150 accounts in the ledger." Do you agree? Explain.

16. In what sequence are accounts listed in the ledger? In a trial balance?

PROBLEMS

A. Hunter Hospital completed the following transactions during the month of October, 1977.

1. New equipment was purchased for $16,000 cash.
2. Supplies were purchased on account for $36,400.
3. Supplies which had cost $31,200 were issued from inventory for use in hospital operations.
4. Payments on accounts payable were $34,700.
5. Services rendered to patients during the month were billed as follows:

Routine services	$ 84,300
Ancillary services	37,900
Total	$122,200

6. Collections on patients' accounts totaled $105,750.
7. Other revenues collected in cash amounted to $13,600.
8. Operating expenses were paid as follows:

Salaries and wages	$ 82,400
Utilities	8,700
Insurance	2,900
Repairs	1,600
Other expenses	7,300
Total	$102,900

9. A short-term, 9% loan of $15,000 was obtained from a local bank (disregard interest).

Required. Using the chart of accounts provided at page 46, prepare in good form general journal entries for each of the above transactions.

B. Hopeful Hospital began its corporate existence on January 1, 1977. During the ensuing year, it completed the following transactions.

1. The hospital received initial capital of $250,000 from a fund-raising committee established by the citizens of Hopeful. This money was deposited in a bank checking account opened in the name of Hopeful Hospital.

2. The hospital issued $150,000 of 6%, 10-year bonds at face value. Interest on these bonds is payable annually on December 31.
3. Plant assets were purchased for cash, as follows:

Land	$ 35,000
Building	200,000
Equipment	125,000
Total	$360,000

4. Purchases of supplies on account totaled $37,500.
5. Supplies which had cost $32,000 were issued from inventory for use in hospital operations.
6. Services were billed to patients as follows:

Routine services	$ 81,000
Ancillary services	56,700
Total	$137,700

7. Cash collections on patients' accounts, amounted to $121,600.
8. Payments on accounts payable came to $24,900.
9. Other revenues received in cash totaled $9,350.
10. Payments of operating expenses were as follows:

Salaries and wages	$ 79,250
Utilities	11,600
Insurance	4,200
Repairs	3,100
Other expenses	2,300
Total	$100,450

11. A short-term, 12% loan of $20,000 was obtained from a local bank.
12. On December 31 the following expense was paid:

Interest on bonds	$ 9,000
Interest on bank loan	600
Total	$ 9,600

Required. Using the chart of accounts provided at page 46, (1) journalize the 1977 transactions, (2) post the transaction entries to the general ledger, (3) prepare a trial balance at December 31, 1977, (4) prepare an income statement for 1977, and (5) prepare a balance sheet at December 31, 1977.

C. Hasty Hospital's trial balance at January 1, 1978, includes the following accounts:

Cash	$ 10,500	
Accounts receivable	24,800	
Inventory	5,700	
Land	19,000	
Building	73,000	
Equipment	27,000	
Accounts payable		$ 6,600
Bank loan payable		15,000
Bonds payable		60,000
Hospital equity		78,400
	$160,000	$160,000

The hospital completed the following transactions during the month ended January 31, 1978:

1. Purchases of supplies on account were $4,900.
2. Supplies which had cost $5,200 were issued from inventory for use in hospital activities.
3. Services billed to patients were

Routine services	$40,800
Ancillary services	21,600
Total	$62,400

4. Cash collections on patients' accounts amounted to $59,100.
5. Payments on accounts payable totaled $5,070.
6. Other revenues received in cash amounted to $7,300.
7. Payment of operating expenses involved

Salaries and wages	$53,200
Utilities	1,900
Insurance	1,200
Repairs	1,100
Other expenses	600
Total	$58,000

8. Payment of interest on bonds and bank loan, $870.

Required. Using the chart of accounts provided at page 46, (1) enter the January 1, 1978, balances in ledger accounts, (2) journalize the January, 1978, transactions, (3) post the transaction entries to the ledger accounts, (4) prepare a trial balance at January 31, 1978, (5) prepare an income statement for January, 1978, and (6) prepare a balance sheet at January 31, 1978.

D. Hangout Hospital's trial balance at November 30, 1977, which includes data accumulated since December 31, 1976, is provided below:

Cash	$ 14,700	
Accounts receivable	34,900	
Inventory	7,400	
Land	30,000	
Building	200,000	
Equipment	105,000	
Accounts payable		$ 11,200
Bank loan payable		25,000
Bonds payable		75,000
Hospital equity		274,300
Routine services revenue		85,800
Ancillary services revenue		31,300
Other revenues		9,400
Salaries and wages expense	95,000	
Supplies expense	13,000	
Utilities expense	3,600	
Insurance expense	1,200	
Repairs expense	1,700	
Interest expense	4,500	
Other expenses	1,000	
	$512,000	$512,000

The hospital completed the following transactions during the month of December, 1977:

1. Purchases of supplies on account amounted to $2,300.

2. Supplies which had cost $1,100 were issued from inventory for use in hospital operations.
3. Payments on accounts payable totaled $3,060.
4. Services billed to patients were

Routine services	$ 9,300
Ancillary services	4,070
Total	$13,370

5. Cash collections on patients' accounts totaled $16,140.
6. Other revenues received in cash totaled $980.
7. Payment of operating expenses involved

Salaries and wages	$ 9,100
Utilities	300
Insurance	150
Repairs	240
Other expenses	80
Total	$ 9,870

8. Payment of interest on bonds and bank loan amounted to $850.

Required. Using the chart of accounts provided at page 46, (1) enter the November 30, 1977, balances in ledger accounts, (2) journalize the December, 1977, transactions, (3) post the transaction entries to the ledger accounts, (4) prepare a trial balance at December 31, 1977, (5) prepare an income statement for the year ended December 31, 1977, and (6) prepare a balance sheet at December 31, 1977.

4
Worksheet, Financial Statements, and Closing Entries

In the previous chapter, you had an opportunity to examine 3 of the initial steps involved in the accounting process: the recording of transaction entries in a general journal, the posting of these entries to a general ledger, and the preparation of a trial balance. The discussion centered around the business transactions completed by a hypothetical Smalltown Hospital during 1977, the first year of that hospital's economic life. We will continue that illustration in this chapter.

Here, we want to illustrate a simplified version of the *worksheets* (or, as they are sometimes called, "working papers") widely used by accountants as a device to facilitate the preparation of financial statements. The worksheet we develop will lead us into an illustration and discussion of Smalltown Hospital's 1977 income statement and December 31, 1977, balance sheet. In the last section of this chapter, the procedures performed in a closing of the books for Smalltown Hospital will be described and demonstrated.

General Worksheet

After transaction entries have been journalized and posted, a trial balance is prepared of the ledger account balances. Financial statements often can be prepared directly from the trial-balance listing of accounts. In certain cases, where a large number of accounts is involved, the development of the statements can be facilitated by the preparation of a *general worksheet*. A major purpose of the worksheet is to classify and segregate the trial-balance figures according to the financial statements in which they will be presented. Other purposes of the worksheet will be seen in subsequent chapters. Later chapters will introduce you, in addition, to special-purpose worksheets.

A worksheet to develop financial statements for 1977 for Smalltown Hospital is illustrated in figure 15. Note the following points:

1. The trial balance at December 31, 1977, is entered on the left-hand side, with the dollar amounts being shown in the first

Figure 15

Smalltown Hospital
Worksheet to Develop Financial Statements
Year Ended December 31, 1977

Acct. No.	Account Title	12/31/77 Trial Balance Dr.	12/31/77 Trial Balance Cr.	Income Statement Dr.	Income Statement Cr.	Equity Statement Dr.	Equity Statement Cr.	Balance Sheet Dr.	Balance Sheet Cr.
101	Cash	9,500						9,500	
102	Accounts receivable	25,800						25,800	
103	Inventory	6,700						6,700	
110	Land	25,000						25,000	
111	Building	67,000						67,000	
112	Equipment	45,000						45,000	
201	Accounts payable		5,600						5,600
202	Bank loan payable		12,000						12,000
210	Bonds payable		50,000						50,000
301	Hospital equity		100,000				100,000		
302	Revenue and expense summary		---						
401	Routine services revenue		72,180		72,180				
402	Ancillary services revenue		48,120		48,120				
403	Other revenues		13,800		13,800				
501	Salaries and wages expense	76,400		76,400					
502	Supplies expense	21,500		21,500					
503	Utilities expense	12,700		12,700					
504	Insurance expense	3,600		3,600					
505	Repairs expense	2,900		2,900					
506	Interest expense	4,300		4,300					
507	Other expenses	1,300		1,300					
	Totals	301,700	301,700	122,700	134,100				
	Net income for the year			11,400			11,400		
	Totals			134,100	134,100	–0–	111,400		
	Hospital equity, 12/31/77					111,400			111,400
	Totals					111,400	111,400	179,000	179,000

2 columns. This is the same trial balance that was developed in the preceding chapter and illustrated as figure 14.

2. Next, the individual balances in the trial balance are extended to the appropriate financial statement columns. Debit balances are extended as debits, and credit balances are extended as credits, as follows:
   a. Asset and liability account balances are extended into the balance sheet columns.
   b. The trial-balance figure for hospital equity is extended into the equity statement column. This statement has not been mentioned previously, but it will be discussed in the next section of this chapter.
   c. The revenue and expense summary account has no balance and can be disregarded in the preparation of the worksheet. This account is used only in the process of closing the books, a matter discussed later in this chapter.
   d. Revenue and expense account balances are extended into the income statement columns.

   In this way, the individual trial-balance items are categorized or assembled into groups according to the financial statements in which the items will be presented.
3. Totals now are taken of the debits and credits in the income statement columns; debits total $122,700, and credits total $134,100. Since the debits are expenses and the credits are revenues, the difference is the 1977 net income, or $11,400.

   The net income figure ($11,400) is shown in the income statement section as a debit in order to balance the columns at $134,100. In addition, the $11,400 net income is extended as a credit to the equity-statement section of the worksheet.
4. Then, totals are taken of the debits (none) and credits in the equity-statement section. In certain situations, there could be debits to the equity statement but you need not be concerned with that possibility at this time. The credits to the equity statement include the $100,000 of hospital equity at January 1, 1977, and the $11,400 net income for 1977. This credit total of $111,400 is the amount of the hospital equity at December 31, 1977.

   The $111,400 figure is entered in the equity statement section as a debit in order to balance the columns; the figure also is extended to the balance sheet columns as a credit item.
5. A final step in completion of the worksheet is the totaling of the debits and credits in the balance sheet columns. Notice that these columns balance with totals of $179,000.

Thus, a primary function of the worksheet is to assemble the account balances in financial statement groupings. This, of course, facilitates preparation of the statements.

Financial Statements

The assembled data provided by the worksheet now are used in the preparation of 1977 financial statements for Smalltown Hospital.

These statements, in the order in which they usually are prepared, are as follows:

1. An *income statement* for the year ended December 31, 1977, illustrated in figure 16
2. A *statement of hospital equity* for the year ended December 31, 1977, in figure 17
3. A *balance sheet* at December 31, 1977, in figure 18

As previously stated, financial statements are the end product of the accounting process. They are the means by which financial information is communicated to hospital management and interested external parties for use in making economic decisions.

INCOME STATEMENT

The heading of the income statement (figure 16) identifies the accounting entity as Smalltown Hospital, indicates that the statement is an income statement, and specifies the time period covered by the statement as being the year ended December 31, 1977. This statement presents the operating results of the hospital for 1977 in terms of revenues earned and expenses incurred. The net result of operations, measured as the difference between revenues earned and expenses incurred, is the *net income* (or *net loss*, in some cases).

Smalltown Hospital's income statement has been prepared in accordance with the *accrual basis of accounting*. Under this system of accounting, revenues are recognized and recorded in the time period in which they are earned by the hospital in rendering services and selling products to patients and others, regardless of when (if ever) the related inflow of cash occurs. Expenses are recognized and recorded in the time period in which they are incurred or consumed in revenue-producing activities of the hospital, regardless of when (if ever) the related outflow of cash occurs. The accrual basis is a generally accepted accounting principle which should be employed by all hospitals.

The alternative to the accrual system is the *cash basis of accounting*. In this system of accounting, revenues are recognized and recorded in the time period in which they are received in cash; expenses are recognized and recorded in the time period in which they are paid in cash. An income statement prepared on a cash basis, then, is little more than a statement of cash receipts and cash disbursements (and an incomplete statement at that, since not all cash receipts are revenues and not all disbursements expenses); so, the cash basis of accounting is not recommended for hospitals.

Smalltown Hospital's income statement, then, is a statement of revenues earned and expenses incurred during 1977. It is not a statement of cash received and disbursed. The term *revenues* does not mean cash receipts, nor is the term *expenses* synonomous with cash disbursements. Notice, for example, that the income statement of Smalltown Hospital reports $120,300 of revenues earned from patient services. How much of this amount has been received in cash? Having seen the 1977 transactions, you know that only $94,500 was collected during the year on patients' accounts. And where is the other $25,800? It is presented in the balance sheet as accounts receivable (see figure 18)! Thus, $120,300 of patient services were rendered by Smalltown Hospital during 1977, and this is the amount reported as revenues for the year, although $25,800 of that amount will not be collected until sometime in 1978.

Or consider the $21,500 supplies expense item in the income statement of Smalltown Hospital. Is this the amount of supplies purchased and paid for during 1977? No! Having worked with the 1977 transactions, you know that $28,200 of supplies were purchased on account during the year and that cash payments of only $22,600 were made to the suppliers of these items. The income statement of the year is charged only for the cost of supplies consumed in operations of the period. As a result of this accrual-basis accounting, the balance sheet reports a $6,700 inventory and $5,600 of accounts payable to suppliers. These items would not appear in the balance sheet if cash-basis accounting were used.

All of this also means that there is no necessary short-run relationship between reported net income and the change in the cash balance during the year. Smalltown Hospital begins the year with $100,000 of cash but ends the year with a cash balance of only $9,500. Thus, in a year when a $11,400 net income is reported, the cash balance decreases by more than $90,000! Do not get the idea, therefore, that the income statement is a presentation of cash flows.

Figure 16
Smalltown Hospital
Income Statement
Year Ended December 31, 1977

Patient Service Revenues:		
Routine Services	$ 72,180	
Ancillary Services	48,120	
Total Patient Service Revenues	120,300	
Other Revenues	13,800	
Total Revenues		$134,100
Less Operating Expenses:		
Salaries and Wages	76,400	
Supplies	21,500	
Utilities	12,700	
Insurance	3,600	
Repairs	2,900	
Interest	4,300	
Other	1,300	
Total Operating Expenses		122,700
Net income for the year		$ 11,400

Cash flows, however, are vitally important in the management of a hospital. In addition to income statements and balance sheets, accountants also prepare statements of cash receipts and disbursements ("cash-flow" statements) for internal management purposes. A discussion of such statements will appear at a subsequent point in this book.

You should understand that the 2-column format of the income statement in no way implies a debit-and-credit relationship. The left-hand column is not a debit column, nor is the right a credit column. There are no debit or credit columns in financial statements. The number of columns employed is only a matter of presentation style.

EQUITY STATEMENT

A statement of hospital equity for the year ended December 31, 1977, is illustrated for Smalltown Hospital in figure 17. The statement begins with the equity figure at January 1. To this figure we add the 1977 net income as indicated by the income statement. (If a net loss had been reported, the net loss would be subtracted for the January 1 equity.) The resulting figure is the amount of hospital equity at December 31. This figure, of course, is the equity balance to be reported in the December 31, 1977, balance sheet.

Figure 17
Smalltown Hospital
Statement of Hospital Equity
Year Ended December 31, 1977

Hospital Equity, January 1*	$100,000
Add Net Income for the Year	11,400
Hospital Equity, December 31	$111,400

*This represents the contribution of initial equity funds received on January 1, 1977, from the Smalltown Civic Improvement Committee, when the hospital began its operations.

For our present purposes, we are assuming that a hospital's equity is affected (changed) only by the net income or net loss of the period. Further on we will see, however, that the hospital equity balance is increased and decreased by other factors, particularly when a fund-accounting system is used. When these factors are introduced into the discussion, a more sophisticated equity statement will be illustrated.

The equity statement provides a connection between the income statement and the balance sheet. It also explains the change in the equity balance from one balance sheet to the next. It is an essential financial statement, one which all hospitals should prepare and include in their annual financial reports.

BALANCE SHEET

Smalltown Hospital's December 31, 1977, balance sheet is illustrated in figure 18. Notice that the heading provides the name of the accounting entity, the name of the statement, and the date of the statement. Unlike the dating of the other statements, the dating of the balance sheet specifies a particular point in time (rather than a period of time). The figures in the balance sheet apply only to the financial position of the hospital at the "close of business" on December 31, 1977. Most of the balance sheet figures were different on the preceding day, and also will be different on the following day. The balance sheet is somewhat like a photographic snapshot, whereas the income and capital statements are more like *moving* pictures covering a period of time.

Figure 18
Smalltown Hospital
Balance Sheet
December 31, 1977

Assets		
Cash	$ 9,500	
Accounts Receivable	25,800	
Inventory	6,700	
Total Current Assets		$ 42,000
Land	25,000	
Building	67,000	
Equipment	45,000	
Total Plant Assets		137,000
Total Assets		$179,000
Liabilities and Equity		
Accounts Payable	5,600	
Bank Loan Payable	12,000	
Total Current Liabilities		$ 17,600
Long-Term Debt (8% Bonds Payable)		50,000
Total Liabilities		67,600
Hospital Equity		111,400
Total Liabilities and Equity		$179,000

The financial position of Smalltown Hospital is presented in terms of its assets, liabilities, and equity at December 31, 1977. *Assets* are the economic resources of the hospital that are recognized and measured in conformity with generally accepted accounting principles. *Liabilities* are the economic obligations of the hospital that are recognized and measured in conformity with generally accepted accounting principles. *Equity*, sometimes called "capital" or "net worth," is the excess of assets over liabilities. Since most of the assets are carried in the balance sheet at cost rather than at what they are "worth," however, the use of the term *net worth* can be misleading. So, we will use the term *equity*.

Smalltown Hospital's assets are listed in the sequence usually seen in actual practice. The assets are classified into 2 main groups: current assets and noncurrent assets (which, in this situation, consist only of plant assets). The current assets consist of cash plus those other assets which are likely to be converted into cash within a short period (one year or less). Normally, the plant assets would be reduced by depreciation, but we are disregarding the recording of depreciation for the time being.

Smalltown Hospital's liabilities and equity also are listed in the usual sequence. Like the assets, the liabilities are classified into 2 categories: current liabilities and noncurrent (or "long-term") liabilities. The current liabilities consist of debts which ordinarily will be paid within a short time (one year or less). In this example, the noncurrent liabilities are comprised of a single item, the 8% bonds due in 9 more years. A total of liabilities is obtained, and to it is added the hospital equity balance as reported in the equity statement. Then, of course, you see that total assets equal the total of liabilities and equity (the accounting equation).

As this book unfolds, more-sophisticated financial statements will be developed. Many additional accounts will be introduced into the statements, and the impact of fund accounting and responsibility accounting on the statements will be described. We also must probe more deeply into problems of terminology, classification, valuation, and disclosure. The subject of financial analysis and interpretation also is covered in subsequent chapters.

Closing the Books

Once the financial statements are prepared, the accountant can proceed to the last step in the accounting process. This procedure is known as "closing the books." It consists of the closing of revenue and expense accounts in the hospital's ledger, and of the adjustment of the hospital equity to the balance at which it is stated in the year-end balance sheet. The balances of revenue and expense accounts in Smalltown Hospital's ledger relate only to the 1977 year. These balances therefore must be eliminated in order to prepare the ledger for the next accounting period and to avoid the commingling of revenue and expense balances of one year with those of the next year.

Balance sheet accounts, which are called *real* (permanent) accounts, are not closed. The balances of these accounts—assets, liabilities, and equity—are carried over into the next year as the opening balances for that year. The accounts to be closed are the income statement accounts, often called *nominal* (temporary) accounts. Thus, all revenue and expense account balances are closed; these accounts begin the next year with zero balances.

A closing of the books is accomplished by making what are called *closing entries* in the hospital's journal and by posting these entries to the ledger accounts. Figure 19 presents the closing entries for Smalltown Hospital for 1977.

The first closing entry is one to eliminate the revenue account balances. As you will recall, all revenue accounts have *credit*

Figure 19
Smalltown Hospital
1977 Journal
Closing Entries

Entry No.	Accounts and Explanations	Acct. No.	Debit	Credit
13	Routine Services Revenue	401	72,180	
	Ancillary Services Revenue	402	48,120	
	Other Revenues	403	13,800	
	Revenue and Expense Summary	302		134,100
	To close revenue accounts.			
14	Revenue and Expense Summary	302	122,700	
	Salaries and Wages Expense	501		76,400
	Supplies Expense	502		21,500
	Utilities Expense	503		12,700
	Insurance Expense	504		3,600
	Repairs Expense	505		2,900
	Interest Expense	506		4,300
	Other Expense	507		1,300
	To close expense accounts.			
15	Revenue and Expense Summary	302	11,400	
	Hospital Equity	301		11,400
	To close revenue and expense summary, and to add net income for the year to the hospital equity.			

balances. The closing entry, therefore, *debits* each revenue account for its credit balance as shown in the hospital's ledger. A credit is made in this entry to the revenue and expense summary account for the total revenues of the period. This credit balances the entry which we have numbered as entry 13.

A second closing entry is made to remove the expense account balances from the ledger. Since the expense accounts have *debit* balances, this entry *credits* each of the expense accounts for its debit balance. The total of these credits (total expenses for the period) is debited to the revenue and expense summary. This is entry 14.

The third and last closing entry (number 15) is one to close the revenue and expense summary account and to add the net income for the period to the hospital equity account. Since the revenue and expense summary account has been debited (entry 14) for total expenses and credited (entry 13) for total revenues, that account now has a credit balance in the amount of the net income for the period. The debit to the summary account in entry 15 for the net income therefore will close that account. If the hospital had a net loss for the period, of course, the debit and credit in this entry would be reversed.

The posting of these 3 closing entries from Smalltown Hospital's journal to its ledger accounts is shown in figure 20. It is suggested that you trace the individual postings into the ledger; the postings, of course, are referenced as numbers 13, 14, and 15. Notice also that the closing of the revenue accounts, expense accounts, and the revenue and expense summary account is indicated in the ledger by the "double-ruling" of the individual accounts.

Smalltown Hospital's ledger now contains balance sheet accounts only; all other accounts have been closed. These remaining ledger balances are left open to become the beginning ledger balances of the ensuing year. None of the revenue or expense accounts have balances, so these accounts are ready to receive postings of the next year's revenues and expenses. In this way, the revenues and expenses of one year are not mixed up with the revenues and expenses of the next year. This facilitates the measurement of net income for each year.

Figure 20
Smalltown Hospital
1977 Ledger
(With Closing Entries)

Cash 101

(1) 100,000	(3) 137,000
(2) 50,000	(8) 22,600
(7) 94,500	(10) 96,900
(9) 13,800	(12) 4,300
(11) 12,000	
(B) 9,500	

Accounts Receivable 102

(6) 120,300	(7) 94,500
(B) 25,800	

Inventory 103

(4) 28,200	(5) 21,500
(B) 6,700	

Land 110

(3) 25,000	

Building 111

(3) 67,000	

Equipment 112

(3) 45,000	

Accounts Payable 201

(8) 22,600	(4) 28,200
	(B) 5,600

Bank Loan Payable 202

	(11) 12,000

Bonds Payable 210

	(2) 50,000

Figure 20 (continued)

Hospital Equity 301

		(1)	100,000
		(15)	11,400
		(B)	111,400

Revenue and Expense Summary 302

(14)	122,700	(13)	134,100
(15)	11,400		

Routine Services Revenue 401

(13)	72,180	(6)	72,180

Ancillary Services Revenue 402

(13)	48,120	(6)	48,120

Other Revenues 403

(13)	13,800	(9)	13,800

Salaries and Wages Expense 501

(10)	76,400	(14)	76,400

Supplies Expense 502

(5)	21,500	(14)	21,500

Utilities Expense 503

(10)	12,700	(14)	12,700

Insurance Expense 504

(10)	3,600	(14)	3,600

Repairs Expense 505

(10)	2,900	(14)	2,900

Interest Expense 506

(12)	4,300	(14)	4,300

Other Expenses 507

(10)	1,300	(14)	1,300

At this point, another trial balance may be taken of the ledger to determine whether the accounts are in balance after the closing of the books. This trial balance is called a *postclosing* trial balance; the trial balance illustrated in chapter 3 as figure 14 is referred to as a *preclosing* trial balance. A postclosing trial balance for Smalltown Hospital is presented in figure 21. Notice that it contains balance sheet account balances *only*. These are the balances with which Smalltown Hospital will begin 1978.

Summary of Accounting Procedure

It would be useful at this time to present a summary of the operations we have covered so far in our discussion. All of the procedures or operations performed during the annual accounting period

Figure 21
Smalltown Hospital
Postclosing Trial Balance
December 31, 1977

Acct. No.	Account Titles	Dr.	Cr.
101	Cash	$ 9,500	
102	Accounts Receivable	25,800	
103	Inventory	6,700	
110	Land	25,000	
111	Building	67,000	
112	Equipment	45,000	
201	Accounts Payable		$ 5,600
202	Bank Loan Payable		12,000
210	Bonds Payable		50,000
301	Hospital Equity		111,400
302	Revenue and Expense Summary		
401	Routine Services Revenue		
402	Ancillary Services Revenue		
403	Other Revenues		
501	Salaries and Wages Expense		
502	Supplies Expense		
503	Utilities Expense		
504	Insurance Expense		
505	Repairs Expense		
506	Interest Expense		
507	Other Expenses		
	Totals	$179,000	$179,000

are together called the *accounting cycle*. The steps in this cycle that we have discussed and illustrated up to this point are summarized in the diagram in figure 22.

Assuming the existence of documentary evidences of transactions and a well-designed chart of accounts, the steps in the accounting cycle are as follows:

1. Journalizing transaction entries in the journal
2. Posting transaction entries from the journal to the ledger and determining individual account balances
3. Entering the preclosing trial balance on a worksheet and completion of the worksheet
4. Preparing financial statements from the information provided on the worksheet
5. Journalizing closing entries in the journal
6. Posting closing entries from the journal to the ledger

7. Preparing a postclosing trial balance of the account balances now remaining in the ledger

There are, however, additional steps involved in a complete accounting cycle. One of these additional steps is the journalizing and posting of another kind of journal entry called the *adjusting entry*. This procedure, often a matter of considerable difficulty for introductory accounting students, is treated in detail in the next 3 chapters.

Figure 22
Summary of Accounting Procedure

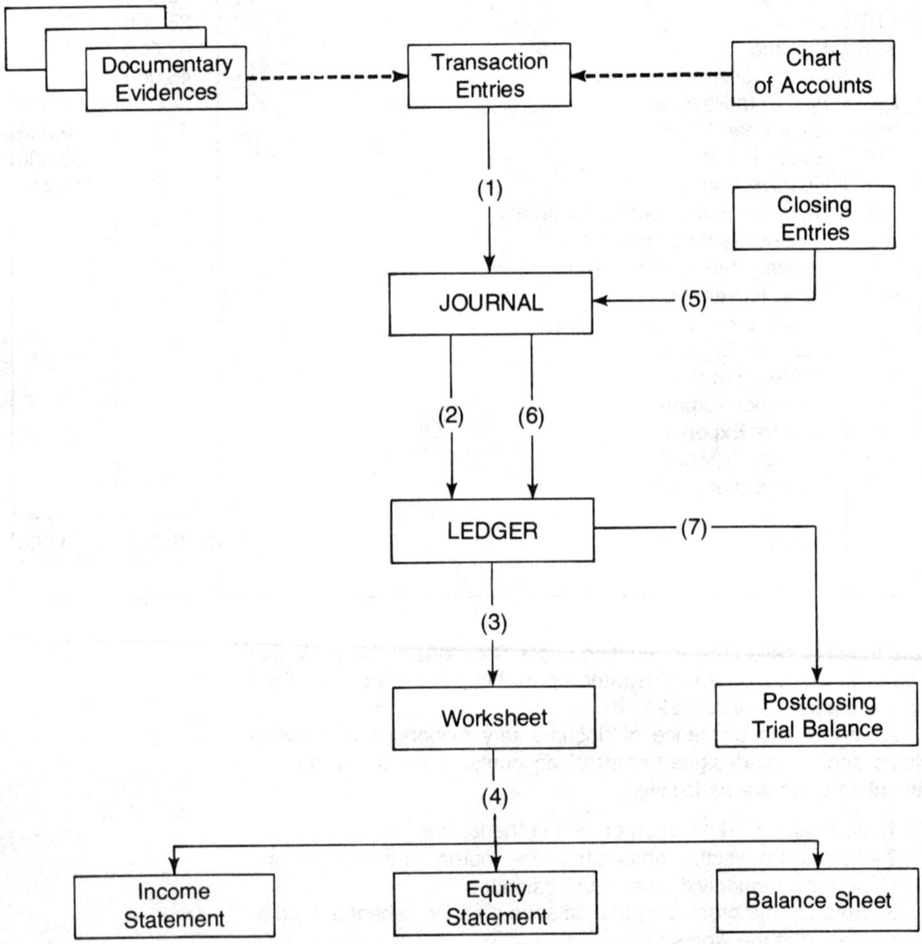

QUESTIONS

1. What is the major purpose of a general worksheet?

2. Distinguish between the cash basis and the accrual basis of accounting.

3. Distinguish between revenues and cash receipts.

4. Distinguish between expenses and cash disbursements.

5. Why should the cash basis of accounting *not* be employed by hospitals?

6. What is the purpose of the statement of hospital equity?

7. Define briefly each of the following terms: (a) *assets,* (b) *liabilities,* and (c) *equity.*

8. Describe briefly the procedure known as "closing the books."

9. Distinguish between "real" and "nominal" accounts.

10. Distinguish between a preclosing trial balance and a postclosing trial balance.

11. List, in the sequence normally completed, the steps involved in a complete accounting cycle.

12. What is the significance of "double rulings" in ledger accounts?

PROBLEMS

A. The following balances, among others, appeared in the general ledger of Kent Hospital at the end of its fiscal year:

Acct. No.		
301	Hospital equity	$143,674
302	Revenue and expense summary	–0–
401	Routine services revenue	85,375
402	Ancillary services revenue	52,939
403	Other revenues	21,655
501	Salaries and wages expense	101,488
502	Supplies expense	22,475
503	Utilities expense	13,880
504	Insurance expense	4,203
505	Repairs expense	1,922
506	Interest expense	3,077
507	Other expenses	1,249

Required. Prepare, in good form, general journal entries to close the books of Kent Hospital for the year.

B. Following is the preclosing trail balance of Winston Hospital at December 31, 1977:

Acct. No.		Dr.	Cr.
101	Cash	$ 11,200	
102	Accounts receivable	27,400	
103	Inventory	7,300	
110	Land	15,000	
111	Building	80,000	
112	Equipment	35,000	
201	Accounts payable		$ 6,900
202	Bank loan payable		14,000
210	Bonds payable		60,000
301	Hospital equity		96,900
302	Revenue and expense summary		–0–
401	Routine services revenue		86,400

Acct. No.		Dr.	Cr.
402	Ancillary services revenue		41,700
403	Other revenues		19,200
501	Salaries and wages expense	94,600	
502	Supplies expense	28,700	
503	Utilities expense	13,400	
504	Insurance expense	3,100	
505	Repairs expense	2,700	
506	Interest expense	4,400	
507	Other expenses	2,300	
		$325,100	$325,100

Required. (1) Prepare a general worksheet to develop financial statements for the year ended December 31, 1977. (2) Prepare, in good form, financial statements for 1977. (3) Prepare, in general journal form, closing entries for 1977.

C. The following balances, among others, appeared in the general ledger of Jackson Hospital at the end of its fiscal year:

Acct. No.		
301	Hospital equity	$294,600
302	Revenue and expense summary	–0–
401	Routine services revenue	121,800
402	Ancillary services revenue	87,500
403	Other revenues	26,300
501	Salaries and wages expense	155,400
502	Supplies expense	31,400
503	Utilities expense	18,700
504	Insurance expense	6,400
505	Repairs expense	3,900
506	Interest expense	7,500
507	Other expenses	3,300

Required. (1) Enter the above balances in ledger accounts. (2) Journalize the necessary closing entries for the year. (3) Post the closing entries to the ledger accounts.

D. The following balances appeared in the general ledger of Gowdy Hospital at December 31, 1977:

Acct. No.		
101	Cash	$ 31,100
102	Accounts receivable	89,700
103	Inventory	11,200
110	Land	25,000
111	Building	240,000
112	Equipment	114,000
201	Accounts payable	22,800
202	Bank loan payable	28,000
210	Bonds payable	75,000
301	Hospital equity	372,300
302	Revenue and expense summary	–0–
401	Routine services revenue	140,700
402	Ancillary services revenue	79,900
403	Other revenues	21,300

Acct. No.		
501	Salaries and wages expense	150,800
502	Supplies expense	38,500
503	Utilities expense	22,100
504	Insurance expense	4,700
505	Repairs expense	3,200
506	Interest expense	7,900
507	Other expenses	1,800

Required. (1) Prepare a general worksheet to develop financial statements for the year ended December 31, 1977. (2) Prepare, in good form, financial statements for 1977. (3) Prepare, in general journal form, closing entries for 1977.

II
Periodic Adjustments and Summary

5
Prepaid and Accrued Expenses

In the 2 preceding chapters, we illustrated the journalizing and posting of Smalltown Hospital's 1977 transaction entries. A trial balance of the ledger accounts was then prepared. We assumed that the figures in this trial balance were the correct account balances at the end of the year, and these figures were used for financial statement purposes. In actual practice, however, many of the account balances in this trial balance are likely to be incorrect! This means that financial statements cannot be prepared until the incorrect balances in the trial balance are adjusted to the correct amounts. The necessary corrections are accomplished by journalizing and posting *adjusting entries.* All of the required adjustments must be made before the financial statements can be prepared.

Incorrect account balances will appear in the trial balance regardless of the amount of care exercised in recording the transactions of the period. Some of the reasons for this are listed below:

1. *Prepaid and Accrued Expenses.* The trial balance may include expense accounts that are either overstated or understated because of
   a. the prepayment of expenses during the period or
   b. the failure to recognize expenses that were incurred during the current period but which will not be paid until the next period.

   Adjustments for prepaid and accrued expenses are illustrated and discussed in this chapter.
2. *Deferred and Accrued Revenues.* The trial balance may include revenue accounts that are either overstated or understated because of
   a. the receipt of revenues in advance or
   b. the failure to recognize revenues that were earned during the current period but which will not be received until the next period.

   Adjustments for deferred and accrued revenues are illustrated and discussed in chapter 6.

3. *Revenue Deductions.* The trial balance may include incorrect balances in accounts representing revenue deductions, such as charity service and bad debts. Chapter 7 will deal with adjustments of this type.
4. *Depreciation.* The trial balance may not reflect the correct amount of depreciation for hospital buildings and equipment. Depreciation adjustments too will be discussed in chapter 7.

These are the types of adjusting entries we will consider in this chapter and chapters 6 and 7. After this is accomplished, all of the adjustments will be brought together in a single illustration in chapter 8.

MATCHING PRINCIPLE

In chapter 4, a very important distinction was made between cash-basis accounting and accrual-basis accounting. You have seen that the business life of the hospital is divided into time segments called accounting periods. So far in our discussion, we have assumed that these accounting periods are calendar years, that is, the 12 months from January 1 through December 31. This is the fiscal year employed by Smalltown Hospital. Many, perhaps most, hospitals use a fiscal year accounting period, however, which ends June 30 or September 30. Such a fiscal period sometimes is called the *natural business year*. No matter what the annual period may be, it usually is broken into monthly reporting periods. Financial statements are prepared monthly as well as annually.

Regardless of the period involved, a major accounting objective is the determination of the net income for the period. How is this determination made? Under the *cash-basis* method, the revenues of the period are considered to be only those received in cash during the period; the expenses of the period are only those paid in cash during the period. The cash-basis procedure, however, is not a generally accepted method of accounting for hospitals.

Under the *accrual-basis* method of accounting, the revenues of the period are considered to be those which were earned during the period, regardless of whether the related cash was received during the same period. The expenses of the period primarily are those incurred in the production of the revenue of the period, regardless of whether the related cash was expended during the same period. In addition, certain other expenses may be recognized during the period by a process of systematic and rational allocation even though those expenses cannot be directly associated with the revenues of that period. The accrual basis is a generally accepted accounting principle upon which the financial statements of hospitals must be based.

This brings us to the *matching principle*. The revenues of the hospital are "matched" with the accounting period during which they are *earned*. To put it another way, revenues must be recognized and recorded in the time period during which they are earned by the hospital through the provision of services and the sale of goods to patients and others. Revenues are earned when a hospital renders services to patients, when assets are sold, and when the hospital rents its assets to others. The hospital may receive cash prior to the earning of the revenue, at the time the revenue is earned, or after the earning of the revenue. Unfortunately hospitals also earn revenues for which they are never paid. Revenue adjustments related to the matching principle are treated in chapter 6.

The matching principle also has important implications for the recognition of hospital expenses. The expenses of the hospital are "matched" to the extent practicable with the revenues to which they are related. In other words, expenses are incurred in the production of revenues. Once the revenues of a given time period are measured and recorded, the expenses incurred in the production of those revenues should be recognized and recorded *in the same period*. There is, then, a "matching" of expenses with revenues in each accounting period so as to permit a meaningful and useful measurement of periodic net income.

Not all hospital costs, however, can be directly and easily associated with specific revenues, yet these costs must be charged as expenses to one or more accounting periods at one time or another. Where no direct association of expenses with revenues can be made, the costs are "matched" with the accounting period or periods which they benefit. If more than one accounting period benefits from a cost expenditure, the cost is allocated to expense on some systematic and rational basis. If a cost expenditure is made during the current period and no future benefit is expected, that cost is charged in its entirety to expense of the current period. Expense adjustments related to the matching principle are treated in the present chapter and in chapter 7.

Prepaid Expenses

Prepaid expenses, sometimes called deferred expenses or deferred charges, are expenditures made by the hospital for goods and services not yet consumed or used in hospital operations; they are therefore chargeable as expenses in a *future* accounting period (or periods). Since these cost expenditures benefit one or more future accounting periods, they are appropriately classified in the balance sheet as assets. Prepaid expenses, then, may be referred to as unexpired or "unexpensed" costs. Some examples of prepaid expenses are prepaid insurance, prepaid rent, and prepaid interest.

At the end of each accounting period, the trial balance must be scanned to determine the need for adjustments arising because of prepayments of expenses by the hospital. An analysis often must be made of the debits and credits in some of the accounts to develop the necessary adjusting entry. As a basis for illustration, we will assume a hypothetical Hoosier Hospital at the end of its first year of operations. This hospital's December 31, 1977, trial balance is shown in figure 23. From this point on, the trial balance taken after all transaction entries have been journalized and posted will be called a *preadjusted* trial balance (to distinguish it from an adjusted trial balance and from a postclosing trial balance). Certain of the accounts included in figure 23 have not been discussed before, but their nature and use will soon become apparent to you.

Figure 23
Hoosier Hospital
Preadjusted Trial Balance
December 31, 1977

Acct. No.	Account Titles	Dr.	Cr.
101	Cash	$ 38,300	
102	Temporary Investments	12,000	
103	Accrued Interest Receivable	---	
104	Accounts Receivable	96,600	
105	Allowance for Uncollectible Accounts		$ ---
106	Inventory	10,500	
107	Prepaid Insurance	3,600	
108	Prepaid Rent	1,080	
109	Prepaid Interest	720	
150	Land	25,000	
160	Building	180,000	
161	Accumulated Depreciation—Building		---
170	Equipment	60,000	
171	Accumulated Depreciation—Equipment		---
201	Accounts Payable		29,840
202	Notes Payable		18,000
203	Accrued Interest Payable		---
204	Accrued Salaries and Wages Payable		---
205	Deferred Rental Income		4,200
206	Deferred Tuition Income		2,160
250	Bonds Payable		80,000
301	Hospital Equity		225,000
302	Revenue and Expense Summary		---
401	Routine Services Revenue		151,300
402	Ancillary Services Revenue		137,400
403	Interest Income		---
404	Rental Income		---
405	Tuition Income		---
406	Other Revenues		27,100
501	Charity Service	29,200	
502	Contractual Adjustments	19,400	
503	Bad Debts	---	
601	Salaries and Wages Expense	139,600	
602	Supplies Expense	28,600	
603	Utilities Expense	14,400	
604	Insurance Expense	---	
605	Repairs Expense	8,300	
606	Rent Expense	---	
607	Depreciation Expense	---	
608	Interest Expense	---	
609	Other Expenses	7,700	
	Totals	$675,000	$675,000

PREPAID INSURANCE

Observe that Hoosier Hospital's preadjusted trial balance includes a prepaid insurance account (number 107) with a debit balance of $3,600. Normally, we would expect Hoosier Hospital also to have some amount of insurance expense for the 1977 year, but the insurance expense account (number 604) has no balance whatever! It would seem clear that an adjustment is needed here.

To determine the necessary adjustment, we would have to examine copies of the hospital's insurance policies. Let us assume that we discover a single comprehensive insurance policy for which the hospital paid a 3-year premium in advance on January 1, 1977. The amount of the premium was $3,600, meaning that the hospital's insurance expense is $1,200 per year; that is, a third of the insurance premium expired in 1977. The *transaction entry* made by Hoosier Hospital on January 1, 1977, when the premium was paid, must have been the following:

Prepaid Insurance	107	$3,600	
Cash	101		$3,600
Payment of 3-year premium in advance on comprehensive insurance policy.			

At the end of the year, however, $1,200 of this prepayment has expired and should be included in the hospital's 1977 expenses. Also at year's end, the amount of prepaid insurance to be reported as an asset is only $2,400—or $3,600 − $1,200.

An adjusting entry therefore must be made in Hoosier Hospital's journal at December 31, 1977. The required entry is as follows:

Insurance Expense	604	$1,200	
Prepaid Insurance	107		$1,200
Adjustment for portion of prepaid premium which expired during 1977.			

This entry, when posted, will correct the 2 account balances in the ledger of the hospital. The $1,200 of insurance expense will appear among the expenses in Hoosier Hospital's 1977 income statement. The $2,400 adjusted balance of prepaid insurance will be presented as an asset in the hospital's December 31, 1977, balance sheet. It is an asset because the insurance company "owes" Hoosier Hospital insurance protection for the next 2 years (1978 and 1979), and this asset is valued at the unexpired cost of the insurance.

The same adjusting entry will be required at the end of 1978 and at the end of 1979. Then, of course, it will be time to renew the insurance and pay the premium again. In this way, a $3,600 expenditure on January 1, 1977, is charged to expense over the 3-year period benefiting from the expenditure at the rate of $1,200 per year. Had the entire $3,600 been charged to 1977 expense, this would have resulted in an overstatement of 1977 expense and an understatement of 1978 and 1979 expenses. This is accrual-basis accounting: expenses are recognized in the period in which they are *incurred*, regardless of when they are *paid*.

Just suppose, however, that the entire $3,600 premium had been charged to insurance expense at the time it was paid. The transaction entry would have been this:

Insurance Expense	604	$3,600	
Cash	101		$3,600
Payment of insurance premium.			

Had this been done, the required adjusting entry at December 31, 1977, would have been as follows:

Prepaid Insurance	107	$2,400	
Insurance Expense	604		$2,400
Adjustment for prepaid insurance premium.			

The result is the same as before: $1,200 of 1977 insurance expense and $2,400 of prepaid insurance for the year-end balance sheet.

It is important that you clearly understand that this discussion of adjusting entries is presented in terms of an *annual* time frame. Well-managed hospitals, of course, prepare monthly income statements and balance sheets. In order for these statements to be functional, all significant adjustments must be made at the end of each month. If we were assuming the preparation of monthly financial statements for Hoosier Hospital, for example, an adjusting entry would be made at the end of each month to recognize $100 (i.e., $1,200/12) of insurance expense and to reduce prepaid insurance by the same amount:

Insurance Expense	604	$100	
Prepaid Insurance	107		$100
Adjustment for monthly expiration of prepaid insurance premiums.			

The illustration presented in chapter 9 assumes monthly adjusting entries, but we will discuss adjustments in annual terms until then.

As you may know, hospitals carry large amounts of many different kinds of insurance. Because of this, and the sizeable number of policies involved, the determination of the monthly and annual insurance-expense figures can be somewhat difficult. It may be necessary to maintain an *insurance register* and perhaps an *insurance expiration schedule* or worksheet. Not only do these specialized records provide the necessary information for accounting adjustments, they also aid in the management of the hospital's insurance requirements to the end that adequate coverages are maintained, that claims for insured losses are promptly reported and recovered, and so on.

PREPAID RENT

Let us assume now that Hoosier Hospital rented certain equipment for use in its business offices on May 1, 1977, making the following transaction entry:

Prepaid Rent	108	$1,080	
Cash	101		$1,080
Payment of a year's rent in advance for office equipment ($90 per month).			

The December 31, 1977, preadjusted trial balance therefore includes $1,080 of prepaid rent (account 108) but no balance in rent expense (account 606).

Since the rent is $90 per month, Hoosier Hospital's expenses for 1977 therefore should include rent expense of $720 (i.e., $90 × 8 months). Prepaid rent at December 31, 1977, should be $360, the rent prepaid for January through April of 1978. This requires the following December 31, 1977, adjusting entry:

Rent Expense	606	$720	
Prepaid Rent	108		$720
Adjustment to record rent expense for May through December, 1977, at $90 per month.			

In 1978, the remaining $360 of prepaid rent will be charged to expense. In this way, the equipment rental cost is charged to expense during the periods in which the equipment is being used by the hospital. Had the entire $1,080 payment been charged to expense in the year of payment, Hoosier Hospital's 1977 expenses would have been overstated and its 1978 expenses understated.

Suppose, however, that the prepayment of the rent on May 1, 1977, had been recorded as a debit to rent expense, as follows:

Rent Expense	606	$1,080	
Cash	101		$1,080
Payment of one year's rent in advance for office equipment ($90 per month).			

Had this been the transaction entry, the December 31, 1977, adjusting entry would be somewhat different. The necessary adjusting entry would be as follows:

Prepaid Rent	108	$360	
Rent Expense	606		$360
Adjustment to record prepaid rent for January through April, 1978, at $90 per month.			

However the transaction entry is handled, the net result at year's end must be to have $720 in expense and $360 in the prepaid rent account.

PREPAID INTEREST

Assume that Hoosier Hospital obtained a 6-month loan of $18,000 from a bank on November 1, 1977. The hospital issued to the bank a promissory note, paying 8% interest in advance for the 6-month term of the note. The hospital's transaction entry on November 1 was the following:

Cash	101	$17,280	
Prepaid Interest	109	720	
Notes Payable	202		$18,000
Proceeds from 6-month note issued to bank, with 8% interest deducted in advance:			

Face amount of note	$18,000
Less interest ($18,000 × 8% × ½)	720
Proceeds of note	$17,280

Interest on the note for a full year would be $1,440—or 8% × $18,000. Since the loan is only for a 6-month period, only a half year's interest is prepaid. The interest, then, is $120 per month ($720/6 months).

At December 31, 1977, November's and December's interest expense has been incurred by the hospital. The necessary adjusting entry is the following:

Interest Expense	608	$240	
Prepaid Interest	109		$240
Adjustment for interest on bank loan for November and December, 1977: $18,000 × 8% × 2/12 = $240.			

The remaining $480 of prepaid interest is an asset at December 31, 1977. The bank "owes" the hospital the use of the borrowed money for another 4 months. This $480 will be charged to interest expense in 1978.

If the interest payment on November 1, 1977, had been charged to interest expense (instead of prepaid interest), the required adjusting entry at December 31 would be as follows:

Prepaid Interest	109	$480	
Interest Expense	608		$480
Adjustment for 4 months' prepaid interest on bank loan at December 31: $18,000 × 8% × 4/12 = $480.			

Again, no matter what debit is made for the prepayment in the transaction entry, we must end up with $240 in interest expense and $480 in prepaid interest at the end of the year.

A hospital likely will have other types of prepaid expenses. Whatever the particular expense item, adjustments are made in the manner shown by the preceding illustrations. The procedure is summarized below.

1. Assuming the prepayment is debited to a prepaid expense account in the transaction entry:

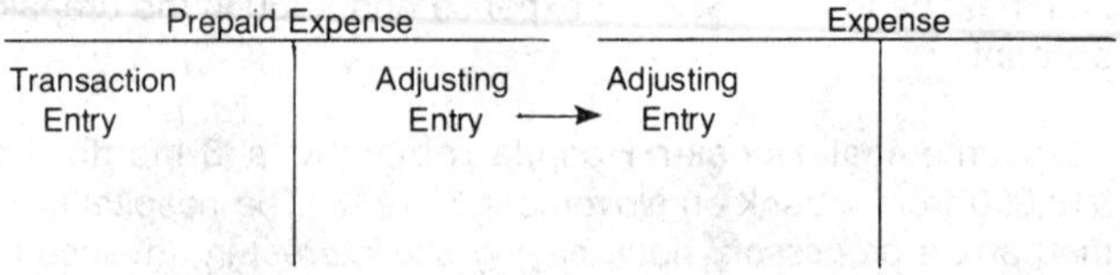

The amount of the adjusting entry is that portion of the prepayment which has expired and is chargeable to expenses of the current period.

2. Assuming the prepayment is debited to an expense account in the transaction entry:

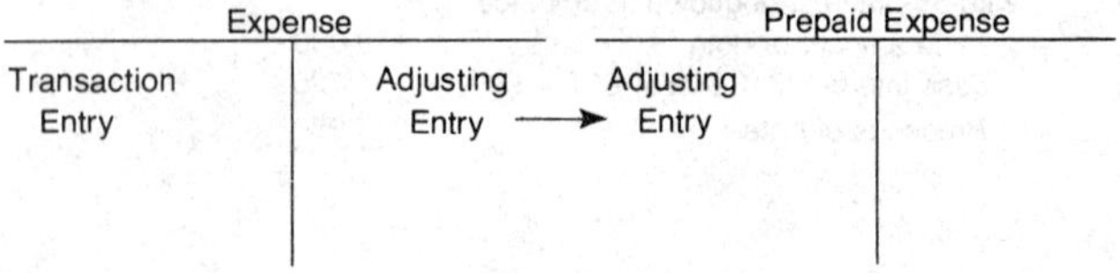

The amount of the adjusting entry is that portion of the prepayment which has *not* expired and is chargeable to expenses of a future period.

Prepaid expenses are assets because they represent unexpired costs—costs which benefit a future accounting period. They represent benefits—insurance protection, use of equipment, use of money—to be received in the future and consequently not to be charged to expense in the present period.

ACCRUED EXPENSES

Accrued expenses are expenses that have been incurred but for which the hospital has not yet paid. Accrued expenses represent the costs of goods and services consumed and used in hospital operations of the current period, but the hospital will not make expenditures for those goods and services until some future accounting period. The liability for these future disbursements is called an "accrued liability," or an "accrued expense payable." In most cases, the liability is presented among the current liabilities in the balance sheet of the hospital. Examples include accrued interest payable and accrued salaries and wages payable (sometimes called "accrued payroll").

At the end of each accounting period, the trial balance accounts must be scanned and analyzed to determine the need for adjustments for accrued expense. Once the necessary adjustments are determined, they are journalized in the hospital's journal and posted to its ledger.

ACCRUED INTEREST

Let us assume that the Hoosier Hospital issued $80,000 of 9%, 15-year bonds on July 1, 1977, at face value. The transaction entry was as follows:

Cash	101	$80,000	
Bonds Payable	250		$80,000
Proceeds from issuance of $80,000 of 9%, 15-year bonds at face value.			

Assume also that interest on these bonds is payable semiannually on January 1 and July 1 of each year, beginning January 1, 1978. These semiannual interest payments therefore will be $3,600—or $\$80,000 \times 9\% \times 1/2$. At the trial balance date, December 31, 1977, no interest has yet been paid on these bonds; the first interest payment is due January 1, 1977.

So, here we have a situation in which expense has been incurred but is unrecorded *and* unpaid. The required December 31, 1977, adjusting entry is the following:

Interest Expense	608	$3,600	
Accrued Interest Payable	203		$3,600
Adjustment for 6 months' interest accrued on bonds since July 1, 1977.			

The money borrowed by the hospital through the issuance of the bonds costs the hospital 9% per year. Since the hospital has had the use of this money for 6 months (July through December, 1977), the cost of using the money for this half-year period is charged to expenses of the period. The fact that this expense has not yet been paid by the hospital has nothing at all to do with the measurement or recognition of the expense in the current period. Because the interest has not been paid, however, the adjusting entry must establish the liability as accrued interest payable.

On January 1, 1978, the first semiannual-interest payment date, the bond interest is paid. The transaction entry will be this:

Accrued Interest Payable	203	$3,600	
Cash	101		$3,600
Payment of semiannual interest on bonds for the 6 months ended December 31, 1977.			

In this way, the bond interest applicable to 1977 was charged to 1977 expenses, although it was not actually paid until 1978. Had the December 31, 1977, adjusting entry not been made, the interest expense for 1977 would have been understated and the 1978 expense overstated.

ACCRUED SALARIES AND WAGES

In Hoosier Hospital's preadjusted trial balance (figure 23), the salaries and wages expense account (number 601) has a debit balance of $139,600. This figure is the amount of 1977 salaries and wages *paid* to the employees of Hoosier Hospital in 1977. But is this the correct amount of salaries and wages *expense* for 1977?

For the purpose of illustration, let us assume that Hoosier Hospital pays all of its employees on the tenth day of each month for salaries and wages they earned in the preceding month. The $139,600 appearing in the trial balance is, therefore, salaries and wages for the first *eleven* months of 1977! Employees' salaries and wages for December, 1977, have not yet been paid and, consequently, are not included in the salaries and wages expense account balance. These December salaries and wages will be paid January 10, 1978, but should be recorded as 1977 expense. At December 31, 1977, the hospital employees have earned their December pay. The hospital has received the benefit of their time and labors during the month. The December payroll is a cost that has been incurred by the hospital, but that cost is unrecorded and unpaid. It is an expired cost which must be recognized as a 1977 expense, and as a December 31, 1977, liability of the hospital to its employees.

Assume that the December, 1977, payroll is determined to be $13,000. (In actual practice, the accrued-payroll figure sometimes must be estimated. Much more will be said about this in a later chapter.) This will be the necessary adjusting entry at December 31, 1977:

Salaries and Wages Expense	601	$13,000	
Accrued Salaries and Wages Payable	204		$13,000
Adjustment for accrued payroll for the month of December, 1977.			

This entry puts salaries and wages into the expense of the period during which they were incurred as hospital expenses. It also establishes a liability for unpaid salaries and wages for inclusion in the hospital's December 31, 1977, balance sheet.

On January 10, 1978, the December (1977) payroll will be paid. Assuming that the amount actually disbursed on that date is the same as the amount that was accrued in the adjusting entry above, the transaction entry will be the following:

Accrued Salaries and Wages Payable	204	$13,000	
Cash	101		$13,000
Payment of December, 1977, accrued salaries and wages.			

Thus, the salaries and wages are recorded as expenses of the period in which they are incurred as expenses rather than in the period in which they are paid.

Now, a complication should be introduced. Disregard the above situation and assume instead that Hoosier Hospital pays its employees every 2 weeks, that is, every 14 days. Let us say that the last payroll period in 1977 was the 14-day period ending December 27, 1977. On the following day, December 28, employees received their pay checks for that 14-day period. What this means is that the trial-balance figure for salaries and wages expense of $139,600 represents 361 days of payroll expense (not 365 days). Employees have presumably worked another 4 days in 1977 (December 28–31) for which they have not yet been, and will not be, paid until January 10, 1978 (the end of the next 14-day payroll period). These 4 days of payroll, however, must be recorded as 1977 expense!

Let us assume that these 4 days of payroll are computed (estimated in some way) to be $3,700. The necessary December 31, 1977, adjusting entry is

Salaries and Wages Expense	601	$3,700	
Accrued Salaries and Wages Payable	204		$3,700
Adjustment for accrued payroll for the last 4 days of December, 1977.			

Now assume that the actual payroll for the 14-day period ending January 10, 1978, turns out to be $13,000. When this is paid, perhaps on January 11, 1978, the transaction entry will be

Accrued Salaries and Wages Payable	204	$3,700	
Salaries and Wages Expense	601	9,300	
Cash	101		$13,000
Payment of payroll for the 14-day period ending January 10, 1978.			

This entry records the payment of 2 things: (1) the 4 days of payroll for 1977 which was recorded previously as a liability and as 1977 expense, and (2) the 10 days of payroll for 1978 which is debited to 1978 expense. In this way, employees' salaries and wages are recorded as expenses of the period in which they are incurred by the hospital, and not necessarily in the period in which they are paid.

Hospitals, of course, have many types of expense accruals other than those illustrated here. Whatever expense items they might be, they are handled in the manner described for accrued interest and accrued payroll. The required adjusting entry will always be a debit to an expense account and a credit to a liability account. Then, when that liability is paid, the liability account is debited and the cash account credited.

Reversing Entries

In some accounting systems, what are known as *reversing entries* are prepared on the first day of each new accounting period. They are called reversing entries because they "reverse" certain previously recorded adjusting entries. Reversing entries are made to avoid certain complications in the accounting routine. In this book, however, we will employ reversing entries only in a small number of cases. One of these cases concerns adjusting for accrued payroll. Let us examine the reversing procedure in that area.

Assume the facts of the preceding illustration. Hoosier Hospital had paid $139,600 of salaries and wages during 1977, $3,700 of salaries and wages were accrued at year end, and $13,000 of salaries and wages were paid on January 11, 1978. The (1) summary transaction entry, (2) year-end adjusting entry, (3) December 31, 1977, closing entry, (4) January 1, 1978, reversing entry, and (5) January 11, 1978, transaction entry are shown below:

(1) Salaries and Wages Expense	601	$139,600	
Cash	101		$139,600
Payments of salaries and wages during 1977.			
(2) Salaries and Wages Expense	601	$ 3,700	
Accrued Salaries and Wages Payable	204		$ 3,700
Adjustment for accrued salaries and wages at December 31, 1977.			
(3) Revenue and Expense Summary	302	$143,300	
Salaries and Wages Expense	601		$143,300
To close the expense account.			
(4) Accrued Salaries and Wages Payable	204	$ 3,700	
Salaries and Wages Expense	601		$ 3,700
Reversal of December 31, 1977, adjusting entry.			
(5) Salaries and Wages Expense	601	$13,000	
Cash	101		$13,000
Payment of salaries and wages on January 11, 1978.			

Notice that the reversing entry (number 4) is the "reverse" of the December 31, 1977, adjusting entry (number 2). The reversing entry eliminates the accrued salaries and wages payable account and places a *credit* balance of $3,700 in the *1978* salaries and wages expense account. Entry 5 debits the salaries and wages expense account for $13,000. As a result, the 1978 salaries and wages expense account winds up with a debit balance of $9,300, the correct amount for 1978.

These are the postings of these entries to the ledger accounts for salaries and wages expense and for accrued salaries and wages payable:

Salaries and Wages Expense 601

Debit	Credit
(1) 139,600	(3) 143,300
(2) 3,700	
(5) 13,000	(4) 3,700
(B) 9,300	

Accrued Salaries and Wages Expense 204

Debit	Credit
(4) 3,700	(2) 3,700

Thus, because of the reversing entry, the total amount of salaries and wages paid on January 11, 1978, can be debited to the expense account. There is no need to "break" the debit between the expense account and the accrued liability account. This is the complication that is avoided by reversing entries.

You should not get the idea, however, that all adjusting entries are to be reversed. Some are reversed, some are not. In this book, the use of reversing entries will be limited to a few illustrations concerning accrued expenses (such as salaries and wages) and accrued revenues (seen in the following chapter).

QUESTIONS

1. What is the purpose of adjusting entries? Distinguish between transaction and adjusting entries.

2. Describe briefly the "matching principle."

3. Define *prepaid expense*. Give 3 examples of hospital expense items which may be prepaid.

4. Define *accrued expense*. Give 3 examples of hospital expense items which often must be accrued at the end of an accounting period.

5. Distinguish between prepaid and accrued expenses.

6. Distinguish among (a) preadjusted trial balance, (b) adjusted trial balance, (c) preclosing trial balance, and (d) postclosing trial balance.

7. Why are prepaid expenses reported in a balance sheet as assets?

8. Why are accrued expenses reported in a balance sheet as liabilities?

9. What is the purpose of reversing entries? Distinguish between adjusting entries and reversing entries.

10. Henry Hospital paid a 3-year insurance premium of $1,350 in advance on January 1, 1977. What amount should Henry Hospital report as prepaid insurance in its December 31, 1978, balance sheet?

11. Hartland Hospital paid a 3-year insurance premium in advance on January 1, 1977. The hospital's adjusted trial balance at December 31, 1978, included a prepaid insurance account with a balance of $1,400. What was the amount of the insurance premium paid on January 1, 1977?

12. Hadley Hospital rented certain equipment for use in its business offices on October 1, 1977, paying one year's rent of $1,800 in advance. What amount should appear as prepaid rent in Hadley Hospital's postclosing trial balance at December 31, 1977?

13. Homely Hospital obtained a 6-month loan of $24,000 from a bank on August 1, 1977, paying 10% interest in advance. The interest payment was debited to interest expense. Assuming that adjustments are made annually on December 31 only, prepare the necessary adjusting entry at December 31, 1977.

14. Refer to the data of question 13, but assume that the August 1, 1977, transaction entry debited the interest payment to prepaid interest expense. If adjustments are made annually on December 31 only, what is the necessary adjusting entry at December 31, 1977?

15. Homestead Hospital issued $100,000 of 6%, 20-year bonds on July 1, 1977, at face value. Interest on these bonds is payable semiannually on January 1 and July 1 of each year, beginning January 1, 1978. Assuming that adjustments are made annually on December 31 only, prepare the necessary adjusting entry at December 31, 1977.

16. Happy Hospital's preadjusted trial balance at December 31, 1977, includes a salaries and wages expense account with a debit balance of $805,200. It is determined, however, that employees have earned an additional $38,900 of salaries and wages in 1977 which have not yet been paid to them. Prepare the necessary adjusting entry at December 31, 1977.

17. Hopewell Hospital's 1977 income statement reports salaries and wages expense of $699,400. The hospital's balance sheets include the following accounts:

12/31/76 Accrued salaries and wages payable	$41,600
12/31/77 Accrued salaries and wages payable	38,400

What was the amount of salaries and wages actually paid in cash during 1977?

18. Welcome Hospital paid $355,100 of salaries and wages during 1977. Its balance sheets reported accrued salaries and wages payable as follows:

12/31/77	$28,300
12/31/76	25,700

What amount should be reported as salaries and wages expense in Welcome Hospital's 1977 income statement?

19. Wallace Hospital's 1977 income statement reported insurance expense as $8,000. Its balance sheets reported prepaid insurance as follows:

12/31/76	$1,400
12/31/77	1,100

What was the amount of insurance premiums actually paid in cash during 1977?

20. Walter Hospital paid $4,600 of rent expense during 1977. Its balance sheets reported prepaid rent expense as follows:

12/31/76	$1,300
12/31/77	900

What amount should be reported as rent expense in Walter Hospital's 1977 income statement?

PROBLEMS

A. Wilson Hospital's preadjusted trial balance at December 31, 1977, included the following accounts, among others:

Acct. No.		
107	Prepaid insurance	$5,040
108	Prepaid rent	2,100
109	Prepaid interest	1,200
604	Insurance expense	–0–
606	Rent expense	–0–
608	Interest expense	–0–

The hospital paid a 3-year insurance premium in advance on January 1, 1977. On August 1, 1977, a year's rent was paid in advance. A $20,000, 12% loan for 6 months was obtained from a bank on November 1, 1977, and the interest was paid in advance by the hospital.

Required. Prepare, in general journal form, the necessary adjusting entries at December 31, 1977.

B. Williams Hospital's preadjusted trial balance at December 31, 1977, included the following accounts, among others:

Acct. No.		
203	Accrued interest payable	$ –0–
204	Accrued salaries and wages payable	–0–
601	Salaries and wages expense	245,600
608	Interest expense	–0–
202	Notes payable	120,000

On September 1, 1977, the hospital issued its $120,000, 8%, 6-month note to a local bank in connection with a short-term loan. An analysis indicated that employees had earned $33,600 of salaries and wages during 1977 which had not been paid to them at December 31, 1977.

Required. Prepare, in general journal form, the necessary adjusting entries at December 31, 1977

C. Watson Hospital's preadjusted trial balance at December 31, 1977, included the following accounts, among others:

Acct. No.		
107	Prepaid insurance	$ 5,760
108	Prepaid rent	2,700
109	Prepaid interest	3,600
202	Notes payable	80,000
203	Accrued interest payable	–0–
204	Accrued salaries and wages payable	–0–

Acct. No.		
250	Bonds payable	400,000
601	Salaries and wages expense	755,200
604	Insurance expense	−0−
606	Rent expense	−0−
608	Interest expense	−0−

The following additional information is available:

1. A 3-year insurance premium was prepaid on January 1, 1977.
2. One year's rent was paid in advance on June 1, 1977.
3. On December 1, 1977, an $80,000, 9%, 6-month loan was obtained from a local bank. Interest was prepaid.
4. Unpaid salaries and wages at December 31, 1977, totaled $68,700.
5. On October 1, 1977, $400,000 of 6%, 10-year bonds were issued at face value. Interest on these bonds is payable annually on October 1, beginning October 1, 1978.

Required. Prepare, in general journal form, the necessary adjusting entries at December 31, 1977.

D. The following accounts appeared in the adjusted trial balance of Wilmington Hospital at December 31, 1977:

Cash	$ 26,300
Accounts receivable	105,900
Inventory	14,700
Prepaid insurance	1,800
Prepaid rent	900
Prepaid interest	500
Plant and equipment	575,000
Accounts payable	29,700
Notes payable	125,000
Accrued interest payable	2,300
Accrued salaries and wages payable	9,800
Bonds payable	350,000
Hospital equity	193,600
Routine services revenue	135,000
Ancillary services revenue	75,800
Other revenues	30,900
Salaries and wages expense	140,000
Supplies expense	31,000
Utilities expense	29,000
Insurance expense	8,200
Repairs expense	5,400
Rent expense	7,100
Interest expense	4,900
Other expenses	1,400

Required. Prepare, in good form, a balance sheet at December 31, 1977, and an income statement for the year then ended.

E. Washington Hospital's preadjusted trial balance at December 31, 1977, included the following accounts, among others:

Acct. No.		
107	Prepaid insurance	$ −0−
108	Prepaid rent	−0−
109	Prepaid interest	−0−
202	Notes payable	80,000

Acct. No.		
203	Accrued interest payable	–0–
204	Accrued salaries and wages payable	–0–
250	Bonds payable	100,000
601	Salaries and wages expense	399,500
604	Insurance expense	5,760
606	Rent expense	2,700
608	Interest expense	4,800

The following additional information is available:

1. A 3-year insurance premium was prepaid on January 1, 1977.
2. One year's rent was paid in advance on June 1, 1977.
3. On December 1, 1977, an $80,000, 12%, 6-month loan was obtained from a local bank. Interest was prepaid.
4. Unpaid salaries and wages at December 31, 1977, amounted to $27,400.
5. On April 1, 1977, 6%, 15-year bonds valued at $100,000 were issued at face value. Interest on these bonds is payable annually on April 1, beginning April 1, 1978.

Required. Prepare, in general journal form, the necessary adjusting entries at December 31, 1977.

6 Deferred and Accrued Revenues

This chapter introduces some additional adjustments of Hoosier Hospital's December 31, 1977, trial balance (see figure 23 at page 88). These adjustments are of 2 major types:

1. *Deferred Revenues.* Certain revenues have been received in cash, but as yet these revenues have not been earned by the hospital.
2. *Accrued Revenues.* Certain revenues have been earned but as yet have not been received in cash by the hospital.

The adjustments required for these items are similar to those illustrated in the preceding chapter for prepaid and accrued expenses. In this chapter, however, we are concerned with revenues, not expenses. The accrual-basis objective of the adjustments described here is to give accounting recognition to revenues in the accounting period in which they are earned, regardless of when the related cash receipt occurs. While hospital revenues are for the most part received in cash in the period earned, a substantial amount of revenues is earned prior to the receipt of cash. Less frequently, certain other revenues may be earned in an accounting period subsequent to the period in which the related cash receipt occurs.

DEFERRED REVENUES

Deferred revenues, sometimes called "deferred income," "prepaid income," or "revenues received in advance," consist of revenue items for which cash has been received but which the hospital has not yet earned. Because of the cash receipt, the hospital is obligated to provide certain goods and services in some future accounting period (or periods). Examples of deferred revenues include rentals received in advance and advance receipts of tuition for educational programs to be conducted by the hospital. More-complicated deferred revenue situations will be discussed at later points in this book.

DEFERRED RENT

Let us assume that Hoosier Hospital rents office space in its building to certain physicians on its medical staff. This practice began on August 1, 1977, when a year's rent of $4,200 ($350 per month) was received in advance. At that time, Hoosier Hospital made the following transaction entry:

Cash	101	$4,200	
Deferred Rental Income	205		$4,200
Receipt of one year's rent in advance for office space provided for staff physicians ($350 per month).			

On August 1, 1977, then, the hospital has a liability to the physicians to provide office space for their use during the next 12 months. The deferred rental income account reflects that liability.

At December 31, 1977, the hospital has provided the office space for 5 months (August through December). The hospital therefore has *earned* $1,750 of rental income ($350 × 5 months). Since this income has not been recorded by the hospital, an adjusting entry is required as follows:

Deferred Rental Income	205	$1,750	
Rental Income	404		$1,750
Adjustment for 5 months of rental income earned from provision of office space for physicians.			

This entry recognizes the rental income earned in 1977 and reduces the deferred rental income account to the correct December 31, 1977, balance of $2,450. In other words, at December 31 the hospital has a remaining liability to furnish office space for 7 months in 1978. This liability is measured at $350 per month ($350 × 7 months = $2,450).

Thus, $2,450 of rental income received in 1977 is *deferred* to 1978, the year in which it will be earned by the hospital. Were this not done, the income of 1977 would be overstated and the 1978 income understated. The accrual basis of accounting avoids such misstatements.

Suppose, however, that the August 1, 1977, transaction entry credited the $4,200 to rental income rather than to deferred rental income. This would have been the transaction entry:

Cash	101	$4,200	
Rental Income	404		$4,200
Receipt of a year's rent for office space to be provided to physicians.			

In scanning the trial balance at the end of the year, the accountant must be alert in order to recognize the need for an adjustment of the rental income account. Perhaps this would come to the accountant's attention through his examination of rental agreements, leases, and other documents. In any event, the following adjustment is required at December 31, 1977:

Rental Income	404	$2,450	
Deferred Rental Income	205		$2,450
Adjustment for 7 months' rental income to be deferred to 1978.			

So, regardless of the credit made in the transaction entry, we must wind up 1977 with $1,750 in rental income and $2,450 in deferred rental income.

There is another possibility that might be mentioned here, although it is not likely to be seen in actual practice. The transaction entry could be as follows:

Cash	101	$4,200	
Rental Income	404		$1,750
Deferred Rental Income	205		2,450
Receipt of a year's rentals of which 5 months is income of the current year; the remainder is deferred to 1978.			

If this transaction entry is made on August 1, 1977, no adjusting entry will be necessary at the year's end. For various reasons, however, this procedure may be undesirable or unworkable in actual practice. It is mentioned here only to assist you in understanding adjustment procedures.

Income also may arise from the rental of space in the hospital as sleeping quarters for interns and residents. Or the hospital may own separate buildings which are used as residences for nurses and other personnel. Space in the hospital's lobby and public areas may be rented to private concerns for gift shops and newsstands. A hospital-operated television service also may produce rental income. In any of these cases, adjusting entries may be appropriate at the end of each accounting period.

DEFERRED TUITION

Assume that Hoosier Hospital operates an educational program such as, for example, a school of nursing or a school for laboratory technologists. Let us further assume that, on September 1, 1977, the hospital received $2,160 of fees and tuition for the 9-month school year which ends May 31, 1978. For this transaction, Hoosier Hospital made the following entry:

Cash	101	$2,160	
Deferred Tuition Income	206		$2,160
Receipt of tuition ($240 per month) for the 9-month school year ending May 31, 1978.			

Here again, the hospital has received revenue in advance. The hospital has an obligation to the students in the program to provide educational services over the next 9 months. This liability is represented by the above credit to the deferred tuition income account. When the tuition is received, the hospital has earned no income.

By the end of 1977, however, the school presumably has been operating for 4 months (September through December), and the hospital therefore has earned $960 of tuition income ($240 × 4 months, or $^4/_9$ × $2,160). The following adjusting entry is required at December 31, 1977:

Deferred Tuition Income	206	$ 960	
Tuition Income	405		$ 960
Adjustment for tuition income earned in 1977 (4 months @ $240 per month).			

This entry gives accounting recognition to the tuition income earned during the current year and *defers* recognition of the remaining tuition revenue to 1978. Hoosier Hospital will report $960 of tuition income in its 1977 income statement and $1,200 of deferred tuition income (a liability) in its December 31, 1977, balance sheet.

Now assume that the September 1, 1977, transaction entry credited all of the tuition received to income as follows:

Cash	101	$2,160	
Tuition Income	405		$2,160
Receipt of tuition ($240 per month) for the 9-month school year ending May 31, 1978.			

Had this been done, the December 31, 1977, trial balance would have $2,160 in the tuition income account (rather than in the deferred tuition income account). In this event, the following adjusting entry would be required at December 31, 1977:

Tuition Income	405	$1,200	
Deferred Tuition Income	206		$1,200
Adjustment for tuition income to be deferred to 1978 (5 months @ $240 per month).			

Thus, we again produce the necessary account balances at December 31, 1977: $960 of tuition income and $1,200 of deferred tuition income.

Let us now summarize the accounting procedure followed with respect to deferred revenues. The entries in T-account form are:

1. Assuming the transaction entry credited the cash received to a deferred revenue account:

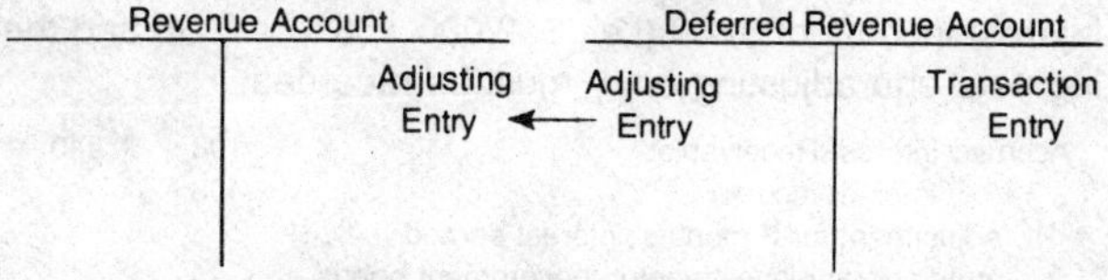

   The adjusting entry transfers the amount of revenue earned during the current period from the liability account to the revenue account.

2. Assuming the transaction entry credited the cash received to a revenue account:

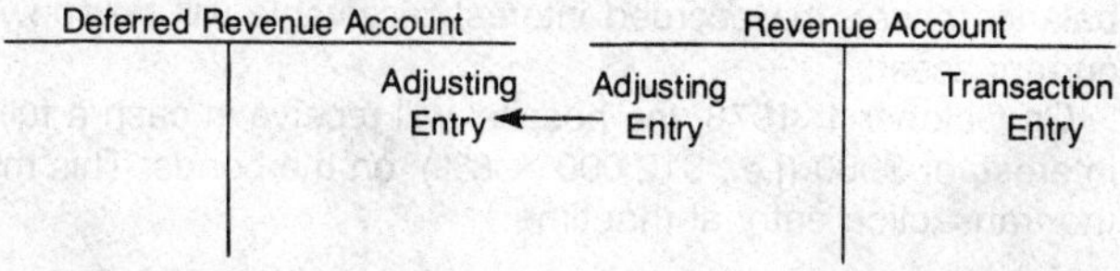

   The adjusting entry transfers the amount of unearned revenue from the revenue account to the deferred revenue account.

The nature and amount of the required adjusting entry depends on the account initially credited in the transaction entry.

ACCRUED REVENUES

Accrued revenues consist of revenue items which the hospital has earned but for which the hospital has not recorded a receivable or collected cash. The hospital, of course, routinely provides goods and services to patients and has a claim against them for the value of those goods and services. These claims are recorded as receivables (assets), as we have previously indicated. In addition, the hospital provides other types of services which produce revenues and require the recognition of related receivables. Some examples of these items, called accrued revenues, are accrued interest receivable, accrued rent receivable, and accrued tuition receivable. We will illustrate the accrual of interest revenues and receivables.

Let us say that Hoosier Hospital invested $12,000 in 8% government bonds on October 1, 1977. These bonds, purchased at face value, pay interest annually on October 1, commencing October 1, 1978. This was the transaction entry:

Temporary Investments	102	$12,000	
Cash	101		$12,000
Purchase of $12,000 (face value) of 8% government bonds as a temporary investment.			

Perhaps at this time Hoosier Hospital had a cash balance in excess of its then-current needs. In accordance with good business practice, it was decided to invest those funds for a short period of time in order to obtain interest income. Although the bonds may be 5- or 10-year bonds, the hospital intends to hold them only as a temporary or short-term investment. As a result, they will be classified as a current asset in Hoosier Hospital's balance sheet.

At December 31, 1977, Hoosier Hospital has held this investment for 3 months (October through December). The hospital has earned interest income of $240 (i.e., $12,000 $\times$ 8% $\times$ 3/12), and the following year-end adjusting entry must be recorded:

Accrued Interest Receivable	103	$ 240	
Interest Income	403		$ 240
Adjustment for 3 months' interest earned on temporary investment in government bonds.			

This entry gives accounting recognition to interest income earned (but not yet received) during 1977. The interest, however, will be received at the next annual interest payment date, October 1, 1978. So, the entry makes a debit to the appropriate asset account, accrued interest receivable. In Hoosier Hospital's December 31, 1977, balance sheet, the accrued interest receivable will be shown as a current asset.

On October 1, 1978, the hospital will receive in cash a full year's interest, or $960 (i.e., $12,000 $\times$ 8%), on the bonds. This might be the transaction entry at that time:

Cash	101	$ 960	
Accrued Interest Receivable	103		$ 240
Interest Income	403		720
Receipt of a year's interest on temporary investment in 8% government bonds, of which $240 was recognized as income in 1977.			

Notice that, while all of the interest income was received in cash in 1978, $240 of it was recorded as 1977 income and $720 was recognized as 1978 income. Thus, income is recorded in the year in which it is earned, and not necessarily in the year in which it is received in cash.

Hoosier Hospital might have chosen to make a reversing entry on January 1, 1978. In addition, if the hospital prepared monthly financial statements, adjusting entries would have been made monthly. We will get to monthly adjustment procedures in chapter 9. So, assuming annual adjustments only, Hoosier Hospital might have made the following reversing entry on January 1, 1978:

Interest Income	403	$ 240	
Accrued Interest Receivable	103		$ 240
Reversal of December 31, 1977, entry for accrued interest on temporary investment in government bonds.			

This entry eliminates the balance in the accrued interest receivable account and places a *debit* balance in the 1978 interest income account. Then, when the annual interest is received on the investment on October 1, 1978, the following transaction entry is made:

Cash	101	$ 960	
Interest Income	403		$ 960
Receipt of a year's interest on temporary investment in 8% government bonds.			

When this $960 credit is posted to the interest income account, the account then will have the proper $720 balance: the $960 credit posting minus the $240 debit posting from the reversing entry above. Compare this transaction entry (assuming a reversing entry was made) with the previously illustrated transaction entry (assuming no reversing entry was made) for October 1, 1978. Thus, the use of reversing entries tends to simplify subsequent transaction entries.

Summary of Adjustments for Prepayments and Accruals

This chapter has illustrated adjusting entries for deferred and accrued revenues; the preceding chapter illustrated adjustments for prepaid and accrued expenses. Now, let us bring these adjustments together as they would appear in Hoosier Hospital's general journal for 1977. In figure 24, the adjusting journal entries (sometimes called "AJEs") numbered 1 through 5 were discussed in the preceding chapter; those numbered 6 through 8 are those which were described earlier in the present chapter.

Entries 1, 2, and 3 are the adjustments arising from the prepayment of expenses during 1977. In each case, an expense account is debited, and an asset account is credited. This is because we have assumed that the hospital has an accounting policy of debiting prepaid expense accounts in the initial transaction entry. For example, when insurance premiums are paid, a debit is made to prepaid insurance, not to insurance expense.

Adjusting entries 4 and 5 are those necessary to give accounting recognition to accrued expenses, expenses incurred during 1977

Figure 24
Hoosier Hospital
1977 Journal
(Adjusting Entries)

Entry No.	Accounts and Explanations	Acct. No.	Debit	Credit
1	Insurance Expense	604	1,200	
	Prepaid Insurance	107		1,200
	Adjustment for portion of prepaid premium which expired during 1977. (Chapter 5, page 89.)			
2	Rent Expense	606	720	
	Prepaid Rent	108		720
	Adjustment to record rent expense for May through December, 1977, at $90 per month. (Chapter 5, page 91.)			
3	Interest Expense	608	240	
	Prepaid Interest	109		240
	Adjustment for interest on bank loan for November and December, 1977. (Chapter 5, page 92.)			
4	Interest Expense	608	3,600	
	Accrued Interest Payable	203		3,600
	Adjustment for 6 months' interest accrued on bonds since July 1, 1977. (Chapter 5, page 93.)			
5	Salaries and Wages Expense	601	13,000	
	Accrued Salaries and Wages Payable	204		13,000
	Adjustment for accrued payroll for the month of December, 1977. (Chapter 5, page 94.)			
6	Deferred Rental Income	205	1,750	
	Rental Income	404		1,750
	Adjustment for 5 months of rental income earned from provision of office space for physicians. (Page 103 of this chapter.)			
7	Deferred Tuition Income	206	960	
	Tuition Income	405		960
	Adjustment for tuition income earned in 1977. (Page 104 of this chapter.)			
8	Accrued Interest Receivable	103	240	
	Interest Income	403		240
	Adjustment for 3 months' interest on temporary investment in government bonds. (Page 106 of this chapter.)			

but not yet paid. In each case, the entry debits an expense account and credits a liability account. This will always be true for adjustments for accrued expenses.

Entries 6 and 7 are adjusting entries for deferred (prepaid) revenues. Each of these entries debits a liability account and credits a revenue account. This is because we have assumed that it is Hoosier Hospital's accounting policy to credit a deferred revenue account whenever revenue items are received in advance. For example, when rental prepayments are received, a credit is made to the deferred rental income account, not to the rental income account.

Entry 8 relates to the accrual of income that was earned during 1977 but which had not been received in cash by the end of the year. The entry debits an asset account and credits an income account. This will always be true of adjustments for accrued revenues.

All of these adjusting entries, of course, will be posted in due course to Hoosier Hospital's ledger. When this is accomplished, most of the ledger accounts will have correct balances in terms of accrual-basis accounting. These 8 entries, however, are not all of the adjusting entries normally required at the end of a fiscal year. In the next chapter, 2 additional types of adjustments will be considered. These adjustments will relate to revenue deductions and to depreciation.

QUESTIONS

1. Define *deferred revenue*. Give 2 examples of deferred revenue.

2. Define *accrued revenue*. Give 2 examples of accrued revenue.

3. Why is deferred revenue reported in a balance sheet as a liability?

4. Why is accrued revenue reported in a balance sheet as an asset?

5. Castor Hospital received a year's rent in advance on May 1, 1977. The hospital's December 31, 1977, balance sheet reported deferred rental income of $580. What was the amount of rent received on May 1, 1977?

6. Crosstown Hospital received $1,800, representing a year's rent in advance, on November 1, 1977. In the transaction entry, $1,800 was credited to the deferred rental income account. Assuming that adjustments are made annually on December 31 only, what adjusting entry should be made on December 31, 1977?

7. Refer to the data of question 6, but assume that the rental income account was credited for $1,800 in the transaction entry. Assuming that adjustments are made annually on December 31 only, what adjusting entry should be made on December 31, 1977?

8. Carson Hospital's 1977 income statement reported rental income of $8,200. The hospital's balance sheets reported deferred rental income as follows:

12/31/76	$1,700
12/31/77	1,300

What was the amount of rent actually received in cash during 1977?

9. Carter Hospital received in cash rental payments of $10,700 during 1977. Its balance sheets reported deferred rental income as follows:

12/31/77	$2,600
12/31/76	1,800

What amount should be reported as rental income in Carter Hospital's 1977 income statement?

10. On September 1, 1977, Carbondale Hospital received $10,620 of fees and tuition for one of its educational programs which has a 9-month school year ending May 31, 1978. What amount should be reported as deferred tuition income in the hospital's December 31, 1977, balance sheet?

11. Cabot Hospital invested $60,000 in 8% government bonds on August 1, 1977. These bonds, which were purchased at face value, pay interest annually on August 1, commencing August 1, 1978. Assuming that adjustments are made annually on December 31 only, prepare the necessary adjusting entry for accrued interest at December 31, 1977.

12. Capital Hospital received interest payments of $8,600 during 1977. Its balance sheets reported accrued interest receivable as follows:

12/31/76	$1,100
12/31/77	1,400

What amount should be reported as interest income in the hospital's 1977 income statement?

PROBLEMS

A. Caspar Hospital's December 31, 1977, preadjusted trial balance included the following accounts, among others:

Acct. No.		
102	Temporary investments	$24,000
103	Accrued interest receivable	–0–
205	Deferred rental income	5,400
206	Deferred tuition income	4,320
403	Interest income	–0–
404	Rental income	–0–
405	Tuition income	–0–

The following additional information is available:

1. On September 1, 1977, the hospital invested $24,000 (face value) in 8% government bonds which pay interest annually on September 1, commencing September 1, 1978.
2. On June 1, 1977, the hospital received a year's rent in advance.
3. On September 1, 1977, the hospital received 9 months' tuition in advance for one of its educational programs.

Required. Prepare, in general journal form, the necessary adjusting entries at December 31, 1977.

B. Cantor Hospital's December 31, 1977, preadjusted trial balance included the following accounts, among others:

Acct. No.		
102	Temporary investments	$30,000
103	Accrued interest receivable	−0−
205	Deferred rental income	−0−
206	Deferred tuition income	−0−
403	Interest income	−0−
404	Rental income	5,400
405	Tuition income	4,320

The following additional information is available:

1. On April 1, 1977, the hospital invested $30,000 (face value) in 8% government bonds which pay interest annually on April 1, commencing April 1, 1978.
2. On June 1, 1977, the hospital received a year's rent in advance.
3. On September 1, 1977, the hospital received 9 months' tuition in advance for one of its educational programs.

Required. Prepare, in general journal form, the necessary adjusting entries at December 31, 1977.

C. The following is Captain Hospital's preadjusted trial balance at December 31, 1977:

Acct. No.			
101	Cash	$ 34,900	
102	Temporary investments	60,000	
103	Accrued interest receivable	−0−	
104	Accounts receivable	172,000	
106	Inventory	15,000	
107	Prepaid insurance	6,480	
108	Prepaid rent	4,500	
109	Prepaid interest	2,400	
150	Plant and equipment	350,020	
201	Accounts payable		$ 28,200
202	Notes payable		48,000
203	Accrued interest payable		−0−
204	Accrued salaries and wages payable		−0−
205	Deferred rental income		3,600
206	Deferred tuition income		4,900
250	Bonds payable		200,000
301	Hospital equity		335,300
302	Revenue and expense summary		−0−
401	Routine services revenue		97,500
402	Ancillary services revenue		58,200
403	Interest income		−0−
404	Rental income		−0−
405	Tuition income		−0−
406	Other revenues		19,300
601	Salaries and wages expense	100,000	
602	Supplies expense	25,000	

Acct. No.			
603	Utilities expense	12,000	
604	Insurance expense	-0-	
605	Repairs expense	9,000	
606	Rent expense	-0-	
608	Interest expense	-0-	
609	Other expenses	3,700	
		$795,000	$795,000

The following additional information is available:

1. On August 1, 1977, the hospital invested $60,000 (face value) in 8% government bonds which pay interest annually on August 1, commencing August 1, 1978.
2. On January 1, 1977, a 3-year insurance premium was paid in advance.
3. One year's rent was received in advance on March 1, 1977.
4. One year's rent was paid in advance by the hospital on May 1, 1977.
5. On November 1, 1977, the hospital issued its 6-month, 10% note for $48,000 to a local bank in connection with a short-term loan. The interest was prepaid by the hospital.
6. On October 1, 1977, the hospital issued $200,000 of 6%, 10-year bonds at face value. These bonds pay interest semiannually on October 1 and April 1, commencing April 1, 1978.
7. Unpaid salaries and wages at December 31, 1977, amounted to $16,800.
8. On September 1, 1977, the hospital received 9 months' tuition in advance for one of its educational programs.

Required. (1) Enter the preadjusted December 31, 1977, balances in general ledger accounts. (2) Prepare, in general journal form, the necessary adjusting entries at December 31, 1977. (3) Post the adjusting entries to the ledger accounts and prepare an adjusted trial balance at December 31, 1977. (4) Prepare an income statement for 1977 and a balance sheet at December 31, 1977. (5) Prepare, in general journal form, the necessary closing entries at December 31, 1977. (6) Post the closing entries to the ledger accounts. (7) Prepare a postclosing trial balance at December 31, 1977.

7
Depreciation and Revenue Deductions

Adjustment procedures for prepaid expenses, accrued expenses, deferred revenues, and accrued revenues were covered in the 2 preceding chapters. In this chapter we want to describe and illustrate 2 additional types of adjustments that are required at the end of the accounting period. The first of these has to do with depreciation of the hospital's plant assets; the second relates to the problem of revenue deductions: charity service, contractual adjustments, and bad debts. When this chapter is concluded, you will have been exposed to a majority of the adjusting entries which are found in hospital accounting.

DEPRECIATION

Hoosier Hospital's December 31, 1977, trial balance (see figure 23 at page 88) includes the following account balances to which your attention should now be directed:

Acct. No.	Account Titles	Dr.	Cr.
150	Land	$ 25,000	
160	Building	180,000	
161	Accumulated Depreciation—Building		$ ---
170	Equipment	60,000	
171	Accumulated Depreciation—Equipment		---
507	Depreciation Expense	---	

Accounts 150, 160, and 170 are asset accounts whose debit balances represent the original, historical costs of the hospital's plant assets: land, buildings, and equipment used in hospital operations (and not held for investment purposes or for sale in the ordinary course of business). Accounts 161 and 171 are called *contra-asset* accounts, that is, *negative* asset accounts. As you learned in chapter 1, these accounts reflect the amount of plant asset cost which has been charged to expense (depreciation) in the hospital's income statements of the current and prior accounting periods. Account 507 reports the amount of depreciation allocated to the current period. Depreciation therefore enters the accounting records through adjusting entries which debit depreciation expense and credit the accumulated depreciation accounts.

Let us assume, for purposes of illustration, that Hoosier Hospital acquired all its plant assets in a cash transaction on January 1, 1977.

Land	150	$ 25,000	
Building	160	180,000	
Equipment	170	60,000	
Cash	101		$265,000
Purchase of plant assets for cash.			

These plant assets were used throughout 1977. Since the activities of the year were made possible by, and benefited from, the use of these assets, is it not logical to presume that some part of the cost of the assets should be charged as expense against the revenues of the period?

NATURE OF DEPRECIATION

Depreciation is an accounting procedure by which the cost (less salvage value, if any) of certain plant assets is allocated to expense over the estimated useful lives of such assets in a systematic and rational manner. The amount of plant-asset cost allocated to a particular accounting period is called *depreciation* expense. A fundamental point to remember is that depreciation is a process of *cost allocation*, not of *valuation.* Depreciation, in the accounting sense, is not a measurement of the loss in market value of an asset during a given period.

Consider, for example, an item of equipment used in the radiology department of the hospital. This equipment cost, say, $4,000 when acquired on January 1, 1977. Obviously, the equipment will not last forever; it eventually will wear out and/or become obsolete, with time, use, and changes in technology. When the equipment reaches the point at which it is no longer useful to the hospital, it will be discarded (either sold or scrapped) and perhaps replaced by new equipment. The amount, if any, for which the old equipment can be sold at the end of its useful life is called *salvage value*, or *scrap value*.

In order to compute depreciation on this radiology equipment, we must estimate its useful life (usually in *years*) and its salvage value (if any). These estimates must be made when the equipment is acquired; hence, they must be based on informed judgment and experienced opinion. (We will probe more deeply into this matter in a subsequent chapter.)

So, let us assume that we estimate a useful life of 6 years and a salvage value of $400 for the equipment. This means that we expect the equipment to be used over a 6-year period from the beginning of 1977 to the end of 1982, at which time it may be sold for $400. Then, subtracting the salvage value from the cost of the equipment, we obtain $3,600 (i.e., $4,000 − $400), the *depreciation base*, or *depreciable cost.* This is the net cost (acquisition cost minus salvage value) to the hospital for the use of the equipment over its 6-year life. We can depreciate no more than $3,600.

Now, we divide the $3,600 depreciable cost by the estimated useful life of 6 years to determine annual depreciation expense: $3,600/6 = $600 annual depreciation expense. This method of computing depreciation is known as *straight-line depreciation*; it is perhaps the most widely used depreciation method. Other depreciation methods may be used, but we will confine this discussion to the straight-line procedure.

At the end of 1977, then, $600 of the cost of the radiology equipment must be recognized as depreciation expense. This is accomplished by an adjusting entry such as the following:

Depreciation Expense	$600	
Accumulated Depreciation		$600
Adjustment for depreciation of radiology equipment for 1977.		

The 1977 income statement will reflect $600 of depreciation expense. In the balance sheet at December 31, 1977, the presentation is the following:

Equipment, at cost	$4,000	
Less Accumulated Depreciation	600	
Equipment, net		$3,400

Note that accumulated depreciation, the contra-asset account, is shown in the balance sheet as a deduction from the asset account. The resulting $3,400 figure is the undepreciated cost of the equipment; it also is referred to as the "book value" of the equipment. It is not, however, the "market value" of the equipment; that is, it is not the price for which the equipment could be sold by the hospital on December 31, 1977.

Each year, for the next 5 years, $600 will be recorded as annual depreciation expense. That is, depreciation will *accumulate* at the rate of $600 per year. In the December 31, 1979, balance sheet, for example, the presentation will be as follows:

Equipment, at cost	$4,000	
Less Accumulated Depreciation	1,800	
Equipment, net		$2,200

Here, depreciation has accumulated for 3 years, 1977–1979, to a total of $1,800 (i.e., $600 × 3 years). This will continue until the end of 1982, at which time the equipment will be fully depreciated and, presumably, retired from use by the hospital.

What if the equipment is not retired at the end of 1982? Suppose the useful life and salvage value estimates turn out to be incorrect? What happens if the equipment is sold prior to 1982? These are very interesting questions, but we must defer a consideration of the answers to subsequent chapters.

One additional point, however, should be made here. Assume that the equipment mentioned above was acquired on, say, July 1, 1977. In that case, how much depreciation should be taken on the equipment for 1977? The answer is a half year's depreciation, or $300 (i.e., $600/2), since the hospital had the use of the equipment for only 6 months. (The hospital may adopt a different policy with respect to this matter, but we will not discuss it at this time.) Had the equipment been acquired on December 31, 1977, only a month's depreciation ($600/12 = $50) would be taken in 1977.

ADJUSTING ENTRIES

Returning now to Hoosier Hospital, let us develop the December 31, 1977, adjusting entries for depreciation. Land is non-depreciable, but depreciation must be computed and recorded for the hospital's building and equipment.

• ***Depreciation of Building***. The useful life of Hoosier Hospital's building is estimated to be 50 years. Salvage value is estimated to be 20% of the cost of the building, or $36,000 (i.e., 20% of $180,000). The depreciable cost, then, is $144,000 (i.e., $180,000 − $36,000), and annual depreciation is $2,880 (i.e., $144,000/50). At December 31, 1977, the following adjusting entry is required:

Depreciation Expense		507	$2,880	
Accumulated Depreciation—Building		161		$2,880
Adjustment (for 1977 depreciation of hospital building):				
Cost	$180,000			
Less salvage value (20%)	36,000			
Depreciable cost	$144,000			
Divide by useful life	50			
Annual depreciation	$ 2,880			

If monthly adjustments were made by Hoosier Hospital during 1977, this entry for $240 (i.e., $2,880/12 months) would be made at the end of each month.

The $2,880 of depreciation on the building will appear among the expenses in Hoosier Hospital's 1977 income statement. In the process of closing the books at the end of the year, the depreciation expense account will be closed. The accumulated depreciation account, however, is not closed; it is presented in the hospital's December 31, 1977, balance sheet in the manner described earlier. It also is carried forward into 1978 as one of the opening balances for that year.

• ***Depreciation of Equipment***. Assume that the estimated useful life of Hoosier Hospital's equipment is 10 years and that the salvage value is 10%, or $6,000 (i.e., 10% × $60,000). The required adjusting entry at December 31, 1977, is

Depreciation Expense		507	$5,400	
Accumulated Depreciation—Equipment		171		$5,400
Adjustment for 1977 depreciation of hospital equipment:				
Cost	$60,000			
Less salvage value (10%)	6,000			
Depreciable cost	$54,000			
Divide by useful life	10			
Annual depreciation	$ 5,400			

In actual practice, the computation of depreciation is complicated by the fact that hospitals own many different types of equipment which have been acquired at different dates and which have different useful lives and salvage values. And, of course, different depreciation methods may be applied to different classes of equipment.

Several depreciation expense accounts usually are employed in an actual situation. In order to reduce the amount of detail, however, we are using a single depreciation expense account for depreciation on both buildings and equipment.

REVENUE DEDUCTIONS

Turn your attention now to several other accounts in Hoosier Hospital's December 31, 1977, trial balance (figure 23, page 88). The pertinent accounts are shown below:

Acct. No.	Account Titles	Dr.	Cr.
104	Accounts Receivable	$ 96,600	
105	Allowance for Uncollectible Accounts		$ ---
501	Charity Service	29,200	
502	Contractual Adjustments	19,400	
503	Bad Debts	---	

You know, of course, that account 104 reflects the uncollected billings made to patients for hospital services rendered to them. At December 31, 1977, then, $96,600 of Hoosier Hospital's 1977 revenues remain uncollected and in accounts receivable from patients. Account 104 is always debited (and revenues credited) for *all* services provided at *full*, established rates for those services, regardless of the financial status or medical classification of the patients served by the hospital. This is done to provide an accounting measurement of the monetary value of the hospital services rendered during the period.

It is a fact, however, that hospitals do not always collect their full, established rates for services rendered. There are several reasons for this situation. First, most hospitals provide services to all who are in need of those services, regardless of the recipients' ability to pay. Hospitals render a considerable volume of services to the financially indigent either at nominal service rates or at no charge whatever. The difference between the hospital's established rates for such services and the amount collected (if any) is called *charity service*. The amount of charity service provided by the hospital is accumulated and reported as a *revenue deduction* in the charity service account (number 501). Since this account reflects "lost revenues," it has a debit balance.

To illustrate, assume that Hoosier Hospital provides certain ancillary services to a group of charity patients. Established rates for these services total $174, but the hospital receives nothing. Two entries are necessary:

Accounts Receivable	104	$ 174	
Ancillary Services Revenue	402		$ 174
Services rendered to charity patients.			
Revenue Deductions—Charity Service	501	$ 174	
Accounts Receivable	104		$ 174
Write-off of patients' accounts to charity service.			

Periodic Adjustments and Summary

In subsequent discussion, the "revenue deductions" prefix to the charity service account will be omitted for ease of presentation. It is, however, an account to be reported in the income statement as a deduction from patient service revenues.

A second reason why hospitals often do not collect their full rates has to do with certain third-party contracts. Under these contracts, the hospital has agreed to provide certain services to a particular group of patients at contract rates which are less than the hospital's full rates. The difference typically is not collectible by the hospital from those patients. This uncollectible difference is accumulated in another revenue deduction account called *contractual adjustments* (account 502).

To illustrate, assume that Hoosier Hospital provides $10,000 of services to certain third-party patients under a contract which provides for 90% reimbursement to the hospital. The entries are as follows:

Accounts Receivable	104	$10,000	
Routine Services Revenue	401		$ 6,000
Ancillary Services Revenue	402		4,000
Services rendered to patients.			
Cash	101	$ 9,000	
Contractual Adjustments	502	1,000	
Accounts Receivable	104		$10,000
Collection of third-party patients' accounts			

The $1,000 of lost revenue (10% of $10,000) is debited to the contractual adjustments account which, like charity service, will be included in the income statement as a deduction from gross patient service revenues.

A third reason why hospitals fail to collect their revenues is that some patients simply do not pay their hospital bills just as they may not pay their other bills. If these patients' accounts remain uncollected after the hospital's best collection efforts, they are written off as bad debts. These uncollectibles are accumulated in another revenue deduction account: *bad debts* (account 503). It is very important that bad debts not be confused with charity service. At the time of admission, or as soon thereafter as possible, patients' financial status should be clearly established so as to permit accurate accounting classifications of all transactions with patients.

In addition to accounting recognition of charity service, contractual adjustments, and bad debts *during* an accounting period, adjusting entries for these revenue deductions also are necessary at the *end* of the period. These entries consist of estimates of charity service, contractual adjustments, and bad debts related to services rendered during the period and included in the end-of-period accounts receivable. This estimated portion of accounts receivable likely to prove uncollectible in the next accounting period is debited to the revenue deduction accounts and credited to the allowance for uncollectible accounts account (number 105). This is done to "match" revenues with related revenue deductions in the same accounting period. It is the same principle described in chapter 5 as the matching of revenue and expense.

The allowance for uncollectible accounts is a contra-asset account. It is presented in the hospital's balance sheet as a deduction from accounts receivable in much the same manner that accumulated depreciation is deducted from the hospital's plant assets. Journal entries relating to the allowance account are illustrated later in this chapter.

CHARITY SERVICE

Recall that Hoosier Hospital's December 31, 1977, trial balance includes account 501, charity service, with a debit balance of $29,200. This indicates that the hospital, in a series of journal entries, gave accounting recognition to $29,200 of charity service rendered during 1977. In a single summary entry, this is what was recorded:

Charity Service	501	$29,200	
Accounts Receivable	104		$29,200
Write-off of patients' accounts to charity service.			

Prior to this, when the services were provided to charity patients, entries were made to record the revenues and establish the accounts receivable.

At year's end, however, there are $96,600 of accounts receivable. How much of this $96,600 will not be collected by reason of charity? If it is possible and practicable to identify specific accounts (or portions of specific accounts) as charity, such accounts (or portions of them) should be written off immediately and directly to the charity service account. This procedure is frequently feasible. If not, an estimate generally is made of the percentage of accounts receivable likely not to be collected by reason of charity. Assuming this percentage to be 5%, the necessary adjusting entry at December 31, 1977, is

Charity Service	501	$4,830	
Allowance for Uncollectible Accounts	105		$4,830
Adjustment for estimated portion of accounts receivable to prove uncollectible by reason of charity (5% of $96,600 = $4,830).			

This entry matches the charity service revenue deduction with the related revenues recorded during 1977. The entry also establishes the allowance account so that the accounts receivable will be reported in the December 31, 1977, balance sheet at *net realizable value*, or *collectible value*.

In 1978, when it is determined that a 1977 patient account of, say, $700 is deemed uncollectible by reason of financial indigency, the following entry will be made:

Allowance for Uncollectible Accounts	105	$ 700	
Accounts Receivable	104		$ 700
Write-off of 1977 charity accounts against the allowance for uncollectibles.			

Had the adjusting entry not been made at the end of 1977 to establish the allowance account for estimated charity service, the 1978 write-off would have been debited to the 1978 charity service (revenue deduction) account. And this would have put the debit to charity service in the wrong year! The charity service, you see, was performed in 1977, not in 1978.

CONTRACTUAL ADJUSTMENTS

Hoosier Hospital's December 31, 1977, trial balance includes account 502, contractual adjustments, which has a debit balance of $19,400. All of these revenue deductions were recorded by the hospital in a series of entries, but the following entry summarizes them:

Contractual Adjustments	502	$19,400	
Accounts Receivable	104		$19,400
Write-off of patients' accounts to contractual adjustments.			

This entry records the contractual adjustments given accounting recognition during 1977. At December 31, however, how much of the $96,600 of accounts receivable will prove to be uncollectible by reason of contractual adjustments?

If it is possible to identify the contractual-adjustment portion of individual accounts, such amounts should be written off immediately and directly to the contractual adjustments account. This procedure generally is not feasible. Instead, an estimate is made of the percentage of accounts receivable likely to prove uncollectible because of contractual adjustments. Let us assume that only $20,000 of year-end accounts receivable are subject to contractual adjustment, and that an estimated 12% of these balances probably will be uncollected because of such adjustments. The required December 31, 1977, adjusting entry is

Contractual Adjustments	502	$ 2,400	
Allowance for Uncollectible Accounts	105		$ 2,400
Adjustment for estimated portion of accounts receivable to prove uncollectible by reason of contractual adjustments (12% of $20,000).			

This entry matches the revenue deduction for contractual adjustments with the related revenues recorded during 1977.

In 1978, when (say) $1,900 of 1977 accounts receivable are found to be uncollectible by reason of contractual adjustments, the following entry will be made:

Allowance for Uncollectible Accounts	105	$1,900	
Accounts Receivable	104		$1,900
Write-off of a portion of 1977 accounts receivable against the allowance for uncollectibles.			

Had the allowance account not been established by the December 31, 1977, adjusting entry, the 1978 write-off above would have been made to revenue deductions (contractual adjustments) of 1978. This would have produced a mismatching of revenues and revenue deductions.

A third revenue deduction account, bad debts (account 503), appears in the December 31, 1977, trial balance of Hoosier Hospital. Since this account has no balance, it can be correctly assumed that the hospital has not recognized any bad debts during 1977. At December 31, however, the hospital has $96,600 of accounts receivable. How much of these receivables will prove to be uncollectible by reason of bad debts?

BAD DEBTS

If it can be determined that specific accounts are bad debts at December 31, those particular accounts should be written off immediately and directly to the bad debts account; in other words, debit bad debts and credit accounts receivable. This procedure, however, often is not feasible, particularly with respect to those accounts which have been on the books only a short time and for which additional collection efforts will be made in the future; so an estimate must be made as to the amount of bad debts likely to arise out of the December 31 accounts receivable.

This estimate may be developed as a percentage of accounts receivable or as a percentage of patient service revenues for the period. It also may be determined through the preparation of a so-called aging schedule for the year-end accounts receivable. These methods of estimating bad debts are described fully in another chapter. Until we consider them in detail we will estimate bad debts simply as a percentage of year-end accounts receivable, recognizing that this procedure is not entirely appropriate.

Let us assume, then, that Hoosier Hospital estimates its bad debts at 10% of December 31, 1977, accounts receivable. The required adjusting entry is as follows:

Bad Debts	503	$ 9,660	
Allowance for Uncollectible Accounts	105		$ 9,660
Adjustment for estimated portion of accounts receivable to prove uncollectible by reason of bad debts (10% of $96,600 = $9,660).			

This entry puts the revenue deduction (bad debts) in the same year in which the related revenues and accounts receivable arose.

In 1978, when an individual patient's account of (say) $950 is adjudged to be a bad debt and therefore uncollectible, the entry will be the following:

Allowance for Uncollectible Accounts	105	$ 950	
Accounts Receivable	104		$ 950
Write-off of a patient's account deemed to be a bad debt.			

Had the allowance account not been established at the end of 1977, the write-off in 1978 necessarily would have been charged to bad debts of 1978 (the wrong year in that the related revenues were recognized in 1977).

ALLOWANCE FOR UNCOLLECTIBLE ACCOUNTS

The assumed December 31, 1977, adjusting entries for charity service, contractual adjustments, and bad debts are repeated in the following:

Charity Service	501	$ 4,830	
Allowance for Uncollectible Accounts	105		$ 4,830
Adjustment for estimated charity service in year-end accounts receivable.			
Contractual Adjustments	502	$ 2,400	
Allowance for Uncollectible Accounts	105		$ 2,400
Adjustment for estimated amount of contractual adjustments in year-end receivables.			
Bad Debts	503	$ 9,660	
Allowance for Uncollectible Accounts	105		$ 9,660
Adjustment for estimated bad debts in year-end accounts receivable.			

While a separate allowance account generally is maintained for each type of revenue deduction, a single allowance account is used here to reduce the amount of detail.

Figure 25
Hoosier Hospital
1977 Journal
(Adjusting Entries)

Entry No.	Accounts and Explanations	Acct. No.	Debit	Credit
9	Depreciation Expense	507	2,880	
	Accumulated Depreciation—Building	161		2,880
	Adjustment for 1977 depreciation of hospital building. (See page 116.)			
10	Depreciation Expense	507	5,400	
	Accumulated Depreciation—Equipment	171		5,400
	Adjustment for 1977 depreciation of hospital equipment. (See page 116.)			
11	Charity Service	501	4,830	
	Allowance for Uncollectible Accounts	105		4,830
	Adjustment for estimated charity service in year-end receivables. (See page 119.)			
12	Contractual Adjustments	502	2,400	
	Allowance for Uncollectible Accounts	105		2,400
	Adjustment for estimated contractual adjustments in year-end receivables. (See page 120.)			
13	Bad Debts	503	9,660	
	Allowance for Uncollectible Accounts	105		9,660
	Adjustment for estimated bad debts in year-end receivables. (See page 121.)			

Taken together, these entries establish a total credit balance of $16,890 (i.e., $4,830 + $2,400 + $9,660) in the allowance account. The situation presented in Hoosier Hospital's December 31, 1977, balance sheet therefore will be as follows:

Accounts Receivable	$96,600
Less Allowance for Uncollectible Accounts	16,890
Accounts Receivable, net	$79,710

The $79,710 figure is the *net realizable value* of the hospital's accounts receivable at December 31. It is the amount of the accounts receivable estimated to be collectible in cash in the future (we hope, early in 1978). This balance-sheet valuation of accounts receivable is a generally accepted accounting principle.

Summary of Adjustments for Depreciation and Revenue Deductions

In the previous chapter (figure 24 at page 108), adjusting journal entries for prepayments and accruals were illustrated in Hoosier Hospital's 1977 journal. Those adjustments were numbered as entries 1 through 8. Figure 25 shows the adjusting journal entries discussed in this chapter as entries 9 through 13. Entries 9 and 10 are for depreciation; entries 11, 12, and 13 are for revenue deductions. In the next chapter, we will pull together all 13 adjusting entries and prepare the 1977 financial statements for Hoosier Hospital.

Questions

1. What is a contra-asset account? Give 2 examples of such an account.

2. Define *depreciation* as that term is used in accounting.

3. With respect to plant assets, what is salvage value? How is the amount of salvage value determined for a particular asset?

4. How is the estimated useful life of a plant asset determined?

5. Norris Hospital purchased a new item of equipment for $15,000 on January 1, 1978. This equipment has an estimated useful life of 10 years and an expected salvage value of 20%. Compute the amount of straight-line depreciation for 1978.

6. With respect to depreciable plant assets, what is meant by the term "book value"?

7. Is land a depreciable asset? Explain.

8. National Hospital purchased a new item of equipment on January 1, 1973. The equipment has an estimated useful life of 10 years and an expected salvage value of 20%. National Hospital's December 31, 1977, balance sheet reports $10,000 of accumulated depreciation on this equipment. What was the cost of the equipment when acquired on January 1, 1973?

9. Nadir Hospital purchased a new item of equipment for $40,000 on May 1, 1977. The equipment has an estimated useful life of 10 years and an expected salvage value of $4,000. What amount should be reported as accumulated depreciation on this equipment in Nadir Hospital's December 31, 1978, balance sheet?

10. Hospitals do not always collect their full, established rates for services rendered. Explain why this situation exists.

11. Distinguish among (a) charity service, (b) contractual adjustments, and (c) bad debts.

12. Natale Hospital provides $1,600 of routine services and $1,400 of ancillary services to a patient under a third-party contract which provides for 85% reimbursement to the hospital. The remaining 15% is not billable to the patient. Make general journal entries to record (1) the services rendered to the patient and (2) the collection of the patient's account.

13. Northeast Hospital has $100,000 of accounts receivable at December 31, 1977. It is estimated that 9% of these accounts will eventually prove to be bad debts and, therefore, uncollectible. During 1978, $8,300 of the 1977 accounts receivable are written off as bad debts. Make general journal entries to record (1) the estimated bad debts at December 31, 1977, and (2) the write-off of bad accounts during 1978.

14. At what amount should accounts receivable be valued in a hospital's balance sheet?

15. Northwest Hospital has $100,000 of accounts receivable at December 31, 1977. It is estimated that 7% of these accounts will be uncollectible by reason of charity service, 10% will be uncollectible because of contractual adjustments, and 4% will prove to be bad debts. Make the necessary adjusting entries at December 31, 1977, and indicate how the receivables should be reported in Northwest Hospital's balance sheet at December 31, 1977.

16. Refer to the data of question 15. Explain why adjusting entries for estimated uncollectible accounts are necessary at the end of the accounting period.

PROBLEMS

A. Northland Hospital's general ledger contains the following unadjusted account balances, among others, at December 31, 1977:

Acct. No.		
104	Accounts receivable	$ 850,000
105	Allowance for uncollectible accounts	−0−
150	Land	25,000
160	Building	3,000,000
161	Accumulated depreciation—building	−0−
170	Equipment	1,800,000
171	Accumulated depreciation—equipment	−0−
501	Revenue deductions—charity service	−0−
502	Revenue deductions—contractual adjustments	−0−
503	Revenue deductions—bad debts	−0−
607	Depreciation expense	−0−

The following additional information is available:

1. Of the December 31, 1977, accounts receivable, it is estimated that 15% will prove to be uncollectible by reason of (a) charity service, 4%, (b) contractual adjustments, 6%, and (c) bad debts, 5%.
2. The hospital building, which was acquired on January 1, 1977, has an estimated useful life of 40 years and an expected salvage value of $200,000.
3. Equipment, which cost $1,500,000, was acquired on January 1, 1977. Additional equipment was acquired on July 1, 1977, for

$300,000. All equipment has a 20% salvage value and an estimated useful life of 10 years.

Required. Prepare, in general journal form, all necessary adjusting entries at December 31, 1977, for the year then ended.

B. Certain of the accounts in Northside Hospital's preadjusted trial balance at December 31, 1977, are provided below:

Acct. No.		
102	Temporary investments	$ 60,000
103	Accrued interest receivable	−0−
104	Accounts receivable	940,000
105	Allowance for uncollectible accounts	3,000
107	Prepaid insurance	1,800
150	Land	50,000
160	Building	4,000,000
161	Accumulated depreciation—building	450,000
170	Equipment	1,900,000
171	Accumulated depreciation—equipment	750,000
202	Notes payable	100,000
203	Accrued interest payable	−0−
205	Deferred rental income	3,000
403	Interest income	2,875
404	Rental income	1,780
501	Charity service	56,290
502	Contractual adjustments	71,300
503	Bad debts	−0−
604	Insurance expense	11,450
607	Depreciation expense	−0−
608	Interest expense	9,230

The following additional information is available:

1. The hospital's temporary investments consist of $60,000 (face value) of 8% bonds which were acquired on October 1, 1977. These bonds pay interest annually on October 1, commencing October 1, 1978.
2. Account 105 is used only for estimated bad debts; charity service and contractual adjustments are charged directly to accounts 501 and 502, respectively. The $3,000 credit balance in account 105 above represents the excess of estimated bad debts at December 31, 1976, over the actual bad debts written off during 1977. It is estimated that all of the December 31, 1977, accounts receivable are collectible except for 5% which probably will prove to be bad debts.
3. Account 107 contains a 3-year insurance premium paid in advance on June 1, 1977.
4. The hospital building, which was acquired on January 1, 1972, has an estimated useful life of 40 years and an expected 10% salvage value.
5. All the equipment was acquired on January 1, 1972. It has an estimated useful life of 12 years and a $100,000 salvage value.
6. Account 202 represents the face amount of a 12%, 6-month bank loan obtained by the hospital on November 1, 1977. Interest on the note was not prepaid.
7. Account 205 represents a year's rent received in advance on March 1, 1977.

Required. Prepare, in general journal form, the necessary adjusting entries at December 31, 1977, for the year then ended.

C. Northville Hospital's general ledger contains the following unadjusted account balances, among others, at December 31, 1977:

Acct. No.		
104	Accounts receivable	$120,000
105	Allowance for uncollectible accounts	–0–
150	Land	15,000
160	Building	900,000
161	Accumulated depreciation—building	80,000
170	Equipment	450,000
171	Accumulated depreciation—equipment	120,000
501	Revenue deductions—charity service	–0–
502	Revenue deductions—contractual adjustments	–0–
503	Revenue deductions—bad debts	–0–
607	Depreciation expense	–0–

The following additional information is available:

1. Of the December 31, 1977, accounts receivable, it is estimated that 17% will prove to be uncollectible by reason of (a) charity service, 6%, (b) contractual adjustments, 7%, and (c) bad debts, 4%.
2. The hospital building was acquired on January 1, 1973. It has an estimated useful life of 40 years and an estimated salvage value of $100,000.
3. On January 1, 1973, the hospital acquired $400,000 of equipment having an estimated useful life of 12 years and an estimated salvage value of 10%. Additional equipment, costing $50,000 and acquired on May 1, 1977, has an estimated useful life of 8 years and an estimated salvage value of $2,000.

Required. (1) Prepare, in general journal form, the necessary adjusting entries at December 31, 1977, for the year then ended. (2) Indicate the presentation of receivables in the hospital's December 31, 1977, balance sheet. (3) Indicate the presentation of plant assets in the hospital's December 31, 1977, balance sheet.

8
Accounting Cycle Summary

Back in chapter 5, we began an illustration relating to the 1977 financial activities of a hypothetical Hoosier Hospital. That illustration was continued in chapters 6 and 7. Now we want to summarize quickly the discussion in those chapters and proceed to complete the accounting cycle for Hoosier Hospital. A summary of all of the procedures involved in the cycle is presented in figure 26. This diagram is quite similar to the one presented in chapter 4 at page 78. Here, however, we had added the adjustment process.

You will recall that Hoosier Hospital began its existence on January 1, 1977. Over the course of the year, thousands of business transactions were completed with patients, third-party payers, suppliers, employees, and others. As these transactions occurred, documentary evidences were used as a basis for the development of transaction entries. These entries were journalized in the hospital's 1977 journal (step 1 in figure 26) to provide a chronological record of the increase and decrease effects of the transactions on the accounting classifications set forth in the hospital's chart of accounts. At the end of the year, the transaction entries were posted from the journal to the ledger (step 2 in figure 26), and the year-end balance of each account was determined. These balances then were arranged in a preadjusted trial balance and entered on a worksheet (step 3 in figure 26). The previously illustrated trial balance is repeated here as figure 27.

Expansion of the Worksheet

Instead of preparing a separate preadjusted trial balance, the trial balance may be entered directly on the worksheet as shown in figure 28. This worksheet, as you can see, is used to develop the necessary adjusting entries. Each of the trial-balance accounts is carefully scrutinized to determine the need for an adjustment of its balance. As these adjustments are determined, they are entered in the adjustments column of the worksheet (and not in the journal at this time). When all of the adjustments have been made, the adjusted balances of the accounts are extended into the columns for adjusted balances of the worksheet. The worksheet then is completed by the extension of the adjusted balances into the appropriate statement columns. In footing the statement columns, the net income for the year and the hospital's year-end equity balance are determined. Naturally, the various columns of the worksheet are balanced.

Figure 26
Summary of Accounting Procedure

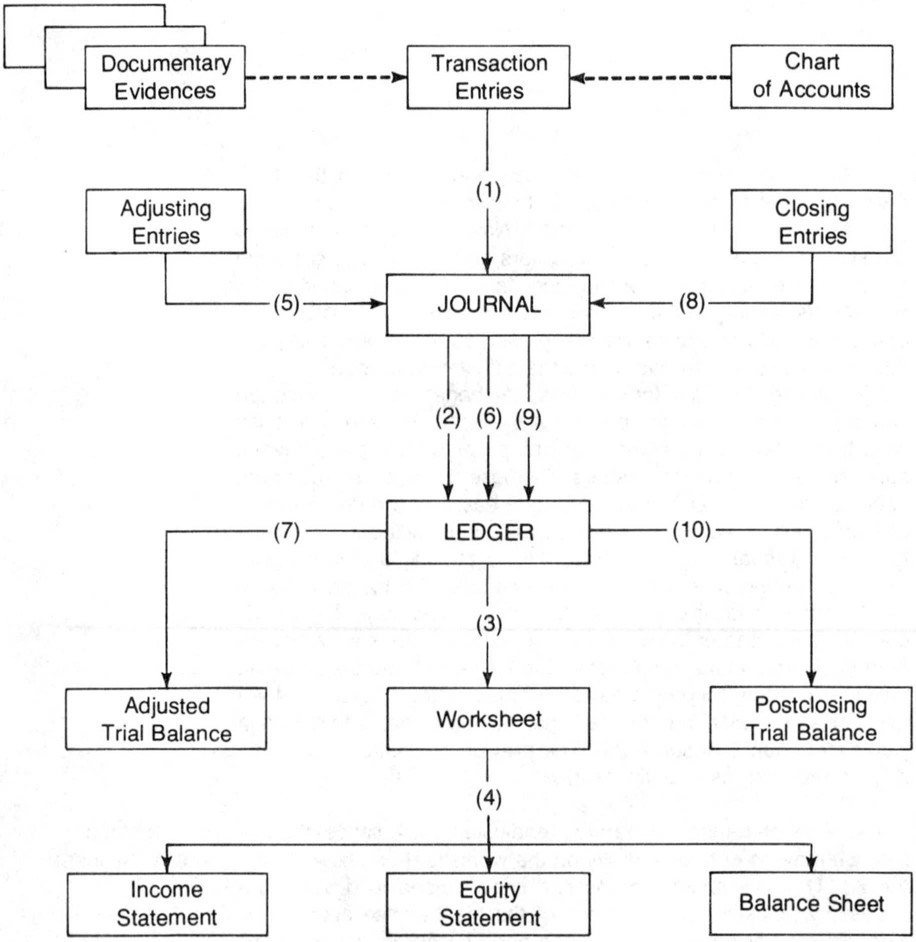

Figure 27
Hoosier Hospital
Preadjusted Trial Balance
December 31, 1977

Acct. No.	Account Titles	Dr.	Cr.
101	Cash	$ 38,300	
102	Temporary Investments	12,000	
103	Accrued Interest Receivable	---	
104	Accounts Receivable	96,600	
105	Allowance for Uncollectible Accounts		$ ---
106	Inventory	10,500	
107	Prepaid Insurance	3,600	
108	Prepaid Rent	1,080	
109	Prepaid Interest	720	
150	Land	25,000	
160	Building	180,000	
161	Accumulated Depreciation—Building		---
170	Equipment	60,000	
171	Accumulated Depreciation—Equipment		---
201	Accounts Payable		29,840
202	Notes Payable		18,000
203	Accrued Interest Payable		---
204	Accrued Salaries and Wages Payable		---
205	Deferred Rental Income		4,200
206	Deferred Tuition Income		2,160
250	Bonds Payable		80,000
301	Hospital Equity		225,000
302	Revenue and Expense Summary		---
401	Routine Services Revenue		151,300
402	Ancillary Services Revenue		137,400
403	Interest Income		---
404	Rental Income		---
405	Tuition Income		---
406	Other Revenues		27,100
501	Charity Service	29,200	
502	Contractual Adjustments	19,400	
503	Bad Debts	---	
601	Salaries and Wages Expense	139,600	
602	Supplies Expense	28,600	
603	Utilities Expense	14,400	
604	Insurance Expense	---	
605	Repairs Expense	8,300	
606	Rent Expense	---	
607	Depreciation Expense	---	
608	Interest Expense	---	
609	Other Expenses	7,700	
	Totals	$675,000	$675,000

Figure 28
Hoosier Hospital
Worksheet to Develop Financial Statements
Year Ended December 31, 1977

Acct. No.	Account Titles	Preadjusted Trial Balance, 12/31/77 Dr.	Preadjusted Trial Balance, 12/31/77 Cr.	12/31/77 Adjustments Dr.	12/31/77 Adjustments Cr.
101	Cash	38,300			
102	Temporary Investments	12,000			
103	Accrued Interest Receivable			(8) 240	
104	Accounts Receivable	96,600			
105	Allowance for Uncollectible Accounts				(11) 4,830
					(12) 2,400
					(13) 9,660
106	Inventory	10,500			
107	Prepaid Insurance	3,600			(1) 1,200
108	Prepaid Rent	1,080			(2) 720
109	Prepaid Interest	720			(3) 240
150	Land	25,000			
160	Building	180,000			
161	Accumulated Depreciation — Building				(9) 2,880
170	Equipment	60,000			
171	Accumulated Depreciation — Equipment				(10) 5,400
201	Accounts Payable		29,840		
202	Notes Payable		18,000		
203	Accrued Interest Payable				(4) 3,600
204	Accrued Salaries and Wages Payable				(5) 13,000
205	Deferred Rental Income		4,200	(6) 1,750	
206	Deferred Tuition Income		2,160	(7) 960	
250	Bonds Payable		80,000		
301	Hospital **Equity**		225,000		
302	Revenue and Expense Summary				
401	Routine Services Revenue		151,300		
402	Ancillary Services Revenue		137,400		
403	Interest Income				(8) 240
404	Rental Income				(6) 1,750
405	Tuition Income				(7) 960
406	Other Revenues		27,100		
501	Charity Service	29,200		(11) 4,830	
502	Contractual Adjustments	19,400		(12) 2,400	
503	Bad Debts			(13) 9,660	
601	Salaries and Wages Expense	139,600		(5) 13,000	
602	Supplies Expense	28,600			
603	Utilities Expense	14,400			
604	Insurance Expense			(1) 1,200	
605	Repairs Expense	8,300			
	Totals Carried Forward	667,300	675,000	34,040	46,880

Adjusted Trial Balance		1977 Income Statement		1977 **Equity** Statement		12/31/77 Balance Sheet	
Dr.	Cr.	Dr.	Cr.	Dr.	Cr.	Dr.	Cr.
38,300						38,300	
12,000						12,000	
240						240	
96,600						96,600	
	16,890						16,890
10,500						10,500	
2,400						2,400	
360						360	
480						480	
25,000						25,000	
180,000						180,000	
	2,880						2,880
60,000						60,000	
	5,400						5,400
	29,840						29,840
	18,000						18,000
	3,600						3,600
	13,000						13,000
	2,450						2,450
	1,200						1,200
	80,000						80,000
	225,000				225,000		
	151,300		151,300				
	137,400		137,400				
	240		240				
	1,750		1,750				
	960		960				
	27,100		27,100				
34,030		34,030					
21,800		21,800					
9,660		9,660					
152,600		152,600					
28,600		28,600					
14,400		14,400					
1,200		1,200					
8,300		8,300					
696,470	717,010	270,590	318,750	-0-	225,000	425,880	173,260

(Figure 28 continued)

Acct. No.	Account Titles		Preadjusted Trial Balance, 12/31/77 Dr.	Preadjusted Trial Balance, 12/31/77 Cr.	12/31/77 Adjustments Dr.	12/31/77 Adjustments Cr.
	Totals Brought Forward		667,300	675,000	34,040	46,880
606	Rent Expense				(2) 720	
607	Depreciation Expense				(9) 2,880	
					(10) 5,400	
608	Interest Expense				(3) 240	
					(4) 3,600	
609	Other Expenses		7,700			
	Totals		675,000	675,000	46,880	46,880
	Net Income for the Year					
	Totals					
	Hospital Equity, December 31, 1977					
	Totals					

FINANCIAL STATEMENTS

The next procedure in the accounting cycle (step 4 in figure 26) is the preparation of financial statements for 1977 for Hoosier Hospital. These statements are prepared directly from the information contained in the worksheet. We illustrate Hoosier Hospital's 1977 financial statements in figure 29 (the income statement), figure 30 (the statement of hospital equity), and figure 31 (the balance sheet). Since these statements are somewhat more sophisticated than the ones previously illustrated, you should give them careful study.

JOURNALIZING AND POSTING ADJUSTING ENTRIES

After the financial statements are distributed to Hoosier Hospital's management, governing board, and other interested parties, the accountant returns to the journal to journalize the adjusting entries for the year (step 5 in figure 26). This is illustrated in figure 32. Once journalized, the adjusting entries are posted to the ledger (step 6 in figure 26). The postings of these entries to Hoosier Hospital's ledger accounts are seen in figure 33. In this illustration, the unadjusted balances in the ledger accounts are labeled *UB*, and the adjusted balances are labeled *AB*. Keep in mind, as you examine figure 33, that the postings of adjusting entries are numbered 1 through 13. You may wish to trace each of these postings from the journal (figure 32).

After the adjusting entries are posted and adjusted balances are

Adjusted Trial Balance		1977 Income Statement		1977 Equity Statement		12/31/77 Balance Sheet	
Dr.	Cr.	Dr.	Cr.	Dr.	Cr.	Dr.	Cr.
696,470	717,010	270,590	318,750	-0-	225,000	425,880	173,260
720		720					
8,280		8,280					
3,840		3,840					
7,700		7,700					
717,010	717,010	291,130	318,750				
		27,620			27,620		
		318,750	318,750	-0-	252,620		
				252,620			252,620
				252,620	252,620	425,880	425,880

obtained in the ledger accounts, the adjusted balances may be arranged in an adjusted trial balance (step 7 in figure 26). Hoosier Hospital's adjusted trial balance is not illustrated here because an adjusted trial balance appears on the worksheet in figure 28.

JOURNALIZING AND POSTING CLOSING ENTRIES

The next procedure in the accounting cycle is the preparation of closing entries. The entries are recorded in the journal (step 8 in figure 26) as shown in figure 34. Notice that the closing entries are numbered 14 through 17. In addition to the closing of revenue and expense accounts, the revenue deduction accounts also must be closed as indicated in entry 15. The closing entries are now posted to the ledger (step 9 in figure 26) as illustrated in figure 35. When this is completed, the revenue, revenue deduction, and expense accounts are double ruled to indicate that those accounts are closed.

The last step in the accounting cycle is the preparation of a postclosing trial balance (step 10 in figure 26). The December 31, 1977, postclosing trial balance for Hoosier Hospital is illustrated in figure 36. Note that the remaining balances are those for asset, liability, and equity accounts only. It is with these balances that Hoosier Hospital will begin the new year, 1978. On January 1, 1978, a new accounting cycle commences.

Figure 29
Hoosier Hospital
Income Statement
Year Ended December 31, 1977

Patient Service Revenues:		
Routine Services	$151,300	
Ancillary Services	137,400	
Total Patient Service Revenues		$288,700
Less Revenue Deductions:		
Charity Service	34,030	
Contractual Adjustments	21,800	
Bad Debts	9,660	
Total Revenue Deductions		65,490
Net Patient Service Revenues		223,210
Other Revenues:		
Interest	240	
Rent	1,750	
Tuition	960	
Other	27,100	
Total Other Revenues		30,050
Total Revenues		253,260
Less Expenses:		
Salaries and Wages	152,600	
Supplies	28,600	
Utilities	14,400	
Insurance	1,200	
Repairs	8,300	
Rent	720	
Depreciation	8,280	
Interest	3,840	
Other	7,700	
Total Expenses		225,640
Net Income for the Year		$ 27,620

Figure 30
Hoosier Hospital
Statement of Hospital Equity
Year Ended December 31, 1977

Hospital Equity, January 1	$225,000
Add Net Income for 1977	27,620
Hospital Equity, December 31	$252,620

Figure 31
Hoosier Hospital
Balance Sheet
December 31, 1977

Assets

Cash			$ 38,300
Temporary Investments			12,000
Accrued Interest Receivable			240
Accounts Receivable		$ 96,600	
Less Allowance for Uncollectible Accounts		16,890	79,710
Inventory			10,500
Prepaid Insurance			2,400
Prepaid Rent			360
Prepaid Interest			480
Total Current Assets			143,990
Land		25,000	
Building	$180,000		
Less Accumulated Depreciation	2,880	177,120	
Equipment	60,000		
Less Accumulated Depreciation	5,400	54,600	256,720
Total Assets			$400,710

Liabilities and Equity

Accounts Payable	$ 29,840	
Notes Payable	18,000	
Accrued Interest Payable	3,600	
Accrued Salaries and Wages Payable	13,000	
Deferred Rental Income	2,450	
Deferred Tuition Income	1,200	
Total Current Liabilities		$ 68,090
Long-Term Debt		
(9% Bonds Payable, Due 1992)		80,000
Total Liabilities		148,090
Hospital Equity		252,620
Total Liabilities and Equity		$400,710

Figure 32
Hoosier Hospital
1977 Journal
(Adjusting Entries)

Entry No.	Accounts and Explanations	Acct. No.	Debit	Credit
1	Insurance Expense	604	1,200	
	Prepaid Insurance	107		1,200
	Adjustment for portion of prepaid premium which expired during 1977. (See chapter 5, page 89.)			
2	Rent Expense	606	720	
	Prepaid Rent	108		720
	Adjustment to record rent expense for May through December, 1977, at $90 per month. (See chapter 5, page 91.)			
3	Interest Expense	608	240	
	Prepaid Interest	109		240
	Adjustment for interest on bank loan for November and December, 1977. (See chapter 5, page 92.)			
4	Interest Expense	608	3,600	
	Accrued Interest Payable	203		3,600
	Adjustment for 6 months' interest accrued on bonds since July 1, 1977. (See chapter 5, page 93.)			
5	Salaries and Wages Expense	601	13,000	
	Accrued Salaries and Wages Payable	204		13,000
	Adjustment for accrued payroll for the month of December, 1977. (See chapter 5 page 94.)			
6	Deferred Rental Income	205	1,750	
	Rental Income	404		1,750
	Adjustment for 5 months of rental income earned from provision of office space for physicians. (See chapter 6, page 103.)			
7	Deferred Tuition Income	206	960	
	Tuition Income	405		960
	Adjustment for tuition income earned in 1977. (See chapter 6, page 104.)			
8	Accrued Interest Receivable	103	240	
	Interest Income	403		240
	Adjustment for 3 months' interest on temporary investment in government bonds. (See chapter 6, page 106.)			

Entry No.	Accounts and Explanations	Acct. No.	Debit	Credit
9	Depreciation Expense	507	2,880	
	Accumulated Depreciation—Building	161		2,880
	Adjustment for 1977 depreciation of hospital building. (See page 116.)			
10	Depreciation Expense	507	5,400	
	Accumulated Depreciation—Equipment	171		5,400
	Adjustment for 1977 depreciation of hospital equipment. (See page 116.)			
11	Charity Service	501	4,830	
	Allowance for Uncollectible Accounts	105		4,830
	Adjustment for estimated charity service in year-end receivables. (See page 119.)			
12	Contractual Adjustments	502	2,400	
	Allowance for Uncollectible Accounts	105		2,400
	Adjustment for estimated contractual adjustments in year-end receivables. (See page 120.)			
13	Bad Debts	503	9,660	
	Allowance for Uncollectible Accounts	105		9,660
	Adjustment for estimated bad debts in year-end receivables. (See page 121.)			

Figure 33
Hoosier Hospital
1977 Ledger
(With Adjusting Entries)

Cash 101

(UB) 38,300	
(AB) 38,300	

Temporary Investments 102

(UB) 12,000	
(AB) 12,000	

Accrued Interest Receivable 103

(8) 240	
(AB) 240	

Accounts Receivable 104

(UB) 96,600	
(AB) 96,600	

Allowance for Uncollectible Accounts 105

	(11) 4,830
	(12) 2,400
	(13) 9,660
	(AB) 16,890

Inventory 106

(UB) 10,500	
(AB) 10,500	

Prepaid Insurance 107

(UB) 3,600	(1) 1,200
(AB) 2,400	

Prepaid Rent 108

(UB) 1,080	(2) 720
(AB) 360	

Prepaid Interest 109

(UB) 720	(3) 240
(AB) 480	

Land 150

(UB) 25,000	
(AB) 25,000	

Building 160

(UB) 180,000	
(AB) 180,000	

Accumulated Depreciation—Building 161

	(9) 2,880
	(AB) 2,880

Equipment 170

(UB) 60,000	
(AB) 60,000	

Accumulated Depreciation—Equipment 171

	(10) 5,400
	(AB) 5,400

Accounts Payable 201

	(UB) 29,840
	(AB) 29,840

Notes Payable 202

	(UB) 18,000
	(AB) 18,000

Accrued Interest Payable 203

	(4) 3,600
	(AB) 3,600

Accrued Salaries and Wages Payable 204

	(5) 13,000
	(AB) 13,000

Deferred Rental Income 205

(6) 1,750	(UB) 4,200
	(AB) 2,450

Deferred Tuition Income 206

(7) 960	(UB) 2,160
	(AB) 1,200

Bonds Payable 250

	(UB) 80,000
	(AB) 80,000

Hospital Equity 301

	(UB)225,000
	(AB)225,000

Revenue and Expense Summary 302

Routine Services Revenue 401

	(UB)151,300
	(AB)151,300

Ancillary Services Revenue 402

	(UB)137,400
	(AB)137,400

Interest Income 403

	(8) 240
	(AB) 240

Rental Income 404

	(6) 1,750
	(AB) 1,750

Tuition Income 405

	(7) 960
	(AB) 960

Other Revenues 406

	(UB) 27,100
	(AB) 27,100

Charity Service 501

(UB) 29,200	
(11) 4,830	
(AB) 34,030	

Contractual Adjustments 502

(UB) 19,400	
(12) 2,400	
(AB) 21,800	

Bad Debts 503

(13) 9,660	
(AB) 9,660	

Salaries and Wages Expense 601

(UB)139,600	
(5) 13,000	
(AB)152,600	

Supplies Expense 602

(UB) 28,600	
(AB) 28,600	

Utilities Expense 603

(UB) 14,400	
(AB) 14,400	

Insurance Expense 604

(1) 1,200	
(AB) 1,200	

Repairs Expense 605

(UB) 8,300	
(AB) 8,300	

Rent Expense 606

(2) 720	
(AB) 720	

Depreciation Expense 607

(9) 2,880	
(10) 5,400	
(AB) 8,280	

Interest Expense 608

(3) 240	
(4) 3,600	
(AB) 3,840	

Other Expenses 609

(UB) 7,700	
(AB) 7,700	

Figure 34
Hoosier Hospital
1977 Journal
(Closing Entries)

Entry No.	Accounts and Explanations	Acct. No.	Debit	Credit
14	Routine Services Revenue	401	151,300	
	Ancillary Services Revenue	402	137,400	
	Interest Income	403	240	
	Rental Income	404	1,750	
	Tuition Income	405	960	
	Other Revenues	406	27,100	
	Revenue and Expense Summary	302		318,750
	To close revenue accounts.			
15	Revenue and Expense Summary	302	65,490	
	Charity Service	501		34,030
	Contractual Adjustments	502		21,800
	Bad Debts	503		9,660
	To close revenue deduction accounts.			
16	Revenue and Expense Summary	302	225,640	
	Salaries and Wages Expense	601		152,600
	Supplies Expense	602		28,600
	Utilities Expense	603		14,400
	Insurance Expense	604		1,200
	Repairs Expense	605		8,300
	Rent Expense	606		720
	Depreciation Expense	607		8,280
	Interest Expense	608		3,840
	Other Expenses	609		7,700
	To close expense accounts.			
17	Revenue and Expense Summary	302	27,620	
	Hospital Equity	301		27,620
	To close revenue and expense summary account and add net income to equity.			

Figure 35
Hoosier Hospital
1977 Ledger
(With Closing Entries)

Cash 101

(UB) 38,300	
(AB) 38,300	

Temporary Investments 102

(UB) 12,000	
(AB) 12,000	

Accrued Interest Receivable 103

(8) 240	
(AB) 240	

Accounts Receivable 104

(UB) 96,600	
(AB) 96,600	

Allowance for Uncollectible Accounts 105

	(11) 4,830
	(12) 2,400
	(13) 9,660
	(AB) 16,890

Inventory 106

(UB) 10,500	
(AB) 10,500	

Prepaid Insurance 107

(UB) 3,600	(1) 1,200
(AB) 2,400	

Prepaid Rent 108

(UB) 1,080	(2) 720
(AB) 360	

Prepaid Interest 109

(UB) 720	(3) 240
(AB) 480	

Land 150

(UB) 25,000	
(AB) 25,000	

Building 160

(UB)180,000	
(AB)180,000	

Accumulated Depreciation—Building 161

	(9) 2,880
	(AB) 2,880

Equipment 170

(UB) 60,000	
(AB) 60,000	

Accumulated Depreciation—Equipment 171

	(10) 5,400
	(AB) 5,400

Accounts Payable 201

	(UB) 29,840
	(AB) 29,840

Notes Payable 202

	(UB) 18,000
	(AB) 18,000

Accrued Interest Payable 203

	(4) 3,600
	(AB) 3,600

Accrued Salaries and Wages Payable 204

	(5) 13,000
	(AB) 13,000

Deferred Rental Income 205

(6) 1,750	(UB) 4,200
	(AB) 2,450

Deferred Tuition Income 206

(7) 960	(UB) 2,160
	(AB) 1,200

Bonds Payable 250

	(UB) 80,000
	(AB) 80,000

(Figure 35 continued)

Hospital Equity 301

	(UB)225,000
	(17) 27,620
	(CB)252,620

Revenue and Expense Summary 302

(15) 65,490	(14)318,750
(16)225,640	
(17) 27,620	

Routine Services Revenue 401

(14)151,300	(UB)151,300

Ancillary Services Revenue 402

(14)137,400	(UB)137,400

Interest Income 403

(14) 240	(8) 240

Rental Income 404

(14) 1,750	(6) 1,750

Tuition Income 405

(14) 960	(7) 960

Other Revenues 406

(14) 27,100	(UB) 27,100

Charity Service 501

(UB) 29,200	(15) 34,030
(11) 4,830	

Contractual Adjustments 502

(UB) 19,400	(15) 21,800
(12) 2,400	

Bad Debts 503

(13) 9,660	(15) 9,660

Salaries and Wages Expense 601

(UB)139,600	(16)152,600
(5) 13,000	

Supplies Expense 602

(UB) 28,600	(16) 28,600

Utilities Expense 603

(UB) 14,400	(16) 14,400

Insurance Expense 604

(1) 1,200	(16) 1,200

Repairs Expense 605

(UB) 8,300	(16) 8,300

Rent Expense 606

(2) 720	(16) 720

Depreciation Expense 607

(9) 2,880	(16) 8,280
(10) 5,400	

Interest Expense 608

(3) 240	(16) 3,840
(4) 3,600	

Other Expenses 609

(UB) 7,700	(16) 7,700

Figure 36
Hoosier Hospital
Postclosing Trial Balance
December 31, 1977

Acct. No.	Account Titles	Dr.	Cr.
101	Cash	$ 38,300	
102	Temporary Investments	12,000	
103	Accrued Interest Receivable	240	
104	Accounts Receivable	96,600	
105	Allowance for Uncollectible Accounts		$ 16,890
106	Inventory	10,500	
107	Prepaid Insurance	2,400	
108	Prepaid Rent	360	
109	Prepaid Interest	480	
150	Land	25,000	
160	Building	180,000	
161	Accumulated Depreciation—Building		2,880
170	Equipment	60,000	
171	Accumulated Depreciation—Equipment		5,400
201	Accounts Payable		29,840
202	Notes Payable		18,000
203	Accrued Interest Payable		3,600
204	Accrued Salaries and Wages Payable		13,000
205	Deferred Rental Income		2,450
206	Deferred Tuition Income		1,200
250	Bonds Payable		80,000
251	Hospital Equity		252,620
	Totals	$425,880	$425,880

QUESTIONS

1. List and describe briefly each of the 10 major steps in a complete accounting cycle.

2. "Annual financial statements cannot be prepared until the books are closed for the year." Do you agree? Explain.

3. Below is a random listing of accounting procedures. Indicate the normal sequence in which these procedures are performed.

a. Prepare financial statements.
b. Journalize closing entries.
c. Post adjusting entries to the ledger.
d. Prepare general worksheet.
e. Journalize transaction entries.
f. Post closing entries to the ledger.
g. Prepare adjusted trial balance.
h. Post transaction entries to the ledger.

i. Prepare postclosing trial balance.
j. Journalize adjusting entries.

4. Garden Hospital paid a 3-year insurance premium of $3,600 in advance on January 1, 1977, debiting the $3,600 to prepaid insurance. At the end of the year, the necessary adjusting entry was not made. The omission was not discovered. What effect would this error have on (a) total assets, (b) total liabilities, and (c) hospital equity, as reported in the hospital's balance sheet at December 31, 1977?

5. Goshen Hospital paid an account payable of $4,500 during December, 1977. In the transaction entry, however, the debit was made erroneously to supplies expense. The error was not discovered until after the financial statements for 1977 were prepared. What effect would this error have on (a) total assets, (b) total liabilities, and (c) hospital equity, as reported in the hospital's December 31, 1977, balance sheet?

6. Gibson Hospital received $2,300 in payment of a patient's account receivable on December 27, 1977. In the transaction entry, however, the credit was made erroneously to routine service revenues. The error was not discovered until after the financial statements for 1977 were prepared. What effect would this error have on (a) the total assets, (b) the total liabilities, and (c) the hospital equity, as reported in the hospital's December 31, 1977, balance sheet?

PROBLEMS

A. Given below is the preadjusted trial balance of Greatville Hospital at December 31, 1977, the end of the hospital's current fiscal year:

Acct. No.		Dr.	Cr.
101	Cash	$ 31,600	
102	Temporary investments	15,000	
103	Accrued interest receivable	–0–	
104	Accounts receivable	102,400	
105	Allowance for uncollectible accounts		–0–
106	Inventory	11,600	
107	Prepaid insurance	1,980	
108	Prepaid rent	2,100	
109	Prepaid interest	1,200	
150	Land	22,000	
160	Building	175,000	
161	Accumulated depreciation—building		–0–
170	Equipment	80,000	
171	Accumulated depreciation—equipment		–0–
201	Accounts payable		31,300
202	Notes payable		20,000
203	Accrued interest payable		–0–
204	Accrued salaries and wages payable		–0–
205	Deferred rental income		1,680

Acct. No.		Dr.	Cr.
206	Deferred tuition income		1,215
250	Bonds payable		100,000
301	Hospital equity		207,085
302	Revenue and expense summary		–0–
401	Routine services revenue		169,300
402	Ancillary services revenue		128,700
403	Interest income		–0–
404	Rental income		–0–
405	Tuition income		–0–
406	Other revenues		29,800
501	Charity service	28,200	
502	Contractual adjustments	20,300	
503	Bad debts	–0–	
601	Salaries and wages expense	141,200	
602	Supplies expense	27,300	
603	Utilities expense	15,100	
604	Insurance expense	–0–	
605	Repairs expense	7,600	
606	Rent expense	–0–	
607	Depreciation expense	–0–	
608	Interest expense	–0–	
609	Other expenses	6,500	
		$689,080	$689,080

The following additional information is available:

1. The temporary investment consists of $15,000 (face value) of 8% bonds acquired by the hospital on October 1, 1977. These bonds pay interest annually on October 1, commencing October 1, 1978.
2. Of the December 31, 1977, accounts receivable, it is estimated that 12% will eventually prove uncollectible by reason of (a) charity service, 4%, (b) contractual adjustments, 5%, and (c) bad debts, 3%.
3. A 3-year insurance premium of $1,980 was paid in advance by the hospital on January 1, 1977.
4. The hospital prepaid a year's rent of $2,100 on June 1, 1977.
5. On November 1, 1977, the hospital borrowed $20,000 from a bank by issuing its 6-month, 12% note. Interest on the note was prepaid.
6. The hospital building, which was acquired on January 1, 1977, has an estimated useful life of 40 years and a salvage value of $15,000.
7. The equipment, which was acquired on January 1, 1977, has an estimated useful life of 8 years and a 10% salvage value.
8. On April 1, 1977, the hospital issued $100,000 of 15-year, 6% bonds at face value. These bonds pay interest annually on April 1, commencing April 1, 1978.
9. Unpaid salaries and wages at December 31, 1977, totaled $15,600.
10. The hospital received one year's rent of $1,680 in advance on March 1, 1977.
11. On September 1, 1977, the hospital received 9 months' tuition in advance in connection with one of its educational programs.

Required. (1) Prepare a worksheet to develop financial statements in the manner illustrated in figure 28 on pages 130-133. (2) Prepare, in good form, a complete set of financial statements for 1977.

B. Certain of the adjusted balances in the ledger of Gatorberg

Hospital at December 31, 1977, the end of the hospital's current fiscal year, are provided in the following:

Acct. No.		
301	Hospital equity	$275,000
302	Revenue and expense summary	–0–
401	Routine services revenue	159,700
402	Ancillary services revenue	101,800
403	Interest income	2,600
404	Rental income	1,900
405	Tuition income	1,500
406	Other revenues	29,800
501	Charity service	31,700
502	Contractual adjustments	42,300
503	Bad debts	11,600
601	Salaries and wages expense	145,900
602	Supplies expense	21,500
603	Utilities expense	12,300
604	Insurance expense	2,300
605	Repairs expense	4,100
606	Rent expense	2,800
607	Depreciation expense	9,400
608	Interest expense	1,400
609	Other expenses	7,200

Required. (1) Prepare, in general journal form, the necessary closing entries for the year ended December 31, 1977. (2) Prepare, in good form, the 1977 income statement for Gatorberg Hospital.

C. Given below is the preadjusted trial balance of Grandtown Hospital at December 31, 1977, the end of the hospital's current fiscal year:

Acct. No.		Dr.	Cr.
101	Cash	$ 37,500	
102	Temporary investments	30,000	
103	Accrued interest receivable	–0–	
104	Accounts receivable	120,000	
105	Allowance for uncollectible accounts		$ –0–
106	Inventory	14,000	
107	Prepaid insurance	3,600	
150	Land	25,000	
160	Building	250,000	
161	Accumulated depreciation—building		–0–
170	Equipment	140,000	
171	Accumulated depreciation—equipment		–0–
201	Accounts payable		37,400
203	Accrued interest payable		–0–
204	Accrued salaries and wages payable		–0–
205	Deferred rental income		2,700
250	Bonds payable		150,000
301	Hospital equity		395,700
302	Revenue and expense summary		–0–

Acct. No.		Dr.	Cr.
401	Routine services revenue		171,200
402	Ancillary services revenue		110,300
403	Interest income		−0−
404	Rental income		−0−
406	Other revenues		23,500
501	Charity service	31,100	
502	Contractual adjustments	22,700	
503	Bad debts	−0−	
601	Salaries and wages expense	155,600	
602	Supplies expense	33,100	
603	Utilities expense	14,900	
604	Insurance expense	−0−	
605	Repairs expense	6,400	
607	Depreciation expense	−0−	
608	Interest expense	4,500	
609	Other expenses	2,400	
		$890,800	$890,800

The following additional information is available:

1. The temporary investment consists of $30,000 (face value) of 8% bonds acquired by the hospital on November 1, 1977. These bonds pay interest annually on November 1, commencing November 1, 1978.
2. Of the December 31, 1977, accounts receivable, it is estimated that 14% will eventually prove uncollectible by reason of (a) charity service, 7%, (b) contractual adjustments, 4%, and (c) bad debts, 3%.
3. A 2-year insurance premium of $3,600 was paid in advance by the hospital on January 1, 1977.
4. The hospital building, which was acquired on January 1, 1977, has an estimated useful life of 50 years and a 20% salvage value.
5. The equipment, which was acquired on January 1, 1977, has an estimated useful life of 12 years and a $20,000 expected salvage value.
6. On January 1, 1977, the hospital issued $150,000 of 20-year, 6% bonds at face value. These bonds pay interest semiannually on January 1 and July 1, commencing July 1, 1977.
7. Unpaid salaries and wages at December 31, 1977, amount to $12,300.
8. The hospital received one year's rent of $2,700 in advance on June 1, 1977.

Required. (1) Prepare a worksheet to develop financial statements in the manner illustrated in figure 28 on pages 130-133. (2) Prepare, in good form, a complete set of financial statements for 1977. (3) Prepare, in general journal form, the necessary adjusting entries at December 31, 1977, for the year then ended. (4) Prepare, in general journal form, the necessary closing entries at December 31, 1977, for the year then ended.

9 Development of Interim Financial Statements

The discussion in all previous chapters has dealt with the accounting process in annual terms—annual posting of transaction entries, annual adjusting entries, and annual financial statements. In this chapter we want to examine the procedures of accounting from a monthly point of view. The preparation of monthly adjusting entries and the development of a set of *interim* financial statements will be given emphasis. As mentioned earlier, interim financial statements are those prepared during the course of a hospital's fiscal year. The illustration presented in this chapter consists of the preparation of an income statement for the month of September, 1977, and for the 9 months ended September 30, 1977. In addition, a September 30, 1977, balance sheet will be constructed.

Interim financial statements are essential to the effective management of hospitals. Important managerial decisions are made during the course of a fiscal year which require the kinds of information provided by monthly income statements and balance sheets. In addition, other types of accounting reports may be prepared on a weekly or daily basis—a cash report, for example. Certain of these special reports are illustrated further on in this book. For now, you are concerned only with the routine income statements and balance sheets prepared at the end of each month.

Monthly Trial Balances

Let us assume a hypothetical Hiowa Hospital which began its corporate existence on January 1, 1975. Financial statements were prepared for 1975 and 1976, and the hospital is now in its third year of operations, 1977. The 1977 transactions have been journalized and posted through September 30. Monthly adjusting entries have been journalized and posted through August 31, and monthly financial statements have been prepared at the end of each month, January through August, 1977. It is now time to prepare financial statements for September and for 9 months ended September 30, 1977.

Hiowa Hospital's trial balances at August 31 and September 30,

1977, are presented in figure 37. Notice that the August 31 trial balance is an *adjusted* trial balance. It includes the adjusted balances, at August 31, of the hospital assets and liabilities. The equity balance is, of course, the opening (January 1, 1977) equity balance for the year, since the books of the hospital have not been closed since December 31, 1976. This trial balance also includes an

Figure 37
Hiowa Hospital
Trial Balances
August 31 and September 30, 1977

Acct. No.	Account Titles	Adjusted Trial Balance, 8/31/77 Dr.	Adjusted Trial Balance, 8/31/77 Cr.	Unadjusted Trial Balance, 9/30/77 Dr.	Unadjusted Trial Balance, 9/30/77 Cr.
101	Cash	$ 30,900		$ 33,200	
102	Accrued Interest Receivable	800		800	
103	Accounts Receivable	84,000		87,100	
104	Allowance for Bad Debts		$ 8,400		$ 8,400
105	Inventory	9,800		11,300	
106	Prepaid Insurance	2,400		2,400	
130	Long-Term Investments	60,000		60,000	
150	Land	23,000		23,000	
160	Depreciable Plant Assets	187,500		187,500	
161	Accumulated Depreciation		20,000		20,000
201	Accounts Payable		18,200		19,400
202	Accrued Salaries and Wages Payable		4,600		−0−
203	Accrued Interest Payable		5,500		5,500
204	Deferred Rental Income		980		980
250	Bonds Payable		100,000		100,000
301	Hospital Equity		219,420		219,420
302	Revenue and Expense Summary		−0−		−0−
401	Inpatient Services Revenue		164,000		187,300
402	Outpatient Services Revenue		96,100		106,800
403	Interest Income		800		800
404	Rental Income		700		700
405	Other Revenues		46,300		52,200
501	Bad Debts	11,400		11,400	
502	Other Revenue Deductions	27,000		31,800	
601	Salaries and Wages Expense	160,000		176,400	
602	Supplies Expense	24,000		26,800	
603	Utilities Expense	16,000		18,100	
604	Insurance Expense	1,200		1,200	
605	Depreciation Expense	5,000		5,000	
606	Interest Expense	4,000		4,000	
607	Other Expenses	38,000		41,500	
	Totals	$685,000	$685,000	$721,500	$721,500

8-month accumulation of revenue, revenue deduction, and expense balances, adjusted through August 31, 1977. In short, these are the figures used in Hiowa Hospital's August 31 balance sheet, and in its income statement for the 8 months ended August 31, 1977. These statements are illustrated in figure 38 and figure 39. (The income statement for the month of August, 1977, is not illustrated, although we assume such a statement was prepared.)

Carefully note that Hiowa Hospital's trial balance at September 30, 1977, is an *unadjusted* trial balance. The figures in this trial balance are those in the August 31 trial balance together with the effects of the September transactions of the hospital. In other words, this trial balance includes the unadjusted asset and liability balances at September 30, the hospital equity balance at January 1, and the unadjusted revenue, revenue deduction, and expense balances at September 30, 1977. So, before financial statements can be prepared for September and for the 9 months ended September 30, the September adjusting entries must be developed.

Figure 38
Hiowa Hospital
Income Statement
Eight Months Ended August 31, 1977

Patient Service Revenues:			
Inpatient Services		$164,000	
Outpatient Services		96,100	
Total Patient Service Revenues		260,100	
Less Revenue Deductions:			
Bad Debts	$ 11,400		
Other	27,000		
Total Revenue Deductions		38,400	
Net Patient Service Revenues			$221,700
Other Revenues:			
Interest		800	
Rent		700	
Other		46,300	
Total Other Revenues			47,800
Total Revenues			269,500
Less Expenses:			
Salaries and Wages		160,000	
Supplies		24,000	
Utilities		16,000	
Insurance		1,200	
Depreciation		5,000	
Interest		4,000	
Other		38,000	
Total Expenses			248,200
Net Income			$ 21,300

Figure 39
Hiowa Hospital
Balance Sheet
August 31, 1977

Assets			
Cash			$ 30,900
Accrued Interest Receivable			800
Accounts Receivable		$ 84,000	
Less Allowance for Bad Debts		8,400	75,600
Inventory			9,800
Prepaid Insurance			2,400
Total Current Assets			119,500
Long-Term Investments			60,000
Land		23,000	
Depreciable Plant Assets	$187,500		
Less Accumulated Depreciation	20,000	167,500	
Net Plant Assets			190,500
Total Assets			$370,000
Liabilities and Equity			
Accounts Payable		$ 18,200	
Accrued Salaries and Wages Payable		4,600	
Accrued Interest Payable		5,500	
Deferred Rental Income		980	
Total Current Liabilities			$ 29,280
Long-Term Debt (6% Bonds Payable, Due 1988)			100,000
Total Liabilities			129,280
Hospital Equity, January 1*		219,420	
Add Net Income for 8 Months Ended August 31		21,300	
Hospital Equity, August 31			240,720
Total Liabilities and Equity			$370,000

*Change in equity balance shown within balance sheet in lieu of separate statement of hospital equity.

SEPTEMBER ADJUSTING ENTRIES

You will have noticed that Hiowa Hospital's account titles and numbers are somewhat different from those used earlier in the Hoosier Hospital illustration. Some of these differences arise from an effort to simplify the illustration (a single account for depreciable plant assets, for example). Other changes were made to introduce new accounts and procedures. While there is a degree of uniformity in charts of accounts from one hospital to another, there also may be considerable differences due to variations in size, organizational structure, and range of services, among other things.

ACCRUED INTEREST RECEIVABLE

Hiowa Hospital's September 30 trial balance includes $60,000 of long-term investments (account 130). This consists of $60,000 (face value) of 8%, 10-year corporate bonds purchased by the hospital at face value on July 1, 1977. These bonds pay interest semiannually on July 1 and January 1, beginning on January 1, 1977. The semiannual interest payments to the hospital will be \$2,400 (i.e., \$60,000 × 8% × ½). So Hiowa Hospital is earning interest income of \$400 per month (\$2,400/6) on these bonds.

On July 31 and August 31, Hiowa Hospital made an adjusting entry to accrue the monthly interest income:

Accrued Interest Receivable	102	\$ 400	
Interest Income	403		\$ 400
Monthly adjustment for accrual of monthly interest income on corporate bonds held as long-term investments.			

Since this entry was made on July 31 and on August 31, Hiowa Hospital's August 31 trial balance includes \$800 of accrued interest receivable and \$800 of interest income. The September 30 (unadjusted) trial balance, of course, includes the same figures because the September 30 adjustment has not yet been made, so the above entry must be repeated at September 30. This will be September 30, 1977, adjusting entry 1. Notice that it has been entered on the worksheet presented in this chapter (pages 154–155) as figure 40. Still later, the adjustment will be entered in Hiowa Hospital's journal.

The same adjusting entry will be made on October 31, November 30, and December 31, to produce a year-end balance of \$2,400 in the accrued interest receivable account. Then, when the interest is received in cash on January 1, 1978, a transaction entry will be made to debit cash and credit the accrued interest receivable account. As a result, the bond interest income is recognized monthly as it is earned, rather than at the time it is received in cash.

BAD DEBTS

At the end of each month since the year began, Hiowa Hospital has been making an adjusting entry to maintain a balance in its allowance for bad debts account (number 104) equal to 10% of month-end accounts receivable. This is an accounting policy which assumes that 10% of the accounts receivable balance will prove to be bad debts. As mentioned before, there are other methods of accounting for bad debts, but this is the method we will use for present purposes.

As specific accounts are adjudged to be worthless, the accounts are written off by a debit to the allowance account. To illustrate, let us assume that the allowance account had a credit balance of \$6,000 to start the 1977 year. At the end of each month from January through August, an adjusting entry has been made to adjust the allowance account credit balance to 10% of receivables. A summary of the 8 entries appears below as a single entry:

Bad Debts	501	\$11,400	
Allowance for Bad Debts	104		\$11,400
Adjustments of allowance account to 10% of month-end receivables.			

We assumed, however, that the year began with a \$6,000 credit balance in the allowance account. The 8 adjusting entries added $11,400 to the account, so why is the August 31 balance only $8,400? It might appear to you that the August 31 balance should be $17,400 (i.e., $6,000 + $11,400).

Well, in an unknown number of journal entries during the first 8 months of 1977, Hiowa Hospital has written off $9,000 of worthless accounts. A summary of these entries is shown as a single entry:

Allowance for Bad Debts	104	$ 9,000	
Accounts Receivable	103		$ 9,000
Write-off of uncollectible receivables during first 8 months of 1977.			

Thus, between January 1 and August 31, the allowance account (which began with a $6,000 credit balance) has been credited with a total of $11,400 and debited for a total of $9,000. The August 31 balance of the allowance account therefore is $8,400 (i.e., $6,000 + $11,400 − $9,000). The August 31 debit balance of the bad debts account is of course the expense recorded during the first 8 months, $11,400 (see the August 31 trial balance).

The balances in the bad debts and the allowance for bad debts accounts have not changed since August 31. This is because the September 30 adjusting entry has not yet been made and because we assume that no accounts have been written off during September. The required September 30 adjusting entry is as follows:

Bad Debts		501	$ 310	
Allowance for Bad Debts		104		$ 310
Adjustment to increase allowance account to 10% of September 30 accounts receivable:				
Allowance balance, 9/30	$8,400			
Desired balance (10% of $87,100)	8,710			
Required increase	$ 310			

This gives the allowance account a credit balance of $8,710 which is the desired 10% of September 30 receivables. This is entry 2 on the worksheet illustrated in figure 40.

PREPAID INSURANCE

Assume a single comprehensive insurance policy on which Hiowa Hospital paid a 2-year premium of $3,600 in advance on January 1, 1977. This means that insurance expense is $150 per month ($3,600/24 months). Assuming that the payment of the premium was recorded as a debit to prepaid insurance (account 106), the following adjusting entry has been made at the end of each of the 8 months starting January 31:

Insurance Expense	604	$ 150	
Prepaid Insurance	106		$ 150
Adjustment for monthly expiration of prepaid insurance premium.			

Since this entry has been made 8 times, the trial balance at August 31 shows $1,200 of insurance expense and $2,400 of prepaid insurance ($3,600 − $1,200). This adjustment is repeated on September 30 as entry 3 in figure 40.

Figure 40
Hiowa Hospital
Worksheet to Develop Financial Statements
Nine Months Ended September 30, 1977

Acct. No.	Account Titles	Unadjusted Trial Balance, 9/30/77 Dr.	Unadjusted Trial Balance, 9/30/77 Cr.	9/30/77 Adjustments Dr.	9/30/77 Adjustments Cr.
101	Cash	33,200			
102	Accrued Interest Receivable	800		(1) 400	
103	Accounts Receivable	87,100			
104	Allowance for Bad Debts		8,400		(2) 310
105	Inventory	11,300			
106	Prepaid Insurance	2,400			(3) 150
130	Long-Term Investments	60,000			
150	Land	23,000			
160	Depreciable Plant Assets	187,500			
161	Accumulated Depreciation		20,000		(4) 625
201	Accounts Payable		19,400		
202	Accrued Salaries and Wages Payable		-0-		(5) 3,100
203	Accrued Interest Payable		5,500		(7) 500
204	Deferred Rental Income		980	(6) 140	
250	Bonds Payable		100,000		
301	Hospital Equity		219,420		
302	Revenue and Expense Summary		-0-		
401	Inpatient Services Revenue		187,300		
402	Outpatient Services Revenue		106,800		
403	Interest Income		800		(1) 400
404	Rental Income		700		(6) 140
405	Other Revenues		52,200		
501	Bad Debts	11,400		(2) 310	
502	Other Revenue Deductions	31,800			
601	Salaries and Wages Expense	176,400		(5) 3,100	
602	Supplies Expense	26,800			
603	Utilities Expense	18,100			
604	Insurance Expense	1,200		(3) 150	
605	Depreciation Expense	5,000		(4) 625	
606	Interest Expense	4,000		(7) 500	
607	Other Expenses	41,500			
	Totals	721,500	721,500	5,225	5,225
	Net Income for 9 Months Ended 9/30/77				
	Totals				
	Hospital Equity, 9/30/77				

Adjusted Trial Balance, 9/30/77		Income Statement		Equity Statement		Balance Sheet	
Dr.	Cr.	Dr.	Cr.	Dr.	Cr.	Dr.	Cr.
33,200						33,200	
1,200						1,200	
87,100						87,100	
	8,710						8,710
11,300						11,300	
2,250						2,250	
60,000						60,000	
23,000						23,000	
187,500						187,500	
	20,625						20,625
	19,400						19,400
	3,100						3,100
	6,000						6,000
	840						840
	100,000						100,000
	219,420				219,420		
	187,300		187,300				
	106,800		106,800				
	1,200		1,200				
	840		840				
	52,200		52,200				
11,710		11,710					
31,800		31,800					
179,500		179,500					
26,800		26,800					
18,100		18,100					
1,350		1,350					
5,625		5,625					
4,500		4,500					
41,500		41,500					
726,435	726,435	320,885	348,340				
		27,455			27,455		
		348,340	348,340	-0-	246,875		
				246,875			246,875
				246,875	246,875	405,550	405,550

DEPRECIATION

Hiowa Hospital, we will assume, purchased all of its depreciable assets on January 1, 1975, for $187,500. Let us say that these assets (buildings and equipment) have a composite useful life of 25 years, but no salvage value is expected. This means that depreciation expense on a straight-line basis is $7,500 annually ($187,500/25), or $625 per month ($7,500/12). So, Hiowa Hospital has been making the following monthly adjusting entry:

Depreciation Expense	605	$ 625	
Accumulated Depreciation	161		$ 625
Adjustment for monthly depreciation.			

Thus, the August 31 trial balance shows $5,000 (i.e., $625 × 8 months) of depreciation expense. The accumulated depreciation balance, however, includes all the depreciation taken since the assets were acquired: depreciation for 12 months in 1975, 12 months in 1976, and 8 months in 1977. This is a total of 32 months, or $20,000 (i.e., $625 × 32) of accumulated depreciation.

The above depreciation adjustment also must be made at September 30. This entry is entry 4 in figure 40. The entry will be repeated every month until the assets are sold or otherwise retired from use by the hospital.

ACCRUED SALARIES AND WAGES PAYABLE

On August 31, Hiowa Hospital obviously made an adjusting entry for $4,600 of accrued salaries and wages (refer to the August 31 trial balance account 202). That entry charged $4,600 of salaries and wages to expense and credited $4,600 to the accrued liability account. When these salaries and wages were paid in early September, the liability was eliminated. This is why no balance appears in the accrued salaries and wages payable account in the September 30 trial balance.

Now assume that, during the latter part of September, Hiowa Hospital employees earned $3,100 of salaries and wages which have not yet been paid. The required September 30, 1977, adjusting entry is

Salaries and Wages Expense	601	$3,100	
Accrued Salaries and Wages Payable	202		$3,100
Adjustment for accrued payroll at September 30, 1977.			

This entry appears on the worksheet in figure 40. It is labeled adjusting entry 5.

As explained in chapter 5, reversing entries sometimes are employed in connection with certain adjustments relating to accrued expenses. Hiowa Hospital, for example, might have made a September 1 reversing entry for the $4,600 adjustment of August 31. Similarly, the above $3,100 adjustment might be reversed on October 1. Whether or not reversing entries are made, however, the interim statements are not affected; the adjusted figures will be the same.

DEFERRED RENTAL INCOME

Assume that a private concern began operating a gift shop in the hospital on April 1, 1977. At that time, Hiowa Hospital received one year's rent ($1,680) in advance. The hospital's rental income, then, is $140 per month ($1,680/12). Assuming that the $1,680 was credited to deferred rental income (account 204) at the time it was received, the hospital has been making a monthly adjustment of $140 to rental income (account 404) for 5 months (April through August). The monthly adjusting entry has been as follows:

Deferred Rental Income	204	$ 140	
Rental Income	404		$ 140
Adjustment to record rental income earned during the month.			

Since this entry has been made 5 times, the August 31 trial balance shows a balance of $700 in the rental income account. The deferred rental income balance, for the same reason, is $980 (i.e., $1,680 − $700).

Now, at September 30, the same adjusting entry is required again. Figure 40 includes this adjustment as entry 6.

ACCRUED INTEREST PAYABLE

Hiowa Hospital issued $100,000 of 6%, 12-year bonds at face value on October 1, 1976. These bonds pay interest annually on October 1, commencing October 1, 1977. At the end of each month, starting October 31, 1976, Hiowa Hospital has been making the following adjusting entry for the monthly accrual of interest expense on these bonds:

Interest Expense	606	$ 500	
Accrued Interest Payable	203		$ 500
Adjustment for monthly accrual of interest on the 6% bonds ($100,000 × 6% × $^1/_{12}$).			

This entry has been made 11 times (October, 1976, through August, 1977) to produce an August 31 trial balance figure of $5,500 in accrued interest payable. The August 31 balance of the interest expense account, however, is only $4,000 because the remaining $1,500 of interest was charged to expense in 1976. That $1,500 was interest expense for October, November, and December of 1976, and was eliminated from the ledger by a December 31, 1976, closing entry.

The above $500 adjustment for interest expense must be made again at September 30, 1977. This adjustment appears in figure 40 as entry 7.

This completes all of the September 30, 1977, adjustments required for Hiowa Hospital. The worksheet (figure 40) is now finished, and a set of interim financial statements can be prepared.

INTERIM STATEMENTS

Based on the information assembled on the worksheet (figure 40), an interim income statement for the 9 months ended September 30, 1977, along with an income statement for the month of September, 1977, can be prepared as illustrated in figure 41. The figures for the September income statement are obtained simply by subtracting the 8-month income statement figures from the 9-month income statement figures. To obtain the salaries and wages expense for September, for example, the $160,000 expense figure in the income statement for the 8 months ended August 31 (figure 38) is subtracted from the $179,500 expense figure in the income statement for the 9 months ended September 30, 1977. In actual practice, of course, the monthly amounts are obtained by summarizing the transactions of each month alone, thus providing an automatic verification of the change in year-to-date totals.

Figure 41
Hiowa Hospital
Income Statements
Month of September, 1977, and 9 Months Ended September 30, 1977

	Month Ended 9/30/77	Nine Months Ended 9/30/77
Patient Service Revenues:		
Inpatient Services	$ 23,300	$187,300
Outpatient Services	10,700	106,800
Total Patient Service Revenues	34,000	294,100
Less Revenue Deductions:		
Bad Debts	310	11,710
Other	4,800	31,800
Total Revenue Deductions	5,110	43,510
Net Patient Service Revenues	28,890	250,590
Other Revenues:		
Interest	400	1,200
Rent	140	840
Other	5,900	52,200
Total Other Revenues	6,440	54,240
Total Revenues	35,330	304,830
Less Expenses:		
Salaries and Wages	19,500	179,500
Supplies	2,800	26,800
Utilities	2,100	18,100
Insurance	150	1,350
Depreciation	625	5,625
Interest	500	4,500
Other	3,500	41,500
Total Expenses	29,175	277,375
Net Income	$ 6,155	$ 27,455

Figure 42 presents the Hiowa Hospital's September 30, 1977, balance sheet, with the necessary figures taken from the worksheet (figure 40). The August 31 balance sheet also is included in this presentation merely to illustrate the manner in which comparative financial data may be reported. Income and other statements, of course, also can be presented in comparative form. Later in this book, we will get into the managerial analysis and interpretation of comparative financial statements.

Figure 42
Hiowa Hospital
Balance Sheets
September 30 and August 31, 1977

	September 30	August 31
Assets		
Cash	$ 33,200	$ 30,900
Accrued Interest Receivable	1,200	800
Accounts Receivable (net of allowance for bad debts of $8,710 at September 30 and $8,400 at August 31)	78,390	75,600
Inventory	11,300	9,800
Prepaid Insurance	2,250	2,400
Total Current Assets	126,340	119,500
Long-Term Investments	60,000	60,000
Land	23,000	23,000
Depreciable Plant Assets (net of accumulated depreciation of $20,625 at September 30 and $20,000 at August 31)	166,875	167,500
Net Plant Assets	189,875	190,500
Total Assets	$376,215	$370,000
Liabilities and Equity		
Accounts Payable	$ 19,400	$ 18,200
Accrued Salaries and Wages Payable	3,100	4,600
Accrued Interest Payable	6,000	5,500
Deferred Rental Income	840	980
Total Current Liabilities	29,340	29,280
Long-Term Debt (6% Bonds Payable)	100,000	100,000
Total Liabilities	129,340	129,280
Hospital Equity, January 1*	219,420	219,420
Add Net Income:		
For 9 Months Ended September 30	27,455	
For 8 Months Ended August 31		21,300
Hospital Equity at Statement Date	246,875	240,720
Total Liabilities and Equity	$376,215	$370,000

*Changes in equity presented within balance sheet in lieu of separate equity statement.

JOURNALIZING AND POSTING ADJUSTING ENTRIES

After the interim financial statements have been prepared, the accountant returns to the journal and records the September 30, 1977, adjusting entries as shown in figure 43. These journal entries then are posted to the ledger accounts (not illustrated here). When the postings are completed, Hiowa Hospital's ledger account balances will agree with the figures in the adjusted trial balance columns of the worksheet. During the following month (October, 1977), the procedures previously described for September are repeated. As a final point, notice that the books are not closed in the interim accounting process; the books are closed annually on the last day of the fiscal year.

Figure 43
Hiowa Hospital
1977 Journal
(September 30 Adjusting Entries)

Entry No.	Accounts and Explanations	Acct. No.	Debit	Credit
1	Accrued Interest Receivable	102	400	
	Interest Income	403		400
	Adjustment for accrual of monthly interest income on corporate bonds held as long-term investments.			
2	Bad Debts	501	310	
	Allowance for Bad Debts	104		310
	Adjustment to increase allowance account to 10% of month-end receivables.			
3	Insurance Expense	604	150	
	Prepaid Insurance	106		150
	Adjustment for monthly expiration of prepaid insurance premium.			
4	Depreciation Expense	605	625	
	Accumulated Depreciation	161		625
	Adjustment for monthly depreciation.			
5	Salaries and Wages Expense	601	3,100	
	Accrued Salaries and Wages Payable	202		3,100
	Adjustment for accrued payroll.			
6	Deferred Rental Income	204	140	
	Rental Income	404		140
	Adjustment to record rental income earned during the month.			
7	Interest Expense	606	500	
	Accrued Interest Payable	203		500
	Adjustment for monthly accrual of interest on 6% bonds payable.			

QUESTIONS

1. What are interim financial statements?

2. Why are interim financial statements prepared?

3. Iowa Hospital's long-term investments consist of $90,000 (face value) of 8%, 15-year bonds purchased by the hospital at face value on January 1, 1977. These bonds pay interest semiannually on January 1 and July 1, beginning on July 1, 1977. Iowa Hospital's

accounting period is the calendar year. What amounts should be reported in the hospital's adjusted trial balance at November 30, 1977, for (a) interest income? (b) accrued interest receivable?

4. Indiana Hospital, whose accounting period is the calendar year, began 1977 with a $10,000 credit balance in its allowance for bad debts account. At the end of each month of the year, an adjusting entry is made to adjust the allowance account credit balance to 10% of receivables. Also at the end of each month of the year, an entry is made to write off accounts receivable deemed to be worthless (bad debts). Indicate the presentation of receivables in Indiana Hospital's balance sheet at March 31, 1977, given the following data:

	January	February	March
Accounts receivable, end of month*	$128,000	$151,000	$147,000
Accounts written off at end of month	8,000	11,000	15,000

*Prior to monthly write-offs.

5. On January 1, 1977, Ivanhoe Hospital paid a 3-year insurance premium of $6,480 in advance. This premium payment was recorded as a debit to prepaid insurance.

a. What amount should be reported as prepaid insurance in the hospital's preadjusted trial balance at August 31, 1977?
b. What amount should be reported as insurance expense in the hospital's income statement for the 9 months ended September 30, 1977?
c. What amount should be reported as prepaid insurance in the hospital's balance sheet at October 31, 1977?

6. Issel Hospital paid $145,700 of salaries and wages during the month of May, 1977. The hospital's balance sheets reported accrued salaries and wages payable as follows:

April 30, 1977	$31,200
May 31, 1977	37,800

What amount should be reported as salaries and wages expense in the hospital's income statement for the month ended May 31, 1977?

7. If a hospital prepares interim financial statements, how often must adjusting entries be made? How often must closing entries be made?

8. A private concern began operating a gift shop in Inverness Hospital on May 1, 1977. At that time, the hospital received a year's rent ($3,000) in advance. The $3,000 was credited to deferred rental income. Assuming that the hospital prepares monthly financial statements, make the necessary adjusting entry at September 30, 1977.

9. Indelible Hospital issued $300,000 of 6%, 15-year bonds at

face value on April 1, 1977. These bonds pay interest semiannually on April 1 and October 1, commencing October 1, 1977. The hospital's fiscal year ends December 31. What amounts should be reported in the hospital's adjusted trial balance at November 30, 1977, for (a) bond interest expense? (b) accrued bond interest payable?

10. Indeed Hospital purchased all its depreciable equipment on January 1, 1975, for $800,000. This equipment has an estimated useful life of 12 years and an estimated salvage value of 10%. The hospital's fiscal year ends on December 31. What amounts should be reported in the hospital's preadjusted trial balance at May 31, 1977, for (a) depreciation expense? (b) accumulated depreciation?

PROBLEMS

A. Illusion Hospital's adjusted trial balance at March 31, 1978, and its unadjusted trial balance at April 30, 1978, are presented below (the hospital's fiscal year ends on December 31):

Acct. No.		Adjusted Trial Balance March 31, 1978 Dr.	Adjusted Trial Balance March 31, 1978 Cr.	Unadjusted Trial Balance April 30, 1978 Dr.	Unadjusted Trial Balance April 30, 1978 Cr.
101	Cash	$ 30,300		$ 25,400	
102	Accrued interest receivable	1,800		1,800	
103	Accounts receivable	80,000		86,000	
104	Allowance for bad debts		$ 8,000		$ 1,400
105	Inventory	11,000		10,300	
106	Prepaid insurance	3,675		3,675	
130	Long-term investments	90,000		90,000	
150	Land	15,000		15,000	
160	Depreciable plant assets	400,000		400,000	
161	Accumulated depreciation		63,000		63,000
201	Accounts payable		21,600		23,900
202	Accrued salaries and wages payable		4,700		-0-
203	Accrued interest payable		2,400		2,400
204	Deferred rental income		2,340		2,340
250	Bonds payable		160,000		160,000
301	Hospital equity		355,235		355,235
302	Revenue and expense summary		-0-		-0-
401	Inpatient services revenue		81,400		115,200
402	Outpatient services revenue		56,100		72,900
403	Interest income		1,800		1,800
404	Rental income		780		780
405	Other revenues		12,120		16,020
501	Bad debts	3,300		3,300	
502	Other revenue deductions	11,500		14,900	
601	Salaries and wages expense	90,600		120,300	
602	Supplies expense	15,100		21,700	
603	Utilities expense	10,200		14,500	
604	Insurance expense	525		525	
605	Depreciation expense	3,000		3,000	
606	Interest expense	2,400		2,400	
607	Other expenses	1,075		2,175	
		$769,475	$769,475	$814,975	$814,975

The following additional information is available:

1. Long-term investments consist of $90,000 (face value) of 8%, 10-

year bonds purchased by the hospital on January 1, 1978. These bonds pay interest semiannually on January 1 and July 1, commencing July 1, 1978.

2. A 2-year insurance premium of $4,200 was paid in advance on January 1, 1978.
3. Depreciable plant assets, all of which were acquired on January 1, 1973, have an estimated useful life of 30 years and a 10% salvage value.
4. On January 1, 1978, the hospital issued $160,000 of 6%, 15-year bonds at face value. These bonds pay interest annually on January 1, commencing January 1, 1979.
5. A year's rent of $3,120 was received in advance on January 1, 1978.
6. At the end of each month, the allowance for bad debts is adjusted to a credit balance equal to 10% of month-end accounts receivable.
7. Unpaid salaries and wages at April 30, 1978, amounted to $3,400.

Required. (1) Prepare a worksheet to develop financial statements for the 4 months ended April 30, 1978, in the manner illustrated in figure 40 on pages 154–155. (2) Prepare, in good form, income statements for the month of April, 1978, and for the 4 months then ended, in the manner illustrated in figure 41 on page 158. (3) Prepare, in good form, balance sheets at April 30 and March 31, 1978, in the manner illustrated in figure 42 on page 159. (4) Prepare, in general journal form, all necessary adjusting entries for the month ended April 30, 1978.

B. Incomparable Hospital's adjusting trial balance at May 31, 1978, and its unadjusted trial balance at June 30, 1978, are presented below (the hospital's fiscal year ends on December 31):

Acct. No.		Adjusted Trial Balance May 31, 1978 Dr.	Adjusted Trial Balance May 31, 1978 Cr.	Unadjusted Trial Balance June 30, 1978 Dr.	Unadjusted Trial Balance June 30, 1978 Cr.
101	Cash	$ 38,400		$ 16,640	
102	Accrued interest receivable	800		800	
103	Accounts receivable	95,000		106,500	
104	Allowance for bad debts		$ 7,600		$ 300
105	Inventory	10,800		12,300	
106	Prepaid insurance	3,420		3,420	
130	Long-term investments	60,000		75,000	
150	Land	14,000		14,000	
160	Depreciable plant assets	480,000		480,000	
161	Accumulated depreciation		82,250		82,250
201	Accounts payable		19,700		24,100
202	Accrued salaries and wages payable		3,900		−0−
203	Accrued interest payable		2,000		2,000
204	Deferred rental income		2,160		2,160
250	Bonds payable		200,000		200,000
301	Hospital equity		356,810		356,810
302	Revenue and expense summary		−0−		−0−
401	Inpatient services revenue		100,200		128,700
402	Outpatient services revenue		78,400		93,500
403	Interest income		800		800
404	Rental income		720		720
405	Other revenues		12,880		15,100
501	Bad debts	2,900		2,900	
502	Other revenue deductions	12,600		15,700	
601	Salaries and wages expense	101,400		122,300	

Acct. No.		Adjusted Trial Balance May 31, 1978 Dr.	Cr.	Unadjusted Trial Balance June 30, 1978 Dr.	Cr.
602	Supplies expense	$ 16,100		$ 19,800	
603	Utilities expense	11,200		13,900	
604	Insurance expense	900		900	
605	Depreciation expense	10,250		10,250	
606	Interest expense	5,000		5,000	
607	Other expenses	4,650		7,030	
		$867,420	$867,420	$906,440	$906,440

The following additional information is available:

1. Long-term investments consist of $60,000 (face value) of 8%, 15-year bonds purchased by the hospital on April 1, 1978 (interest payable annually on April 1) and $15,000 (face value) of 8%, 10-year bonds purchased by the hospital on June 1, 1978 (interest payable annually on June 1).
2. A 2-year insurance premium was paid in advance on January 1, 1978.
3. On January 1, 1975, the hospital purchased $450,000 of depreciable plant assets having an estimated useful life of 15 years and an estimated salvage value of 20%. On May 1, 1978, the hospital purchased additional depreciable plant assets having a cost of $30,000, an estimated useful life of 8 years, and a 20% salvage value.
4. A year's rent was received in advance on March 1, 1978.
5. On April 1, 1977, the hospital issued $200,000 of 6%, 10-year bonds at face value. These bonds pay interest semiannually on April 1 and October 1.
6. At the end of each month, the allowance for bad debts is adjusted to a credit balance equal to 8% of month-end accounts receivable.
7. Unpaid salaries and wages at June 30, 1978, totaled $4,100.

Required. (1) Prepare a worksheet to develop financial statements for the 6 months ended June 30, 1978, in the manner illustrated in figure 40 on pages 154–155. (2) Prepare, in good form, income statements for the month of June, 1978, and for the 6 months then ended, in the manner illustrated in figure 41 on page 158. (3) Prepare, in good form, balance sheets at June 30 and May 31, 1978, in the manner illustrated in figure 42 on page 159. (4) Prepare, in general journal form, all necessary adjusting entries for the month ended June 30, 1978.

III

Extensions of Basic Procedures

10
Expansion of the Chart of Accounts

Illustrations in the preceding chapters were based upon a highly simplified chart of accounts suitable to an introductory discussion of the fundamentals of bookkeeping. Having accomplished this, we now must expand the chart of accounts to permit the introduction of more-realistic accounting techniques and procedures. The expanded chart of accounts we develop in this chapter will serve as a basis for the discussion in the next 4 chapters, but we will make additional refinements at appropriate points throughout the remainder of this book. By the end of your study of this volume, you will have been exposed to a substantially complete chart of accounts such as one would find in actual practice in an average hospital of medium size.

The chart of accounts presented in this chapter conforms closely to the account classifications and numerical coding system recommended for hospitals by the American Hospital Association.[1] We will not attempt here, however, to deal with all of the accounts listed in the AHA publication. Your attention will be directed only to a representative sample of those accounts. While a degree of realism may be lost through limiting the number of accounts involved in our illustrations, your comprehension of the underlying principles and procedures will not be impaired by unnecessary details.

Balance Sheet Accounts

The chart of balance sheet accounts employed by Hartful Hospital is shown in figure 44. You are already acquainted with most of these accounts, but a number of changes and additions require brief explanations. A more-thorough discussion of these accounts will appear in subsequent chapters. Segregation of the balance sheet accounts into self-balancing groups as required by fund

---

[1]American Hospital Association, *Chart of Accounts for Hospitals* (Chicago: AHA, 1976). You are urged to read this important document in its entirety because its content can only be highlighted and summarized within these pages.

Figure 44
Hartful Hospital
Chart of Balance Sheet Accounts

ASSETS

Current Assets
1011 Cash—General Checking Account
1012 Cash—Payroll Checking Account
1014 Petty Cash Fund
1020 Temporary Investments
1029 Accrued Interest Receivable
1031 Inpatient Receivables—Inhouse
1032 Inpatient Receivables—Discharged
1044 Outpatient Receivables
1061 Allowance for Uncollectible Accounts—Bad Debts
1062 Allowance for Uncollectible Accounts—Contractual Adjustments
1066 Allowance for Uncollectible Accounts—Charity Service
1110 Inventories
1120 Prepaid Expenses
---- Other Accounts

Property, Plant, and Equipment
1130 Land
1150 Buildings
1170 Equipment
1250 Accumulated Depreciation—Buildings
1270 Accumulated Depreciation—Equipment
---- Other Accounts

LIABILITIES

Current Liabilities
2010 Notes Payable
2020 Accounts Payable
2031 Accrued Payroll
2035 FIT Withheld
2036 FICA Withheld and Accrued
2051 Accrued Interest Payable
2113 Deferred Rental Income
---- Other Accounts

Noncurrent Liabilities
2190 Bonds Payable
---- Other Accounts

EQUITY

2210 Hospital Equity
2219 Revenue and Expense Summary
---- Other Accounts

accounting will be deferred to chapter 15. The accounts described in the present chapter relate only to the general (unrestricted) fund.

ASSET ACCOUNTS

In the AHA numerical coding system, the hospital's asset accounts are those numbered in the *1000* series. Any account having *1* as the first digit of its number is an asset account. As you shall see in chapter 15, the second digit is used to specify the fund in which the asset is located; the general fund designators are the second digits *0, 1,* or *2*. The third and fourth digits of the account number specify the primary subclassification of assets. Consider, as an example, account 1011:

Digit Position		
First	1	= Asset
Second	0	= General Fund
Third	1	= Cash
Fourth	1	= General Checking Account

In other words, all *101* accounts are general fund cash accounts;

the fourth digit indicates the *type* of cash account. Similarly, all *103* accounts are general fund asset accounts for inpatient receivables; the fourth digit is used to indicate whether the receivables relate to inhouse or discharged patients.

The AHA system also provides for the use of a fifth and even a sixth digit, according to individual hospital needs, for a secondary subclassification of asset accounts. You need not be concerned, however, with this additional detail. Our discussion is limited, at this point, to the 4-digit primary account number. Starting in the next chapter, however, all asset account numbers will have 5 digits to be consistent with the 5-digit revenue and expense account numbers. The fifth digit of all asset account numbers will always be *0* (e.g., 1011.0, 1012.0, 1014.0, etc.), but this is only for the purposes of our discussion.

Notice that there are 2 cash checking accounts. Account 1011 is Hartful Hospital's general checking account into which all cash receipts are deposited. All hospital disbursements, other than employees' individual payroll checks, are made by checks drawn against this account. Account 1012 is used only for payroll checks, as will be discussed in chapter 13. Procedures relating to the uses of account 1014, account 1020, and account 1029 are topics for discussion in chapter 16.

Hartful Hospital employs 3 accounts for receivables from patients. As services are rendered to inpatients, account 1031 is debited; it is credited when payments are received from patients prior to their discharge from the hospital. The account also is credited (and account 1032 is debited) for the unpaid balances of patients' accounts at the time of discharge. Subsequent collections on these accounts are credited to account 1032. Account 1044 is debited for services provided to outpatients and is credited for all collections received on outpatients' accounts. These accounts for receivables are general ledger *control* accounts; they show the *total* amount due collectively from patients in each of the 3 classifications. Information as to the amounts due from individual patients is developed and maintained in separate *subsidiary* ledgers to be illustrated subsequently in chapter 12. At frequent intervals, the sum of the individual account balances in each subsidiary ledger will have to be reconciled to the balance reflected by the related general ledger control account.

Also notice that the chart provides for a classification of the allowance for uncollectible accounts into 3 separate accounts according to the nature or type of the corresponding revenue deductions. Account 1066, for example, will reflect the amount of receivables estimated to prove eventually uncollectible by reason of charity service that has been rendered to financially indigent patients. Similar allowance accounts are maintained for estimated contractual adjustments and for estimated bad debts. All these accounts, although listed in the asset classification, will carry credit balances. Detailed consideration will be given to these accounts in chapters 12 and 16.

Figure 45
Hartful Hospital
Organization Chart

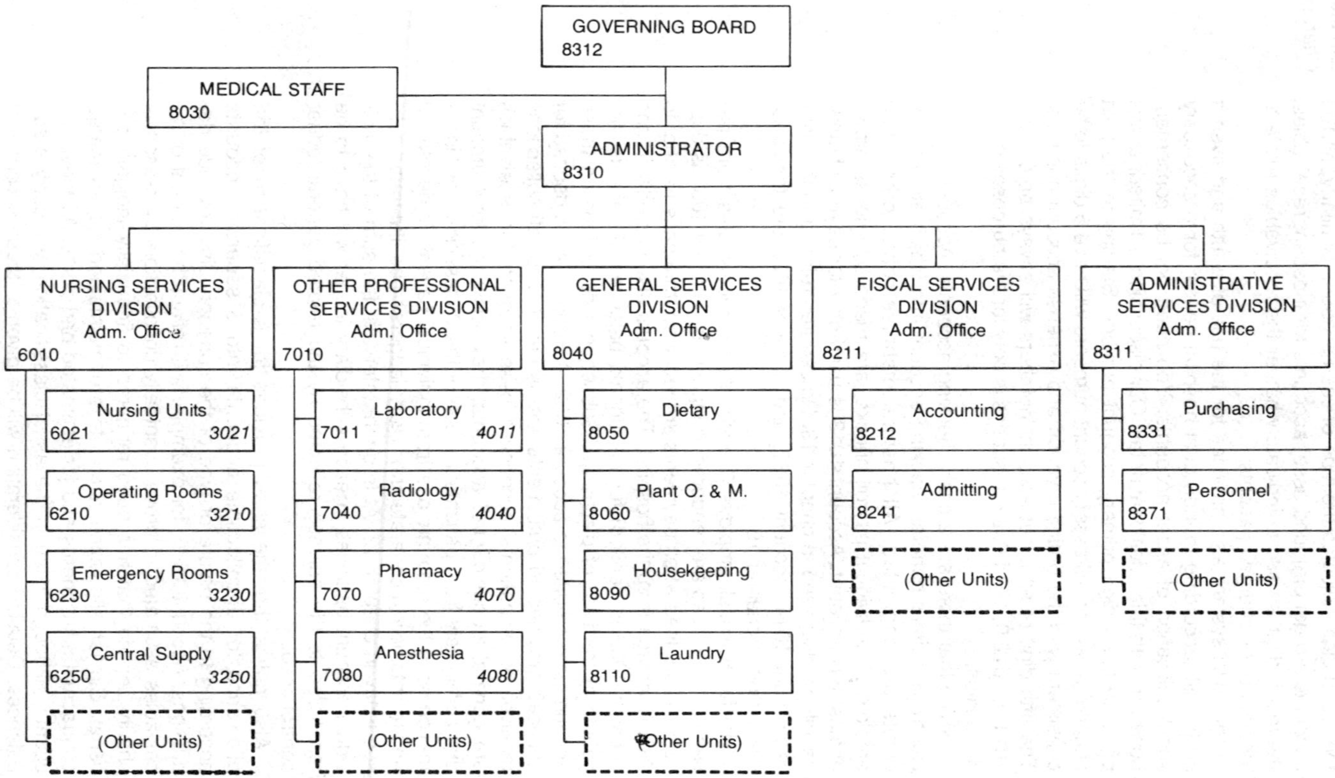

In view of the discussion previously provided in parts 1 and 2 of this book, it is not necessary at this time to comment further on the remaining asset accounts. You will find additional coverage of these accounts in later chapters. Account 1110 (inventories), for example, will be attended to in chapter 17, and the accounts for property, plant, and equipment will be treated fully in chapter 18. Discussions of other asset accounts not included in figure 44 also will be provided at appropriate points in subsequent chapters.

LIABILITY AND EQUITY ACCOUNTS

The liability and equity accounts are numbered in the *2000* series. The liability accounts are numbered 2000 through 2199; the equity accounts are numbered 2200 through 2299. (These numerical codings will be altered somewhat with the introduction of fund accounting in chapter 15.) As was true for the asset accounts, fifth and sixth digits are available for a secondary subclassification of the liability and equity accounts whenever additional detail is required by the individual hospital. The present discussion, however, is confined to the 4-digit primary account numbers. But, commencing with the next chapter, all liability and equity account numbers will consist of 5 digits in order to be consistent with the 5-digit revenue and expense account numbers. The fifth digit of all liability and equity account numbers will always be *0* (e.g., 2010.0, 2020.0, 2031.0, etc.), but this is only for the purposes of our discussion.

Most of Hartful Hospital's liability and equity accounts have been discussed earlier. The 2 accounts you have not previously seen are accounts 2035 and 2036, the payroll tax accounts. The nature and use of these accounts will be described fully in chapters 13 and 17, and you need not be concerned with them at this time. Of course, hospitals typically maintain liability and equity accounts which are not included in figure 44; we will add these accounts to our discussion at suitable times.

INCOME STATEMENT ACCOUNTS

Hartful Hospital's organizational structure is presented in condensed form in figure 45. Notice that the hospital activity is organized into 5 basic divisions, each having an administrative office. The administrative officer of each division often has the title of *director*—"director of nursing services," "director of fiscal services," and so on. The directors report to the hospital administrator to whom they are responsible for the activities organized within their particular divisions.

Figure 45 provides a representative sample of the types of services (or departments) included in each division. It is not feasible in this book to try to deal with a larger number of organizational units. Moreover, you should be aware that a single "box" in the illustrative organizational chart may, in fact, represent 2 or more separately organized units. The nursing units, for example, typically are organized somewhat as follows:

Medical and Surgical Acute Care Units
Pediatric Acute

Psychiatric Acute
Obstetric Acute
Newborn Nursery Acute
Intensive Care
Cardiac Care
Other

The significance of this, in terms of the design of the chart of accounts, is that separate revenue and expense accounts must be provided for each nursing care unit. Only by accumulating and reporting revenues and expenses by individual organizational units can a monetary evaluation of the performance of each unit be made by the hospital's managers. As another example, consider the box labeled *accounting*. This function is generally organized into several different units, as follows:

General Accounting
Budgets and Costs
Payroll Accounting
Accounts Payable
Patient Accounting
Other

While there are no revenues directly associated with these units, the expenses of each unit should be separately accumulated in the accounts. In the interest of brevity, however, we will not do this in our Hartful Hospital illustrations.

In addition to recognizing that the illustrative organization chart in figure 45 is greatly condensed, you also should realize that the chart is not to be regarded as indicative of how all hospitals are, or should be, organized. No 2 hospitals are exactly alike; hospitals differ in size, range of services, management philosophy, and other important ways. These differences have an effect on the manner in which hospitals are organized. What may be a sound organizational pattern for one hospital may not be satisfactory for another.

The important point to recognize is that, however a particular hospital is organized, the hospital's chart of income statement accounts should be designed to conform to that hospital's organizational structure. The basic principle of *responsibility accounting* is that each organized unit (department) of the hospital is a *responsibility center*, for an organized activity or function, headed by an individual responsible for its performance. Each of these individuals is a decision maker who has some degree of control over the amounts of resources employed in his or her center. Since all centers incur expenses, every center is an *expense* (or cost) *center*. Some centers also generate or produce revenues by providing patient services for which a specific charge is made; these centers also are referred to as *revenue centers*. Housekeeping, for example, is an expense center but not a revenue center; radiology, on the other hand, is both an expense center and a revenue center.

Under responsibility accounting, the revenue and expense accounts are classified in a manner to permit the recording of revenues according to the centers responsible for generating them and to permit the recording of expenses according to the centers responsible for their incurrence. Each center is charged only for those expenses which can be directly associated with the activities of that center, however, and over which the center supervisor or manager has decision-making authority. All other expenses, as you will shortly see, are recorded in a special "unassigned" expenses classification.

Hartful Hospital's chart of income statement accounts appears in condensed form in figure 46. Observe here that the classification of the income statement accounts conforms to Hartful Hospital's organizational pattern. This necessary relationship between a hospital's organizational structure and its chart of accounts is indicated by the placement of revenue and expense account numbers in the corresponding "boxes" in the organization chart as shown in figure 45. As you can see, each of the organizational units has its own expense and (where applicable) revenue accounts. Each center is charged with the expenses it incurs and is credited with the revenues (if any) it generates. In this way, relevant expense and revenue data are developed for the purpose of measuring and evaluating the performance of each center and its supervisor or manager.

Figure 46
Hartful Hospital
Chart of Income Statement Accounts

EXPENSES

Nursing Services
6010 Director's Administrative Office
6021 Nursing Units
6210 Operating Rooms
6230 Emergency Rooms
6250 Central Supply
---- Other Units

Other Professional Services
7010 Director's Administrative Office
7011 Laboratory
7040 Radiology
7070 Pharmacy
7080 Anesthesia
---- Other Units

Other Services
8030 Medical Staff
---- Other Units

General Services
8040 Director's Administrative Office
8050 Dietary
8060 Plant Operation and Maintenance

REVENUES

Nursing Services
3021 Nursing Units
3210 Operating Rooms
3230 Emergency Rooms
3250 Central Supply
---- Other Units

Other Professional Services
4011 Laboratory
4040 Radiology
4070 Pharmacy
4080 Anesthesia
---- Other Units

(Figure 46 continued)

8090 Housekeeping
8110 Laundry
---- Other Units

Fiscal Services
8211 Director's Administrative Office
8212 Accounting
8241 Admitting
---- Other Units

Administrative Services
8310 Administrator's Office
8311 Director's Administrative Office
8312 Governing Board
8331 Purchasing
8371 Personnel
---- Other Units

Unassigned Expenses
8510 Depreciation
8610 Insurance
8690 Interest
8710 Employee Benefits
---- Other Accounts

Other Operating Revenues
5061 Cafeteria Sales
5155 Rental Income
5171 Purchase Discounts
---- Other Accounts

Deductions from Revenues
5510 Bad Debts
5520 Contractual Adjustments
5540 Charity Service
---- Other Accounts

Nonoperating Revenues
9041 General Contributions
9051 Interest Income
---- Other Accounts

REVENUE ACCOUNTS

In the AHA numerical coding system, the first digit of revenue (and revenue deduction) accounts may be 3, 4, 5, or 9. Designations for this first digit are as follows:

First Digit		
3	=	Nursing Service Revenues
4	=	Other Professional Service Revenues
5	=	Other Operating Revenues; Deductions from Revenues
9	=	Nonoperating Revenues

Where the first digit of a revenue account number is *3* or *4,* the second, third, and fourth digits provide a classification of revenue by organizational units. Account number 3250, for example, designates the following:

Digit			
First	3	=	Revenues—Nursing Services
Second	2		
Third	5	=	Central Supply
Fourth	0		

In other words, *250* is the numerical code for the central supply department or function. Similarly, *011* is the code for laboratory, *040* is the designation for pharmacy, and so on.

Where a particular service is organized into several subordinate units, as is often true of the laboratory department, the account numbering system provides for a scheme such as the following:

Account No.	
	Laboratory Services
4011	Chemistry
4012	Hematology
4013	Histology
4016	Autopsy
4018	Immunology
4025	Blood Bank

Or even where the laboratory is a single organizational unit, this series of accounts may be used to obtain a classification of laboratory revenues by type of service or examination.

As another example of the use of the second, third, and fourth digits with respect to revenue accounts, observe the following account classifications for revenues derived from acute care nursing units:

Account No.	
	Acute Care Nursing Units
3021	Medical and Surgical—Unit 1
3022	Medical and Surgical—Unit 2
3026	Medical and Surgical—Unit 6
3051	Pediatric—Unit 1
3052	Pediatric—Unit 2
3060	Psychiatric Unit
3080	Obstetric Unit
3090	Newborn Nursery

Extensions of Basic Procedures

While our Hartful Hospital illustration will not include this much detail, it is very important that you keep in mind that detailed revenue information of this kind is essential in actual practice.

Where the first digit of a revenue (or revenue deduction) account is *5* or *9*, the second, third, and fourth digits are used mainly to classify the revenue (or revenue deduction) by type.

The AHA system also calls for the use of a fifth digit in connection with revenue accounts in the *3000* and *4000* series. This fifth digit is employed to classify these patient service revenues by type of patient. The recommended patient classifications are as follows:

Fifth Digit	
0	Inpatient—Acute
1	Inpatient—Long-term
2	Outpatient—Emergency
3	Outpatient—Referred
4	Outpatient—Clinic
5	Day Care
6	Home Health Care
7, 8, 9	Other Classifications

A sixth digit may be used to subclassify further revenues in whatever manner may be desired by the individual hospital. Presumably, this classification could be related to the financial status of the patient (source of payment), the type of hospital accommodation (private, semiprivate, ward), and so on.

Finally, the AHA system also provides for a seventh, eighth, and ninth digit to be used as a 3-digit suffix to classify revenues by functional units for purposes of uniform reporting. If you have a particular interest in this procedure, you will want to refer to chapter 6 of the AHA's *Chart of Accounts for Hospitals* manual. For our present purposes, your attention is directed mainly to the 4-digit revenue account numbers that are included in Hartful Hospital's chart of accounts. Beginning with the next chapter, however, we will add a fifth digit to all patient service revenue account numbers, those in the *3000* and *4000* series. This fifth digit will indicate the following:

Fifth Digit		
1	=	Inpatient Revenues
2	=	Outpatient Revenues

In this way, patient service revenues will be classified by type of patient. All other revenue accounts (those in the *5000* and *9000* series) will always have *0* as a fifth digit.

EXPENSE ACCOUNTS

In the AHA numerical coding system, the first digit of the expense accounts may be *6, 7, 8,* or *9*. Designations for this first digit follow:

First Digit		
6	=	Nursing Service Expenses
7	=	Other Professional Service Expenses
8	=	Other Services Expenses
9	=	Nonoperating Expenses

Where the first digit of an expense account number is *6, 7,* or *8,* the second, third, and fourth digits provide a classification of expense by organizational units. Account number 6250, for example, designates the following:

Digit Position		
First	6	= Expenses—Nursing Services
Second	2	= Central Supply
Third	5	
Fourth	0	

Again, as noted earlier on page 175 in the discussion of revenue accounts, *250* is the numerical code for the central supply department or function. Thus, the central supply revenue account is account 3250; the central supply expense account is account 6250. A similar procedure is followed for all other organized units which incur expenses and generate revenues.

In those situations where a particular service is organized into several subordinate units, as is often true of the laboratory department, the account numbering system for expense accounts parallels that of the revenue accounts in a scheme such as the one in the following:

Expense Account No.		Revenue Account No.
	Laboratory Services	
7011	Chemistry	4011
7012	Hematology	4012
7013	Histology	4013
7016	Autopsy	4016
7018	Immunology	4018
⟆		⟆
7025	Blood Bank	4025

As another example of the use of the second, third, and fourth digits as codes for the various organizational units, observe the following account classifications for expenses and revenues related to the acute care nursing units:

Expense Account No.		Revenue Account No.
	Acute Care Nursing Units	
6021	Medical and Surgical—Unit 1	3021
6022	Medical and Surgical—Unit 2	3022
⟩		⟩
6026	Medical and Surgical—Unit 6	3026
6051	Pediatric—Unit 1	3051
6052	Pediatric—Unit 2	3052
6060	Psychiatric Unit	3060
6080	Obstetric Unit	3080
6090	Newborn Nursery	3090

The Hartful Hospital illustrations to be presented in subsequent chapters will not include quite this much detail, but you should keep in mind that detailed expense information of this kind is required in actual practice.

Where the first digit of an expense account number is *9*, the second, third, and fourth digits are used to classify the expense by major type. You may have noticed that Hartful Hospital's chart of accounts does not include any expense accounts in the *9000* series. At later points in this book, we will introduce a number of expense items which may be recorded in this "nonoperating expense" classification.

For expense accounts in the *6000*, *7000*, and *8000* series, the AHA numbering system provides fifth and sixth digits to be used as indicators for the natural classification of expenses in each organizational unit of the hospital. The suggested natural (or object of expenditure) classification is as follows:

Fifth and Sixth Digits	Major Categories
.00	Salaries and Wages
.15	Employee Benefits
.25	Professional Fees—Medical
.30	Other Professional Fees
.35	Supplies and Materials, Special Departmental
.45	General Supplies
.54	Purchased Services
.65 ⟩ .99	Other Direct Expenses

Within each of the above major categories detailed classifications should be maintained to indicate job classifications, kinds of benefits, types of fees, types of supplies, and so on. A sufficient number of digits is available to permit such breakdowns in each category.

The Hartful Hospital illustrations to follow in the next several chapters will not include this detailed use of the fifth and sixth digits. Instead, we will use only a fifth digit for expense center accounts. The designation of this fifth digit will be as follows:

Fifth Digit	
.1	Salaries and Wages
.2	Supplies and Other Expense

Thus, account 6250.1, for example, will indicate central supply—salaries and wages. Account 6250.2 will designate central supply—supplies and other expense. The fifth digit will have the same meaning in each expense center.

As was noted earlier in connection with revenue accounts, the AHA system also provides for the use of seventh, eighth, and ninth digits for expense accounts. These digits may be used as a 3-digit suffix to the basic account numbers for purposes of uniform reporting. For the time being, however, you need not concern yourself with this matter.

Several accounts are provided for Hartful Hospital's *unassigned expenses*. These expenses are general in nature and, in the regular accounting routine, are not charged or assigned to specific departmental expense centers. The reason for this is that, for the most part, these expenses are not controllable by individual department heads and supervisors. In the periodic cost-finding procedure, however, the unassigned expenses are allocated to the various expense centers to determine the full costs of providing departmental services. Cost-finding procedures will be dealt with in detail in chapter 23 of this book.

In the next chapter, we will incorporate Hartful Hospital's chart of accounts into a journal and ledger system. It is important, therefore, that you have a good understanding of the materials presented in this chapter before moving on to chapter 11. Detailed applications of Hartful Hospital's chart of accounts also will be encountered in chapters 12, 13, and 14.

QUESTIONS

1. What is your understanding of the term *responsibility accounting*?

2. What is a responsibility center? Give an example.

3. Distinguish between an expense center and a revenue center. Give an example of each.

4. What are "unassigned expenses"? Give 4 examples.

5. Why do you think the American Hospital Association publishes a *Chart of Accounts for Hospitals* manual?

6. The AHA *Chart of Accounts* manual contains an account numbered *1031*. Explain briefly what each digit of this account number means.

7. The following account appeared in the ledger of Hartful Hospital on May 31, 1977:

Account Number 2020			
5/31	49,351	5/1	46,877
		5/31	52,308
		(GB)	49,834

Briefly identify each of the figures in the account.

8. The AHA *Chart of Accounts* manual contains an account numbered *3230*. Explain briefly what the digits of this account number mean.

9. In connection with revenue accounts in the *3000* and *4000* series, the AHA *Chart of Accounts* manual provides for the use of a fifth digit. For what purpose is this fifth digit employed?

10. In the AHA *Chart of Accounts* manual, the first digit of expense account numbers may be either *6, 7, 8,* or *9*. Briefly explain the meaning of each of these initial digits.

11. The AHA Chart of Accounts manual contains an account numbered *8212*. Explain briefly what the digits of this account number mean.

12. In connection with expense accounts in the *6000, 7000,* and *8000* series, the AHA *Chart of Accounts* manual provides for the use of fifth and sixth digits. For what purpose are these fifth and sixth digits employed?

13. In the AHA *Chart of Accounts manual,* the first digit of revenue account numbers may be either *3, 4, 5,* or *9*. Briefly explain the meaning of each of these initial digits.

14. In the account numbering system set forth in the AHA *Chart of Accounts* manual, how does one distinguish between a liability account number and a hospital equity account number?

11
Special Journals and Ledgers

In the preceding chapters, all transactions were recorded in one journal: the general journal. All postings of these transaction entries were made to one ledger: the general ledger. Charges to patients for services rendered were debited to a single accounts receivable account; purchases of supplies on account from suppliers were credited to a single accounts payable account. We rather conveniently ignored the need for maintaining a continuous record of the amounts due from each patient or due to each supplier.

These procedures were followed in earlier chapters only to simplify the introductory explanation of the accounting process. In actual practice, using a single journal and ledger is not feasible. Too, the necessity for keeping receivables records for individual patients and records of payables according to individual creditors cannot be avoided. In this chapter, and in the next 3, you will have an opportunity to study a multijournal, multiledger system as it would be maintained on a manual basis. The system overcomes the inefficiency of the single-journal and -ledger procedure, and provides the detailed information that is required with respect to hospital receivables and payables.

The illustrated system assumes that the accounting records are maintained manually (in handwritten form). This assumption is made only for pedagogical reasons. Most hospitals, including smaller ones, have mechanized or automated accounting systems because the volume of transactions prohibits the use of methods which are entirely manual. But your time is not wasted in a study of the manual system illustrated here, since in essence all systems fulfill the same functions. You will learn how an accounting system works, whether machine oriented or not.

Overview of the System

The system of special journals and ledgers described in this chapter, and explored in detail in the next 3 chapters, includes (1) a general journal, (2) 6 special journals, (3) a general ledger, and (4) 2 special (subsidiary) ledgers. The 5-digit numerical coding scheme for the accounts involved in this system was outlined in the previous chapter, you will remember.

Figure 47 summarizes the flow of transaction data through the system. As transactions occur, documentary evidences—charge tickets, purchase orders, cash receipt slips, bank deposit slips, and other business papers—are accumulated. These source documents serve as a basis for transaction entries in the journal system. A separate journal is maintained for each major type of transaction. The cash receipts journal, for example, is used to record all of the hospital's cash receipt transactions, the cash disbursements journal is used to record all cash disbursements, and so on. This permits a division and specialization of labor within the accounting function. In a large office, for example, a different accounting employee may be assigned to each journal. Transactions are likely to be recorded in a more accurate and efficient manner, as a result, than would be possible under a single-journal system.

So, as daily transactions are completed, they are recorded by transaction entries in the appropriate journal. These entries accumulate in the journals day by day over a period of a month. At the end of each month, the accumulated entries in each journal are totaled, and these totals are posted to the hospital's general ledger; individual daily entries are not posted to the general ledger accounts. For example, daily entries are made in the cash receipts journal to record debits to cash. These numerous individual debits are totaled at the end of the month, and *only the total* is posted to the general ledger cash account. This greatly reduces the number of individual postings to be made to the general ledger accounts and eliminates much of the detail which otherwise would be found in the hospital's general ledger.

Certain daily postings, however, are made to the *subsidiary ledgers*. Two of the subsidiary ledgers maintained by Hartful Hospital are included in figure 47. One of these is the accounts receivable subsidiary ledger, sometimes referred to simply as the "patients' ledger" or "receivables ledger." It consists of a ledger account for each patient. These accounts receive daily debit postings from the revenue journal, and daily credit postings come from the cash receipts journal. (Occasional debit and credit postings also may arise from certain transaction entries made in the general journal.) In this way, a continuous daily balance is maintained in each patient's account. The total of these individual balances is reconciled monthly against the balances of the accounts receivable control accounts (accounts 1031.0, 1032.0, and 1044.0) in the general ledger. In addition, a schedule of individual subsidiary ledger balances can be prepared in support of the total of accounts receivable as reported in the month-end balance sheet. These procedures will be described more fully in chapter 12.

The other subsidiary ledger shown in figure 47 is the accounts payable subsidiary ledger, often called simply the "payables ledger." This ledger consists of a separate ledger account for each supplier of goods and services purchased by the hospital. These

Figure 47
Hartful Hospital
Journal and Ledger System

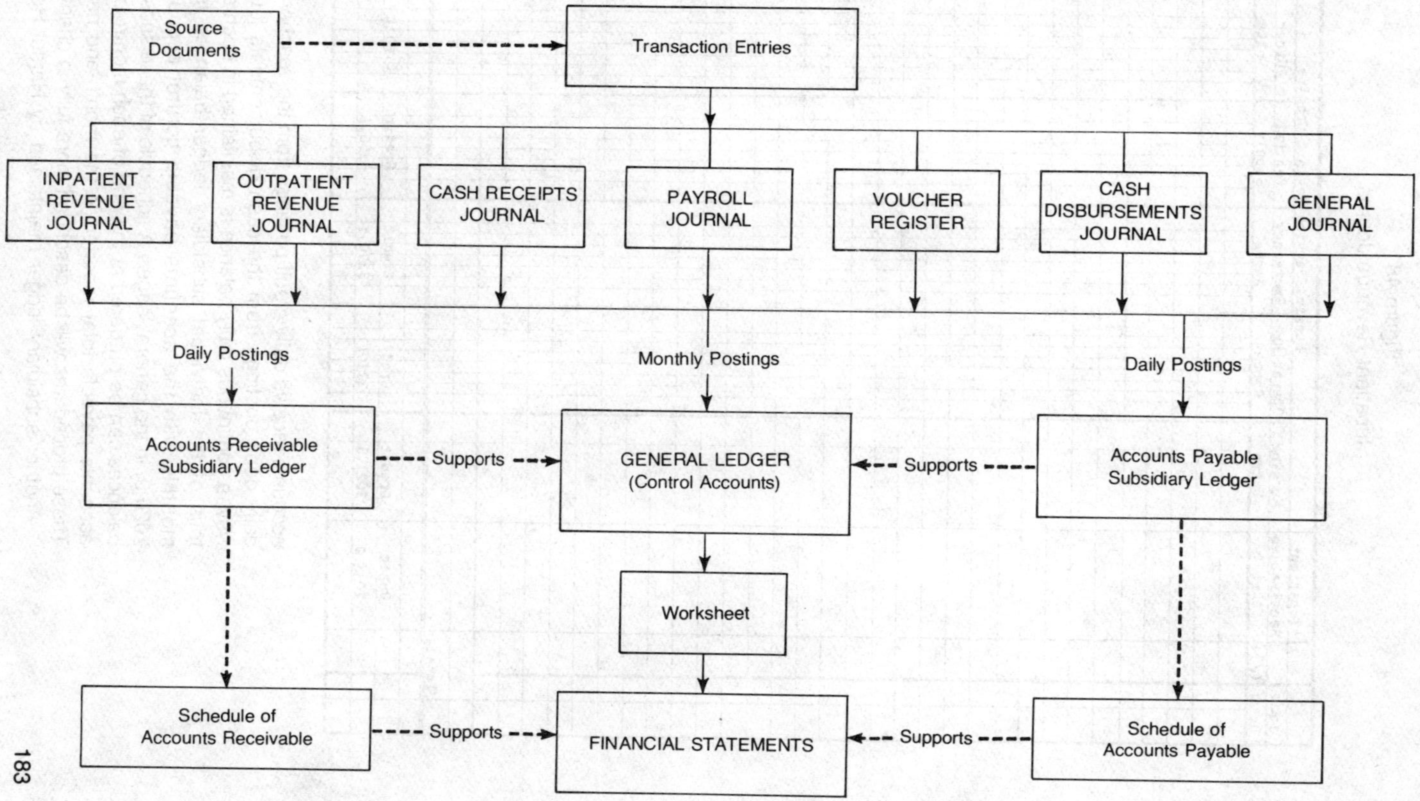

Figure 48
Inpatient Revenue Journal

19-- Date	(√)	Inpatient Receivables Dr.	Nursing Service Revenue Credits					
			Nursing Units	Operating Rooms	Emergency Rooms	Central Supply	Other Units	Other Units
Totals								
		Debit	Credit	Credit	Credit	Credit	Credit	Credit
		1031.0	3021.1	3210.1	3230.1	3250.1		

accounts receive daily credit postings from the voucher register and daily debit postings from the cash disbursements journal. In this way, a continuous daily balance is maintained in each account. The total of the individual subsidiary ledger balances is reconciled monthly with the accounts payable control account (account 2020.0) in the general ledger. A schedule of these subsidiary ledger balances can be prepared at the end of each month to support the accounts payable total reported in the month-end balance sheet. These procedures will be described more fully in chapter 14.

Another subsidiary ledger maintained by Hartful Hospital is the

Other Professional Service Revenue Credits					Sundry Debits and Credits		
Laboratory	Radiology	Pharmacy	Anesthesia	Other Units	Account Numbers	Dr.	Cr.
Credit	Credit	Credit	Credit	Credit			
4011.1	4040.1	4070.1	4080.1				

payroll subsidiary ledger, more often called the "employees' individual earnings record." This ledger is used in connection with the payroll journal and is discussed at length in chapter 13. Subsidiary ledgers for inventories and plant assets will be described and illustrated at subsequent points in this book.

Journal System

Hartful Hospital's journal system is based upon the following classification of the business transactions of the hospital:

1. Charges to inpatients for services rendered
2. Charges to outpatients for services rendered

Figure 49
Outpatient Revenue Journal

19-- Date	(√)	Outpatient Receivables Dr.	Nursing Service Revenue Credits: Operating Rooms	Emergency Rooms	Central Supply	Other Units
Totals						
		Debit	Credit	Credit	Credit	Credit
		1044.0	3210.2	3230.2	3250.2	

3. Cash receipts
4. Purchases of supplies and services
5. Payroll
6. Cash disbursements
7. All other transactions

In the system described here, as noted earlier, a separate journal is maintained for each of these 7 major types of transactions.

INPATIENT REVENUE JOURNAL

The inpatient revenue journal, illustrated in figure 48, is used only to record those transactions which result in charges to inpatients for

Other Professional Service Revenue Credits					Sundry Debits and Credits		
Laboratory	Radiology	Pharmacy	Anesthesia	Other Units	Account Numbers	Dr.	Cr.
Credit 4011.2	Credit 4040.2	Credit 4070.2	Credit 4080.2	Credit			

hospital services provided to them. No other type of transaction should be recorded in this journal, nor should inpatient revenue transactions be recorded in any of the other journals. As hospital services are rendered to inpatients, source documents—census reports and charge tickets, for example—are prepared. Copies of these documents are routed to the hospital's accounting offices where they are turned over to the employee who maintains the inpatient revenue journal. This person uses the source documents as the basis for daily journal entries which debit patients' accounts receivable and credit the various patient service revenue accounts.

Figure 50
Cash Receipts Journal

	Cash		Revenue Deduction	Debits	
19--	Receipt	Cash	Contractual	Charity	
Date	Slip Nos.	Dr.	Adjustments	Service	Other
	Totals				
		Debit	Debit	Debit	Debit
		1011.0	5520.0	5540.0	

The details of this procedure are provided in chapter 12.

These daily entries in the inpatient revenue journal are *not posted* to the hospital's general ledger. Instead, at the end of the month, each column of the journal is totaled, and the totals (except for the sundry debits and credits columns) are posted to the general ledger accounts indicated. Individual entries in the sundry columns have to be individually posted, but entries in these columns will not be frequent or numerous.

Daily postings, however, are made to the accounts receivable subsidiary ledger. These postings consist of debits to individual pa-

Accounts Receivable Credits			Other Credits		Sundry Debits and Credits		
Inpatients							
Inhouse	Discharged	Outpatients	Cafeteria Sales	General Contrbns.	Account Numbers	Dr.	Cr.
Credit 1031.0	Credit 1032.0	Credit 1044.0	Credit 5061.0	Credit 5155.0			

tients' accounts for the services rendered to them each day. Naturally, steps must be taken to insure that the total of these debit postings for each day equals the total debit to accounts receivable entered in the journal for that day. Again, you will find the details of this posting procedure explained in chapter 12.

OUTPATIENT REVENUE JOURNAL

The outpatient revenue journal, illustrated in figure 49, is used only to record those transactions which result in charges to outpatients for hospital services provided to them. No outpatient revenue transactions should be recorded in any of the other journals, nor should any other type of transaction be recorded in this journal. We will assume, for our present purposes, that all services rendered to outpatients at Hartful Hospital are passed through the outpatient receivables account (account 1044.0). This procedure is followed even though payment is received from many outpatients at the time services are rendered to them. The alternative procedure, followed when outpatient services can be provided on a cash basis, is to bypass the receivables account and debit cash directly (crediting the appropriate outpatient revenue accounts). This alternative procedure generally should be discouraged, however, as it tends to weaken internal control over outpatient revenues and cash receipts.

As hospital services are rendered to outpatients, source documents (charge tickets) are prepared in the service-rendering departments. (These departments do not receive cash; outpatients pay for the services at a centralized cash-receiving station as they enter or leave the hospital.) The departments enter the charge tickets in outpatient service logs or reports. Copies of the logs, along with copies of the related charge tickets, are routed to the hospital's accounting offices where they are turned over to the accounting employee who is responsible for maintaining the outpatient revenue journal. These documents are used as the basis for debiting outpatient receivables and crediting the appropriate revenue accounts.

At the end of the month, the journal columns are footed, and the totals are posted to the general ledger. Daily postings of charges to outpatients are made to the accounts receivable subsidiary ledger. You will see the details of the process of journalizing and posting outpatient revenue transactions in chapter 12. The procedure is much the same as for inpatient revenues.

CASH RECEIPTS JOURNAL

Hartful Hospital's cash receipts journal is illustrated in figure 50. It is used to record all cash receipts from whatever source. This hospital, as was noted above, has a centralized cashiering location. As cash is received, either by mail or over the counter, a cash receipt slip is prepared for each item. All cash receipts are deposited intact on a daily basis. Copies of the bank deposit slips, along with copies of the related cash receipt slips, are sent to the hospital's accounting offices each day. Here, the employee in charge of the cash receipts journal uses the source documents to record debits to cash and credits to the receivables accounts.

The journal columns are footed at the end of each month, and the totals are posted to the indicated general ledger accounts. Daily postings are made to the accounts receivable ledger to give individual patients credit for the payments received from them or on their behalf from their third-party sponsors. Details of the procedure of journalizing and posting of cash receipts appear in chapter 12. We also will get into internal control principles and practices with respect to hospital revenues and cash receipts.

PAYROLL JOURNAL

The payroll journal employed by Hartful Hospital is illustrated in figure 51. This journal is used to record the salaries and wages

Figure 51
Payroll Journal

19--			Gross Payroll		Deductions from Payroll Credits				Accrued
Date	Department	Check Numbers	Account Numbers	Amount Dr.	FIT Withheld	FICA Withheld	Other	Total	Payroll Cr.
	Totals								
					Credit 2035.0	Credit 2036.0			Credit 2031.0

Figure 52
Voucher Register

19-- Date	Accounts Payable Credits	(√)	Payroll-Related Debits: Accrued Payroll	FIT Withheld	FICA W/H & Accrued	Nursing Service Expense: Adm. Office	Nursing Units	Operating Rooms
Totals								
	Credit 2020.0		Debit 2031.0	Debit 2035.0	Debit 2036.0	Debit 6010.2	Debit 6021.2	Debit 6210.2

earned by hospital employees during each pay period. As you can see, the journal provides columns for the recording of gross pay, payroll taxes and other withholdings, and the net payroll. The necessary data for the payroll journal entries are compiled from information provided by departmental time reports, personnel department records, time clock cards, and other source documents as will be explained in detail in chapter 13.

Once the net payroll (assume a figure of $116,492) is determined and credited to the accrued payroll liability account (account 2031.0), individual paychecks are written and issued to hospital

Debits	Other Professional Service Expense Debits						
Emergency Rooms	Central Supply	Adm. Office	Laboratory	Radiology	Pharmacy	Anesthesia	Medical Staff Expense
Debit	Debit	Debit	Debit	Debit	Debit	Debit	Debit
6230.2	6250.2	7010.2	7011.2	7040.2	7070.2	7080.2	8030.2

employees. The paychecks are drawn against the hospital's payroll checking account (account 1012.0), but *no entry* is made to credit that account because it is an imprest account. Instead, the amount of the net (accrued) payroll is vouchered through the accounts payable account in the voucher register as follows:

Accrued Payroll	2031.0	$116,492	
Accounts Payable	2020.0		$116,492

The debit closes the accrued payroll account (which previously was established with a credit in the payroll journal), and sets up the amount of the net payroll as an account payable.

(Figure 52 continued)
Voucher Register

General Services Expense Debits					Fiscal Services Expense Debits		
Adm. Office	Dietary	Plant O. & M.	House-keeping	Laundry	Adm. Office	Accounting	Admitting
Debit 8040.2	Debit 8050.2	Debit 8060.2	Debit 8090.2	Debit 8110.2	Debit 8211.2	Debit 8212.2	Debit 8241.2

Then a *single* check is written against the hospital's general checking account (account 1011.0) and is recorded in the cash disbursements journal as follows:

Accounts Payable	2020.0	$116,492	
Cash	1011.0		$116,492

Thus, the payroll checking account is never debited or credited; nor does it ever have a ledger balance (other than perhaps a nominal imprest balance). The $116,492 check drawn on the general checking account, of course, is deposited to the payroll checking account at the hospital's bank. When the individual paychecks are cashed

Administrative Services Expense Debits					Sundry Debits and Credits		
Administrator's Off.	Adm. Office	Governing Board	Purchasing	Personnel	Account Numbers	Dr.	Cr.
Debit 8310.2	Debit 8311.2	Debit 8312.2	Debit 8331.2	Debit 8371.2			

by employees, the payroll checking account is automatically cleared to a zero (or imprest) balance. This procedure removes the large volume of paychecks from the general checking account, thereby facilitating the reconciliation of that account with the monthly bank statement. Another illustration of these procedures will be provided in chapter 14.

All postings from the payroll journal are made on a monthly basis. Hartful Hospital, however, does maintain (as required by law) an "employees' individual earnings record," which in effect is a subsidiary payroll ledger. We will discuss this record in chapter 13.

VOUCHER REGISTER

Hartful Hospital follows an accounting policy which requires that all disbursements be vouchered through accounts payable. In other words, an entry such as the following is *prohibited* by the system:

Dietary—Supplies and Other Expense	8050.2	$1,387	
Cash	1011.0		$1,387

This disbursement or any other disbursement requires preparing a document known as a *voucher*. The vouchering of proposed disbursements involves the auditing of invoices and the securing of various approvals. Once an item is vouchered and approved for payment, the voucher register entry is

Dietary—Supplies and Other Expense	8050.2	$1,387	
Accounts Payable	2020.0		$1,387

Thus, before a check is written, an investigation is made of the proposed disbursement, and (if approved) a credit is made to a liability account (accounts payable). When the check is written, an entry is made in the cash disbursements journal as follows:

Accounts Payable	2020.0	$1,387	
Cash	1011.0		$1,387

This procedure, known as a *voucher system*, provides a high order of accounting control over hospital disbursements. A major portion of chapter 14 will be devoted to a description of the voucher system employed by Hartful Hospital.

Figure 52 presents an illustration of Hartful Hospital's voucher register, which also may be called an accounts payable or purchases journal. As invoices and bills are received by the hospital, they are vouchered (processed for payment) by accounting employees. The vouchers, along with the underlying documents (purchase orders and receiving reports, for example), are turned over to the person who maintains the voucher register. This person enters the vouchers in the register, recording debits to the various accounts indicated by the column headings. In each case the credit is to accounts payable.

At the end of the month, the column totals are posted to the general ledger accounts. Daily postings are made to the accounts payable subsidiary ledger in order to maintain a daily record of the amounts due to individual hospital creditors. This procedure is described more fully in chapter 14.

CASH DISBURSEMENTS JOURNAL

Hartful Hospital's cash disbursements journal is illustrated in figure 53. This journal, which also is known as a cash payments journal or check register, is used to record all hospital disbursements for whatever purpose. Vouchered items, as they become due for payment, are sent to the hospital's disbursing officer; that is, the individual who has authority to sign checks drawn on the hospital's checking account. This person, if satisfied as to the propriety of the disbursements, will sign and mail the related checks. The paid voucher, along with attached underlying documents, is returned to the accounting office where the person in charge of the cash dis-

Figure 53
Cash Disbursements Journal

19-- Date	Description	Check Numbers	Cash Cr.	Purchases Discounts Cr.	Accounts Payable Dr.	Dr.	Sundry Debits and Credits: Account Numbers	Dr.	Cr.
	Totals		Credit 1011.0	Credit 5171.0	Debit 2020.0	Debit			

bursements journal will record the disbursements by debits to accounts payable and credits to cash. The paid vouchers are then placed in a file to be retained for a suitable period of time. Chapter 14 will illustrate these procedures in more detail.

Monthly postings are made to the general ledger of the column totals in the cash disbursements journal. Daily debit postings are made to the accounts payable subsidiary ledger.

Figure 54
General Journal

19-- Date	Accounts and Explanations	Account Numbers	Dr.	Cr.

GENERAL JOURNAL

The general journal used by Hartful Hospital is shown in figure 54. You are already well acquainted with this journal. It is important, however, that you now understand that in a multijournal system the general journal is used sparingly. In Hartful Hospital's system, the general journal is used only to record those transactions for which a special journal has not been provided. It will be used mainly for adjusting and closing entries. Most transaction entries will be recorded in the 6 specialized journals.

LEDGER SYSTEM

If Hartful Hospital maintained only a general ledger, that ledger would have to contain a separate account for each patient and each hospital creditor. As you can imagine, such a ledger would be of immense proportions. It would be cumbersome and unmanageable. For this reason, the individual accounts for hospital patients and creditors are removed from the general ledger and are established as subsidiary ledgers. The general ledger, however, does contain control accounts for patient receivables and accounts payable. As mentioned several times in the preceding discussion, the general ledger control accounts are posted monthly for the accumulated totals provided by the journals; the subsidiary ledgers, on the other hand, are posted daily in the individual amounts of transactions. This requires that the subsidiary ledgers be balanced against, and reconciled with, the month-end balances of the related general ledger control accounts. This is an extremely important feature of a hospital's overall internal control system as you will see in the chapters to follow.

QUESTIONS

1. What are the advantages of maintaining several special journals rather than just a single general journal?

2. Distinguish between the general ledger and a subsidiary ledger. Name 3 kinds of subsidiary ledgers.

3. What is the purpose of having sundry debits and credits columns in a special journal? Describe the posting procedure for the amounts entered in these columns.

4. State 2 advantages of maintaining control accounts in the general ledger of the hospital.

5. How would you determine that a special journal "balances"?

6. "Whenever a debit posting is made to a general ledger control account, one or more credit postings of the same aggregate total must be posted to the related subsidiary ledger." Do you agree? Explain.

7. Why must transactions be posted to the subsidiary ledgers more frequently than to the general ledger?

8. Hartful Hospital employs the 7 journals indicated in figure 47 on page 183. Indicate the name of the journal in which each of the following types of transactions would be recorded:

a. Charges for services rendered to outpatients
b. Purchases of supplies on account
c. Payments made on accounts payable

d. Charges for services rendered to inpatients
e. Issuance of payroll checks to employees
f. Cash collections received on patients' accounts
g. Cash purchases of supplies
h. Sale of long-term investments for cash
i. Purchase of new equipment on account
j. Receipt of interest income from temporary investments

9. Describe briefly the posting procedure for the revenue journals and the cash receipts journal.

10. An inpatient charge ticket for $60 was correctly recorded in the inpatient revenue journal, but the patient's account in the accounts receivable subsidiary ledger was incorrectly debited for only $6. How will this error be discovered?

11. Describe briefly the posting procedure for the payroll journal, voucher register, and the cash disbursements journal.

12. An invoice for the purchase of $150 of supplies was correctly recorded in the voucher register, but the supplier's account in the accounts payable subsidiary ledger was incorrectly credited for $510. How will this error be discovered?

13. Hartful Hospital provides many outpatient services on a cash basis. In such cases, would it be appropriate to bypass the outpatient revenue journal and record the transaction in the cash receipts journal only—that is, to debit cash and credit outpatient revenues?

14. What is the purpose of the check (p) column in the inpatient revenue journal?

15. Describe briefly the use of the imprest payroll checking account (account number 1012).

16. In the accounting system described in chapter 11, is an entry such as the following possible?

Laboratory—Supplies Expense	$259	
Cash		$259
To record cash purchase of supplies for the laboratory department.		

17. The following is a list of general ledger accounts. For each account name the journals from which debit and credit postings would be received.

a. Pharmacy Revenues
b. Accounts Receivable—Outpatients
c. Accounts Receivable—Inpatients
d. Cafeteria Sales
e. Bank Loans Payable

18. The following is a list of general ledger accounts. For each account name the journals from which debit and credit postings would be received.

a. Cash—General Checking Account

b. Pharmacy—Supplies Expense
c. Pharmacy—Salaries and Wages
d. Equipment
e. Accounts Payable

19. The following is a list of general ledger accounts. For each account name the journals from which debit and credit postings would be received.

a. Operating Room Revenues
b. Notes Payable
c. General Contributions
d. Deductions from Revenues—Charity Service
e. Accrued Payroll

20. The following is a list of general ledger accounts. For each account name the journals from which debit and credit postings would be received.

a. Prepaid Expense—Insurance
b. Temporary Investments
c. Allowance for Uncollectible Accounts
d. Land
e. Hospital Equity

12
Revenues, Receivables, and Cash Receipts

This chapter is concerned with the basic procedures involved in recording revenues, receivables, and cash receipts. The discussion and illustrations relate to our hypothetical Hartful Hospital whose chart of accounts was outlined in chapter 10, and whose journal and ledger system was introduced in chapter 11. While the procedures described here are similar to those found in actual practice, you should recognize that there is no "ideal" system that is completely applicable to all hospitals. You should not assume, therefore, that the procedures followed by Hartful Hospital are precisely identical to those of any particular "real-life" hospital. The discussion will, however, give you a reasonable understanding of the accounting requirements as well as an insight into certain methods which have been developed to meet those requirements. These observations also apply to the materials of chapters 13 and 14.

Recording Inpatient Revenues

A large majority of the revenues of a hospital are derived from services rendered to inpatients. These services are of 2 major types: (1) the daily room, board, and routine nursing services and (2) the special professional or ancillary services. The accounting objective is to make a prompt and accurate record, on the accrual basis and at the hospital's established rates, of all services rendered, regardless of the amounts (if any) the hospital actually expects to collect for those services. Sometimes hospitals collect less than their full, established service rates, but this has no bearing on the amount of revenue to be recorded when services are rendered to patients. Any differences between gross revenue (measured at full rates) and collectible revenues are recorded as revenue deductions. This procedure permits monetary measurement of earned revenues, "lost" revenues, and collectible revenues.

Daily Inpatient Services

When a person enters the hospital as an inpatient, several different forms are completed in the admitting process. An illustration of one of these forms is presented in figure 55. It is a multipart form,

Figure 55
Inpatient Ledger Card

Hartful Hospital

37

LAST FIRST M I MAIDEN

DATE	ROOM NO	BEDS	RATE	DAYS

BLUE CROSS CASE NO — TOTAL DAYS: BASIC / SUPPL

COMPLETE FINAL DIAGNOSIS

☐ A DISCHARGED ☐ B STILL HOSPITALIZED ☐ C EXPIRED

PATIENT — HOSP NO
STREET — PHONE
CITY & STATE — MAR STATUS
SEX & AGE — BIRTHDATE — BIRTHPLACE
ADM DATE — TIME — SOC SEC NO
I D NO — STATE — INS OR H I B NO
EFF DATE — INS PAID THRU — DISCHARGE DATE & TIME
GROUP NO — KIND OR BENEFIT CODE — RACE — OCCUPATION
FATHER'S NAME — MOTHER'S MAIDEN NAME
NEAREST REL — RELATION — ADDRESS
RESP PARTY — RELATION — ADDRESS
EMPLOYER — OCCUPATION — ADDRESS
ATTN PHY — RELIGION — CHURCH
PREV ADM YR — PASTOR — ADDRESS
ADM DIAGNOSIS — BABY BIRTHDATE — M ☐ F ☐

MED ☐ SUR ☐ PED ☐ OB ☐ EMERG ☐ URG ☐ ELEC ☐

SERVICE CHARGES									CREDITS		
MISCELLANEOUS SERVICE		SUPPLIES (2)	X-RAY (3)	LAB-PATH. (4)	DRUGS (5)	NURSERY (6)	ROOM, FOOD & NURSING (7)	DATE	CASH UNLESS CODED		BALANCE
CODE	AMOUNT								AMOUNT	CODE	
	(1)	SUPPLIES	X-RAY	LAB PATH	DRUGS	NURSERY	ROOM, FOOD & NURSING	TOTAL	CREDITS		BALANCE
TOTAL CHARGES											

SUMMARY OF BILLING										
BASIC										
SUPPL.										
PATIENT'S PORTION										PATIENT'S PORTION

LEDGER COPY

one part of which is routed to the accounting office where it serves as the patient's individual subsidiary ledger card. It is important that information obtained in the admitting process allow for proper classification of the patient (and the related revenues and receivables) according to financial status, medical category, and so forth.

During the period of stay, the inpatient's ledger card will be charged for the services provided, and the appropriate revenue accounts will be credited. The accounting and control systems must provide detailed written evidence of all hospital services provided as well as documentation of the attending physician's authorizations. This evidence appears in the patient's charts, maintained

Figure 56

DAILY REPORT OF DAY RATE SERVICE

Date ____________________ 19 ____

Room No.	Private	Semi-Private	Ward	Room No.	Private	Semi-Private	Ward	Room No.	Private	Semi-Private	Ward	Room No.	Private	Semi-Private	Ward
												Bed Complement TOTAL			
												Additions			
												Deductions			
												Occupancy TOTAL			
								Bed Complement TOTAL							
								Additions							
								Deductions							
								Occupancy TOTAL							
Bed Complement TOTAL				Bed Complement TOTAL											
Additions				Additions											
Deductions				Deductions											
Occupancy TOTAL				Occupancy TOTAL											

BASSINETS

Location	Number	Rate	Amount

SUMMARY

Location	Private Rooms		Semi-Private Rooms		Wards	
	No.	Amount	No.	Amount	No.	Amount
TOTALS						

FORM 842 DAILY REPORT OF DAY RATE SERVICE
PHYSICIANS' RECORD CO., BERWYN, ILLINOIS · PRINTED IN U.S.A.
PENN-WAY HOSPITAL ACCOUNTING SYSTEM

INSTRUCTIONS:

④ **Occupancy Total:** This represents the total amount of day rate service charges to patients for the day and is the sum of the **Bed Complement Total and Additions minus Deductions.**

③ **Deductions:** Total amount resulting from either unoccupied beds or changes in the number of beds in rooms.

② **Additions:** Total amount due to additional beds being placed in rooms or charges for a part of a day.

① **Bed Complement Total:** Total amount based on 100% occupancy of all available beds.

at the nursing stations, and in supporting source documents which are kept in the accounting department. As you will see shortly, the ledger card will be credited for payments received from or on behalf of the patient. And, in many cases, noncash credits for charity and contractual adjustments may be made to the ledger card. Upon the patient's discharge, the medical documents are filed in the medical records department; the financial documents are retained in the accounting department for billing and collection purposes.

A major portion of the charges to inpatients will arise from the provision of room, board, and routine nursing services. These services sometimes are referred to as *routine services* or *daily patient services*. In any event, these charges (and revenues) are compiled from information obtained from the daily census report. Forms and procedures differ, but the determination of charges and revenues for daily patient services basically is a matter of multiplying occupied rooms (beds) by established daily charges for such accommodations. In the Hartful Hospital system, a form known as a day rate service sheet is used as a combination of census report and revenue-charge summary. This form, shown in figure 56, is a preprinted listing of each room and bed in the hospital. It is classified by nursing unit, including an indication of the daily charge for each type of accommodation. The sheet is pretotaled for 100% occupancy. As a part of the midnight census, a line is drawn through each unoccupied-bed designation. The total revenue represented by these unoccupied accommodations is computed and deducted from the 100%-occupancy figures. This produces the gross earned revenues for the day as well as the charge to each patient's ledger card. The objective is to secure a high degree of assurance that debits are made to the proper patients and that credits are made to the proper revenue accounts in correct amounts for all daily services provided.

SPECIAL PROFESSIONAL (ANCILLARY) SERVICES

Most services rendered to patients must be ordered by a physician. Such orders are written in the patient's chart by attending physicians and prescribe all necessary patient services. The services so prescribed are requisitioned by nurses or nursing station personnel acting under the nurses' supervision. In order to obtain adequate accounting control over the charges and revenues arising from these services, therefore, the full cooperation of all nursing personnel is essential.

As various ancillary services are required for patients, nursing station personnel prepare requisition-charge tickets such as the one illustrated in figure 57. A separate set of tickets may be used for each type of service. Each ticket may be prenumbered, and charge tickets for each service may be of different colors to facilitate identification and sorting procedures.

The charge tickets often are prepared in triplicate. The original and duplicate copies go to the professional department which renders the service, while the triplicate copy remains at the nursing station. The ticket gives the professional department the authority to render the prescribed service. Periodically during each day, the original copies of the charge tickets are collected from the professional departments and are taken to the hospital's accounting offices; the duplicates remain with the professional department. The charge tickets are usually priced either in the professional departments or in the accounting office.

Each day, an accounting employee sorts the charge tickets by color (department). Each color group is then totaled to determine the day's revenue for each departmental service. The same tickets are re-sorted according to individual patient so that appropriate charges can be made to the proper patient's ledger card. Naturally a reconciliation must be made to ascertain that the total debits to the ledger cards equal the total of all tickets and that the total credits to the various revenue accounts equal the total of all tickets. In some systems a worksheet of some kind is prepared to summarize the charge tickets and make the necessary reconciliations.

Figure 57
Requisition-Charge Ticket

LABORATORY

Walk ☐
Chair ☐
Bed ☐

Check If Patient Is Leaving Today ....m. ☐
★ If this is a CREDIT, check here and also circle amount ☐

U 45059

Patient's Name ____________

Room No. ______

If OUT-Patient Address ____________ Age ___

Requested by Dr. ____________ Date ______ 19__

Adm.	Repeat	EXAMINATION OR TEST REQUESTED	CHARGE ★
		Blood Count — Complete ☐ R.B.C. ☐ W.B.C. ☐ Hb. ☐ Diff. ☐	
		Urinalysis — Voided ☐ Catheterized ☐ Time Collected ______.M.	
		Kahn ☐ Kline ☐ Kolmer ☐ Mazzini ☐ Wassermann ☐ ______	
		Special Tests, etc. (Specify) ______	

Medical, etc. ☐ Surgical ☐ Operation Scheduled for—Date ______ 19__ Time ______.M.

Remarks ____________ Signed ____________

1 Please Send 1st and 2nd Copies to Laboratory

Number Checked Off on Control Sheet ☐ Posted to Patient's Account ☐

INPATIENT REVENUE JOURNAL

Whatever the data collection system may be, daily journal entries must be made in the general ledger to record debits to the inpatient receivables control account and credits to the various revenue accounts. We will assume that Hartful Hospital uses the day rate service sheet and the requisition-charge tickets to gather the necessary data. These data are entered in the inpatient revenue journal as indicated in figure 58. This is merely a sample entry to illustrate the manner in which a day's inpatient revenues may be recorded. A similar entry is made each day of the month. You will have to imagine that all 31 lines of the journal are filled. Assume that these 31 daily entries add to the column totals shown in the journal.

It is assumed here that a daily worksheet summary of the day rate service sheet and all charge tickets is prepared in the accounting office. The total of the day rate service sheet and the total of the charge tickets together make up the total $14,645 debit to inpatient receivables (account 1031.0) for May 5, 1977. Similarly, an analysis of the day rate service sheet and of the charge tickets provides the totals credited to each revenue center account for the same day. Each day's entry should be cross-footed to see that the total of credits equals the amount of the debit to inpatient receivables.

Thus, a daily summary of charges and revenues is entered on a single line of the journal. When this procedure is followed, an indication of charge ticket numbers in the journal is not feasible. This requires the retention of the worksheet or other form on which the summary totals were determined, however, as well as retention of the day rate service sheets and charge tickets in appropriate files. In this way the necessary "audit trails" are provided for the hospital's internal and external auditors. In other words, the system must facilitate the auditor's tracing of journal entries to source documents and must provide safeguards against either the omission of transactions or the recording of the same transaction more than once. An alternative would be to journalize the charge tickets individually, but this often is not feasible in a manual system because of the large number of charge tickets issued each day.

Notice the sundry debit and credit columns on the far right-hand side of the journal. These columns are provided for occasional debits or credits that may be required but for which appropriate separate columns have not been included in the journal. The journal should be designed so that the use of these sundry columns will rarely be necessary.

As these daily summaries of charges and revenues are entered in the journal, daily postings of charges are made to the inpatients' subsidiary ledger cards on the basis of the information provided by the day rate service sheet and the individual charge tickets sorted according to patient name, hospital number, or room number. The total of these debit postings, of course, must equal the total debited to inpatient receivables in the journal. When this equality has been established, a check mark (√) is placed in the journal column provided for that indication.

No daily postings are made to the general ledger accounts. At month-end, however, the various columns of the journal are totaled and cross-footed to insure that the total of the debit columns equals the total of the credit columns. Each column total is then posted to the appropriate general ledger account as indicated at the foot of each column.

As noted earlier, the Hartful Hospital procedure is a manual system; it is described here in simplified terms to illustrate easily certain principles. Even a small hospital, however, will find that the use of a posting machine and other accounting equipment is necessary

Figure 58
Inpatient Revenue Journal

1977 Date		(✓)	Inpatient Receivables Dr.	Nursing Service Revenue Credits					
				Nursing Units	Operating Rooms	Emergency Rooms	Central Supply	Other Units	Other Units
5	5	✓	14,645	6,250	900	450	1,100		
	Totals		453,995	187,500	26,100	14,400	34,100		
			Debit	Credit	Credit	Credit	Credit	Credit	Credit
			1031.0	3021.1	3210.1	3230.1	3250.1		

because of the great volume of activity. Posting machines employ carbons and identical columns which allow, in a single operation, the making of the journal entry and a posting to patients' ledger cards. The machine brings forward a new balance on each card and accumulates totals for the various categories of revenue.

Recording Outpatient Revenues

Charges and revenues for departmental services to outpatients also may be determined in much the same way as described above for inpatient accounting. A charge ticket is originated either at a centralized outpatient reception desk or in the professional depart-

Other Professional Service Revenue Credits					Sundry Debits and Credits		
Laboratory	Radiology	Pharmacy	Anesthesia	Other Units	Account Numbers	Dr.	Cr.
1,820	2,135	1,040	950				
56,420	88,835	24,960	21,680				
Credit	Credit	Credit	Credit	Credit			
4011.1	4040.1	4070.1	4080.1				

ments providing the outpatient services. In some cases, the outpatient charge tickets will be summarized by servicing-department personnel in daily service logs. A copy of this log, along with copies of related charge tickets, is collected daily by the accounting department. On the basis of these documents, a daily summary of outpatient charges and revenues is prepared and entered on a single line of the outpatient revenue journal as illustrated in figure 59 for May 5, 1977. The worksheet on which this summary was developed, the logs, and the charge tickets, should be retained in order to provide an appropriate audit trail.

Figure 59
Outpatient Revenue Journal

1977 Date		(√)	Outpatient Receivables Dr.	Nursing Service Revenue Credits: Operating Rooms	Emergency Rooms	Central Supply	Other Units
5	5	√	2,160	150	480	290	
Totals			64,800	3,900	9,000	5,700	
			Debit	Credit	Credit	Credit	Credit
			1044.0	3210.2	3230.2	3250.2	

Daily postings are made of charges to outpatient subsidiary ledger cards. Again, a special column (√) is provided in the journal to indicate that the individual debit postings to the ledger cards equal the total debited to the outpatient receivables column in the journal. At month's end, the various columns are totaled, and the totals are posted to the general ledger accounts. Entries in the sundry columns, however, must be posted individually.

Recording Cash Receipts

An immediate written record should be made of all cash receipts. In many hospital accounting systems, this record is obtained

Other Professional Service Revenue Credits					Sundry Debits and Credits		
Laboratory	Radiology	Pharmacy	Anesthesia	Other Units	Account Numbers	Dr.	Cr.
470	510	210	50				
17,040	21,630	5,880	1,650				
Credit	Credit	Credit	Credit	Credit			
4011.2	4040.2	4070.2	4080.2				

through the preparation of a *cash receipt slip* such as the one illustrated in figure 60. Cash receipts are of 2 types: (1) mail receipts and (2) counter receipts. Two employees may be assigned responsibility for opening incoming mail. Working together, they extract the cash items from the mail and list these items on a mail remittance report. One copy of the report is routed directly to the accounting department, one copy (with the cash items) goes to cashiering, and one copy is retained by the mail openers.

Upon receipt of the cash items from the incoming mail, the cashier issues a cash receipt slip for the total amount. One copy is given to the mail openers, one copy is sent to the accounting department, and one copy is retained by the cashier. For counter receipts, the cashier prepares individual cash receipt slips, again in triplicate. One copy is given to the patient, one copy is sent to the accounting department as a medium for postings to the patients' ledger, and one copy is filed permanently in numerical sequence. All cash items, both mail and counter receipts, should be carefully controlled and should be deposited daily and intact; cash disbursements should never be made from cash receipts. A copy of the bank deposit slip is routed to the accounting office.

At the end of each day, the cash receipt slips are summarized and entered in the cash receipts journal. An accounting employee will compare the cash receipt slips with the mail remittance report and with the duplicate bank deposit slip. The cash receipt slips, sorted by patient name, and the mail remittance report can be used to make the necessary credit postings to the individual patient's ledger card.

Figure 60
Cash Receipt Slip

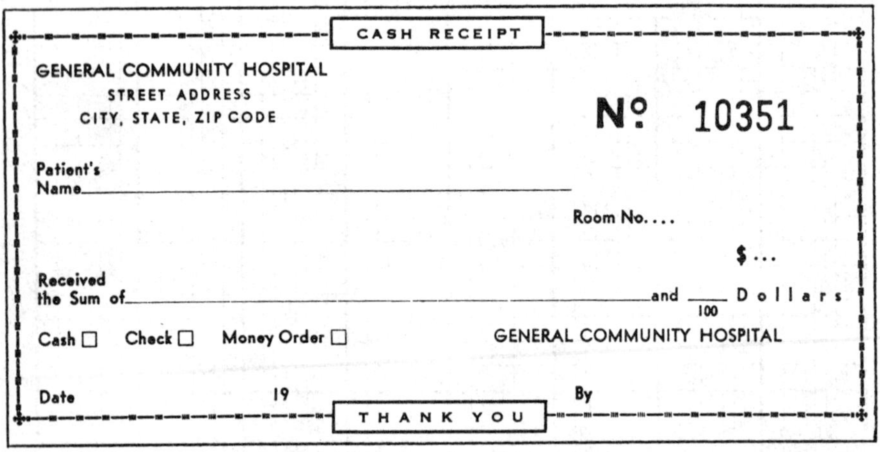
CASH RECEIPT

GENERAL COMMUNITY HOSPITAL
STREET ADDRESS
CITY, STATE, ZIP CODE

Nº 10351

Patient's Name ____________________

Room No. . . .

$ . . .

Received the Sum of ____________________ and ___/100 Dollars

Cash ☐ Check ☐ Money Order ☐

GENERAL COMMUNITY HOSPITAL

Date ______ 19 ___ By ____________________

THANK YOU

Hartful Hospital's cash receipts journal is illustrated in figure 61. A sample entry for May 5, 1977, has been included to indicate how the cash receipt transactions for the day are recorded. If cash receipt slips are issued in several different numerical series concurrently, an indication of cash receipt slip numbers in the journal may not be practicable. Where this is the case, either the slips must be journalized individually or a worksheet summary must be developed to provide an adequate audit trail.

The posting of entries in the cash receipts journal is the same as that for the revenue journals. Daily postings are made to the patients' ledger; monthly postings of column totals are made to the general ledger.

Notice that the cash receipts journal includes columns for debits to the revenue deduction accounts. To describe how these columns are used, assume a discharged patient with an account balance of $1,250. On May 5, 1977, $1,000 is received by the hospital from the patient's third-party sponsor in full payment of the account. The entry to be made by the hospital is as follows:

Cash	1011.0	$1,000	
Contractual Adjustments	5520.0	250	
Inpatient Receivables—Discharged	1032.0		$1,250

It is assumed here that the $250 difference between the patient's hospital bill and the amount reimbursed by the third party is not, under the terms of the contract, recoverable from the patient.

Thus, in Hartful Hospital's system, debits are made to the revenue deduction accounts as patients' accounts are paid. Here the cash receipts journal is designed to provide columns for those debits. In other systems, however, a separate *receivables adjustments and allowances journal* or *revenue deductions journal* is employed to account for these items. But, whatever the procedure may be, it is essential that all noncash credits to receivables be authorized and approved by a responsible hospital official who has no access to the hospital's cash receipts and receivables records. This is necessary in order to protect against a theft of cash receipts which may be covered up by unwarranted write-offs of accounts receivable balances which were really paid.

The method used by Hartful Hospital in accounting for revenue deductions is satisfactory as an accounting routine. Care must be taken, however, to make sure that revenue deductions are recognized on the accrual basis; the deductions must be recognized in the same period as the related revenues. To accomplish this, an adjusting entry is required at the end of each period for which a balance sheet and income statement are prepared. To illustrate the procedure with respect to contractual adjustments, let us assume that a hospital had $3,600,000 of revenues in 1977 and that $600,000 of this total remains in accounts receivable at December 31, 1977. In collecting the $3,000,000 of accounts receivable during the year, assume that contractual adjustments totaling $150,000 were recorded. In other words, contractual adjustments averaged about 5% of receivables.

This means that the year-end accounts receivable probably include $30,000 (i.e., 5% of $600,000) of unrecognized contractual adjustments. This $30,000 must be recognized as revenue deductions in 1977, the year in which the related revenues are recorded. The required December 31, 1977, adjusting entry is

Contractual Adjustments	5520.0	$30,000	
Allowance for Uncollectible Accounts—Contractual Adjustments	1062.0		$30,000

As the $600,000 of accounts receivable are collected in 1978, the actual contractual adjustments on these accounts are recorded in accordance with the routine described for Hartful Hospital, without regard to the adjusting entry. A reversing entry (the reverse of the

Figure 61
Cash Receipts Journal

				Revenue Deduction Credits		
1977		Cash Receipt	Cash	Contractual	Charity	
Date		Slip Nos.	Dr.	Adjustments	Service	Other
5	5	443-657	13,815	1,040	480	
		Totals	477,500	31,600	14,400	
			Debit	Debit	Debit	Debit
			1011.0	5520.0	5540.0	

above adjusting entry) can be made by the hospital on January 1, 1978, to avoid recording the same contractual adjustments twice (in 1977 and 1978). Or, if one prefers, the adjusting entry at the end of the first reporting period in 1978 can merely adjust to the appropriate balance at that time the allowance for uncollectible accounts' contractual adjustments.

A similar procedure can be followed for revenue deductions arising from the provision of charity service. The treatment of bad debts, however, generally is somewhat different, and we will defer a discussion of this matter to chapter 16.

Accounts Receivable		Credits	Other Credits		Sundry Debits and Credits		
Inpatients			Cafeteria	General	Account		
Inhouse	Discharged	Outpatients	Sales	Contrbns.	Numbers	Dr.	Cr.
1,420	11,350	1,930	560	75			
43,020	401,850	57,900	18,480	2,250			
Credit 1031.0	Credit 1032.0	Credit 1044.0	Credit 5061.0	Credit 5155.0			

Reconciling Control Accounts and Subsidiary Records

As you have seen, Hartful Hospital maintains 3 receivables control accounts in its general ledger. These accounts, with assumed May 1, 1977, balances, are as follows:

1031.0 Inpatient Receivables—Inhouse	$110,000
1032.0 Inpatient Receivables—Discharged	800,000
1044.0 Outpatient Receivables	16,000

Hartful Hospital also maintains a separate patients' subsidiary ledger for *each* of these control accounts. Let us assume that the total of the individual debit balances in each subsidiary ledger at

May 1, 1977, agrees with the debit balance of the related control account at May 1, 1977.

During the month of May, as entries were made in the revenue and cash receipt journals, daily postings of charges and credits were made to the patients' subsidiary ledgers. Month-end postings of journal column totals were made to the control accounts in the general ledger as illustrated below:

Inpatient Receivables Inhouse

BB	110,000	CRJ	43,020
IRJ	453,995	GJ	412,975
CB	108,000		

Inpatient Receivables Discharged

BB	800,000	CRJ	401,850
GJ	412,975		
CB	811,125		

Outpatient Receivables

BB	16,000	CRJ	57,900
ORJ	64,800		
CB	22,900		

Posting references:

BB = Beginning balance
IRJ = Inpatient revenue journal
CRJ = Cash receipts journal
GJ = General journal
ORJ = Outpatient revenue journal
CB = Closing balance

All of the postings in this illustration are drawn from the journals shown previously in this chapter, except for postings in the general journal. Not mentioned earlier is the fact that Hartful Hospital, as inpatients are discharged, makes entries in the general journal to transfer the unpaid account balances from the "inhouse" to the "discharged" classification of receivables. That is, during May, patients whose unpaid balances together totaled $412,975 were discharged from the hospital.

Now, after the month-end postings are made as indicated above, we have a May 31, 1977, balance in each of the 3 control accounts for receivables. The individual ledger-card balances in each of the 3 subsidiary ledgers are totaled. In the absence of accounting errors, the tape total of the inhouse inpatient receivables ledger should be $108,000. Similarly, the discharged inpatient receivables ledger cards should total $811,125, and the outpatient ledger cards should total $22,900. If a subsidiary ledger does not reconcile with the corresponding control account, the situation should be thoroughly investigated, and the reasons for the discrepancy identified. Considering the importance of recording hospital receivables accurately and the availability of efficient data processing equipment, there simply is no excuse for a failure to make regular monthly reconciliations of accounts receivable controls and subsidiary ledgers.

You now have seen the Hartful Hospital accounting system as related to its revenue and cash receipt transactions. The next chapter deals with the payroll accounting procedures of the hospital.

QUESTIONS

1. State the basic objective of accounting for services rendered to inpatients and outpatients.

2. Describe briefly how the amounts to be charged to inpatients for services rendered to them generally are determined.

3. Describe briefly how the amounts to be charged to outpatients for services rendered to them generally are determined.

4. How often should postings be made from the inpatient and outpatient revenue journals? Explain.

5. Describe briefly how the daily amounts to be debited to cash and credited to patients' accounts receivable generally are determined.

6. How often should postings be made from the cash receipts journal? Explain.

7. Teeny Hospital's general ledger contained the following receivables control account balances at October 31:

Inpatient receivables—inhouse	$ 57,000
Inpatient receivables—discharged	216,000
Outpatient receivables	19,000

The inpatient receivables column in the November inpatient revenue journal totaled $98,000, and the outpatients receivables column of the November outpatient revenue journal totaled $34,000. The receivables columns of the November cash receipts journal provided the following totals:

Inpatient receivables—inhouse	$ 11,400
Inpatient receivables—discharged	107,600
Outpatient receivables	32,300

The November general journal contained a number of entries which transferred a total of $101,900 in inpatient receivables from the inhouse account to the discharged account.

If you were to prepare adding machine tape totals of the individual patient ledger card balances at November 30, what is the total that you would expect to find in each of the following subsidiary ledgers?

a. Inpatient receivables—inhouse
b. Inpatient receivables—discharged
c. Outpatient receivables

8. James Roe, an inpatient, received the following services on November 7, 1977:

Daily patient service (room and board)	$ 72
Operating room	50
Central supply	24
Laboratory	16
Pharmacy	9
Anesthesia	25
Telephone (long-distance calls)	14

Explain how you would enter this information in the journal and ledger systems described in the text of chapter 12.

9. On October 12, 1978, Dowd Hospital borrowed $50,000 from a local bank by issuance of a 120-day, 9% note. Explain how you would enter this transaction in the hospital's cash receipts journal.

10. Jane Doe, when admitted to Dawson Hospital, was classified as a charity service patient. Jane was admitted on June 1 and was discharged from the hospital on June 8. Services rendered to her during this period totaled $672 in terms of the hospital's full, established rates. What entries should be made by Dawson Hospital (a) to record the services rendered to Jane and (b) to give recognition to the fact that nothing will be collected for those services? Indicate the name of the journal in which these entries will be made.

11. What are some of the basic features of a good system of internal control over revenues and cash receipts?

12. Dodson Hospital's daily patient service (routine service) charge is $72 per day for a private accommodation. On August 29, 1978, these charges were correctly entered in the inpatient revenue journal but, in posting to the accounts receivable subsidiary ledger, a patient's account was inadvertently charged for only $27. How might this error be detected?

13 Payroll Accounting Procedures

The discussion presented in this chapter deals with some of the basic accounting principles and practices relating to the hospital payroll. You may be aware that employee compensation often represents two-thirds or more of the operating expenses of a hospital. That the majority of expense is represented by labor costs, however, should not be surprising in view of these facts:

1. The hospital is largely a personal-service, labor-intensive business which generally requires 2 to 3 employees per patient.
2. The hospital necessarily must employ many highly skilled specialists and professional people who command relatively large salaries.
3. The nature and importance of health care services is such that high-quality, adequately paid personnel should be employed.
4. Competition from industrial and commercial businesses for such personnel has led to an increased general level of wages.

Like any other business, the hospital also is subject to minimum wage laws, a variety of payroll taxes, and other governmental regulations which have added significant amounts to employee compensation costs. In addition, the unionization of hospital workers and the emergence of employee pension plans are 2 relatively recent developments that have had a major impact on hospital payrolls and payroll-related expenditures.

It seems clear, therefore, that particular emphasis must be given in hospitals to personnel management and labor cost control. This requires, among other things, the development of accurate and reliable information about payroll and payroll-related costs through the use of sound accounting methods and practices. In this chapter, through a continuation of the Hartful Hospital illustration, you will have ample opportunity to study some of the procedures that may be followed by hospitals in accounting for employee-compensation costs. If your interest in this topic goes beyond the scope of this chapter, you will find a more advanced discussion of payroll accounting and management in the author's *Hospital Financial Accounting—Theory and Practice*.[1]

Compilation of Gross Payrolls

Hartful Hospital, like most hospitals, maintains a centralized personnel department whose basic functions include the recruitment and orientation of new employees and the keeping of permanent personnel records. In addition to the many records that must be kept for tax purposes, the personnel department keeps a complete, up-to-date employment history or service file for all employees. The centralization of these functions and records localizes responsibility, promotes efficiency, and facilitates control over the size, quality, and cost of the hospital labor force.

Figure 62
Employee Time Record

Name ______________________ Month ____________ 19 ___

Emp. No. or Dept. Floor Position

DATES *		ON	OFF	Hrs.	ON	OFF	Hrs.	ON	OFF	Hrs.	TOTAL HOURS	Employees DO NOT WRITE IN THIS SPACE
1	16											TOTAL ☐ Hours ☐ Days
2	17											Rate per ☐ Hour ☐ Day
3	18											Total Cash Compensation
4	19											Other Compensation
5	20											
6	21											
7	22											TOTAL EARNINGS
8	23											Deductions:
9	24											Withholding Tax
10	25											
11	26											
12	27											
13	28											
14	29											TOTAL DEDUCTIONS
15	30											
	31											AMOUNT OF CHECK

* Cross Out Column of Dates which Does Not Apply

CODE: A—Absent, deduct; AN—Absent, no deduction; V—Vacation, no deduction; S—Sick, deduct; Ⓢ Sick, no deduction

TOTAL ☐ Hours ☐ Days

SUPERVISOR

FORM P-514 PHYSICIANS' RECORD CO., BERWYN, ILLINOIS - PRINTED IN U.S.A. Time and Salary Computation

The personnel department, in cooperation with the accounting department of the hospital, should develop and administer a clear-cut procedure for recording and reporting the time worked by all employees. Some hospitals use time clocks for this purpose; others use manually prepared time reports or time cards such as the one illustrated in figure 62. In either case, the department head or supervisor signs and approves the time records before they are sent to the accounting department's payroll accounting unit for processing. It is essential that these time records be complete and

[1]L. Vann Seawell, *Hospital Financial Accounting—Theory and Practice* (Chicago: The Hospital Financial Management Association, 1975).

accurate as to attendance and hours worked, and that they otherwise provide for full compliance with the provisions of the Fair Labor Standards Act and other laws regulating employment. These records also should be designed to facilitate the computation of the gross payroll and the development of the necessary labor statistics. Analyses of the payroll in terms of hours as well as dollars are extremely important to the financial management of hospitals.

The compilation of the gross payroll is not a particularly difficult task. Accounting employees independent of the timekeeping function examine all time cards for hourly employees to determine that the records are properly executed and approved and that the hours worked by each employee are correctly computed. These must then be multiplied by authorized rates of pay. If overtime hours have been worked, a separate calculation is required. Payment for benefits such as vacations, holidays, and sick pay also affects computation of gross earnings.

To illustrate, let us assume that a particular employee is paid $2.60 per hour for a regular workweek of 40 hours. This employee's gross earnings for a week during which he worked 48 hours ordinarily would be $124.80 (i.e., 48 hours @ $2.60). The Fair Labor Standards Act of 1938 (popularly known as the Wages and Hours Law) provides not only for a minimum hourly wage but also requires that time and a half be paid for hours in excess of 40 hours worked in a given week. The computation of the employee's earnings then becomes

Regular workweek (40 hours @ $2.60)	$104.00
Overtime (8 hours @ $2.60)	20.80
Overtime premium (8 hours @ $1.30)	10.40
Gross earnings	$135.20

Application of the provisions of the Wages and Hours Law to the compensation of hospital employees is substantially more involved than indicated here, but we cannot pursue the matter further in this book. It is important to note, however, that good payroll accounting practice should provide for the separate recording of overtime compensation because such information is useful in evaluating the utilization of personnel by department heads.

For salaried employees, the gross pay per period is a fixed amount which, once determined, does not vary until the salary is changed. All changes in salaries or in hourly rates should enter into the calculation of gross pay only when such changes are authorized in writing by the personnel department. The payroll clerk should not act on the basis of verbal orders. The time records kept for salaried personnel also should be properly executed, approved, and signed by department heads or supervisors.

PAYROLL DEDUCTIONS

Payroll accounting is complicated greatly by the various deductions or withholdings which must be made from employees' gross earnings so as to determine the amounts in which paychecks should be written. Many of these withholdings are required by legislation enacted by the federal, state, and local governments, which impose a number of taxes on salaries and wages paid to hospital personnel. Other deductions arise in connection with group insurance, retirement, and savings-plan agreements with employees. Some of these deductions are described below.

INCOME TAXES

The federal income tax program has operated on a pay-as-you-go basis for more than 30 years. This payment system requires employers to withhold an amount approximating the income tax from employees' wages due on such wages. The amount, generally determined from tax withholding tables furnished by the government, varies according to the amount of taxable wages, the length of the payroll period, the employee's marital status, and the number of dependents (exemptions) claimed by the employee.

The income tax amounts so withheld by the hospital must be remitted to the government at times specified by law. For most hospitals, remittance must often be made within a few days following each pay period. This is accomplished by a deposit of the withheld amounts in an authorized government depository (bank). In addition, a quarterly report must be filed to provide a summary of all wages paid and tax withheld during each quarter. Rather severe penalties and interest charges are imposed on employers who fail to withhold taxes and deposit taxes, or to file payroll returns according to the prescribed manner and times.

Most states and some large cities also levy income taxes. In such cases, hospitals often must withhold these taxes also. Amounts withheld, determined by formulas or tables, are remitted periodically to the governmental units as required by the particular laws.

FICA (SOCIAL SECURITY) TAXES

The Federal Insurance Contributions Act (FICA), popularly called social security, provides for a tax on employees' earnings to finance a federal program of old-age, survivors', disability, and hospital insurance benefits for workers and members of their families. Hospitals and their employees were at first exempt from this law which was originally enacted in 1935, but the basic law has been amended many times to extend its coverage and to increase the tax rate, the amount of wages subject to tax, and benefits provided. The 1965 amendment included enactment of the Federal Hospital Insurance Program, widely known as Medicare.

As is true of income tax, the FICA tax is required to be withheld by the hospital from taxable wage payments to employees. The 1935 Act provided for a 1% tax on the first $3,000 of wages paid to each employee in any one year, but subsequent amendments to the law have increased both the tax rate and the base earnings (maximum annual earnings subject to tax) substantially. For 1977, the FICA tax was 5.85% of the first $16,500 of taxable wages paid to each employee. In other words, the maximum annual tax in 1977 is $965.25 per employee. No doubt this amount will be increased in the future either by increasing the tax rate, base earnings, or both.

So, 5.85% of each employee's salary or wages (until that employee has earned $16,500 in a given year) is withheld by the hospital as FICA taxes. Provisions of the FICA tax legislation, however, also require an equal contribution by the hospital: the hospital must "match" the amount of FICA tax withheld from employees' wages. Thus, a tax is imposed *on the hospital* of 5.85% of the first $16,500 of wages paid to each of its employees. To put it another way, the FICA tax is 11.7%: half is withheld from employees' wages, and half is paid by the hospital. Both the employer's and the employees' FICA taxes are remitted by the hospital to the government at the same time as and together with the federal income tax (FIT) withholdings.

Entries for the withholding of FIT and FICA, and for the accrual of the hospital's share of FICA, are illustrated later in this chapter for Hartful Hospital, but a simpler example might be useful at this point. Let us assume that a single employee earns a salary of $1,175 per month (less than $16,500 per year), all of which is subject to tax. The monthly entries for this employee would be as follows:

Salaries and Wages Expense	$1,175.00	
FICA Withheld and Accrued		$ 68.74
FIT Withheld		235.00
Accrued Payroll Liability		871.26
To record payroll, assuming 20% FIT and 5.85% FICA withholdings.		
Accrued Payroll Liability	$ 871.26	
Cash		$ 871.26
To record issuance of paycheck.		
Employee Benefits (expense)	$ 68.74	
FICA Withheld and Accrued		$ 68.74
To accrue hospital's share of FICA tax.		
FICA Withheld and Accrued	$ 137.48	
FIT Withheld	235.00	
Cash		$ 372.48
To record remittance of payroll taxes withheld and accrued.		

You should recognize that the matching FICA tax imposed on the hospital represents a significant item of expense. Too, there also is the considerable clerical expense involved in computing and recording withholdings, in preparing the many payroll tax reports, and in keeping the detailed payroll records required by these laws.

OTHER DEDUCTIONS

In addition to the compulsory tax withholdings, a variety of other items may be withheld from salary and wage payments to employees. These withholdings usually require the written consent of the employee. Included in this category are deductions for government savings bonds or tax-sheltered annuity programs; premiums for health, accident, hospital, and life insurance; deductions for union membership dues; deductions for the employee's share of pension- and retirement-plan costs; withholdings related to employee credit union savings or debts; and withholdings representing employees' voluntary contributions to the Community Chest or other charities. At specified intervals, the hospital must summarize these withholdings in appropriate reports and remit the amounts withheld to the proper agencies.

RECORDING THE PAYROLL

On the basis of time cards, time reports, and other source documents that have been collected from the various departments, the payroll clerk is able to compute the gross pay of each employee for the pay period involved. The payroll tax deductions then are calculated for each employee by the application of tax rates and the use of tax tables. Other deductions are determined on the basis of written agreements and authorizations obtained from employees. A final step is the subtraction of total deductions from gross pay to arrive at net pay for each employee. All of these data then are entered on the face of the time card or record (refer again to figure 62) for each employee.

Next, a payroll check is prepared for each employee in the net pay amount indicated on the employee's time card. A sample payroll check is illustrated in figure 63. Notice that the upper portion is a stub which provides, for the employee's personal records, complete information as to gross earnings, deductions, and net pay.

Figure 63
Employee Payroll Check

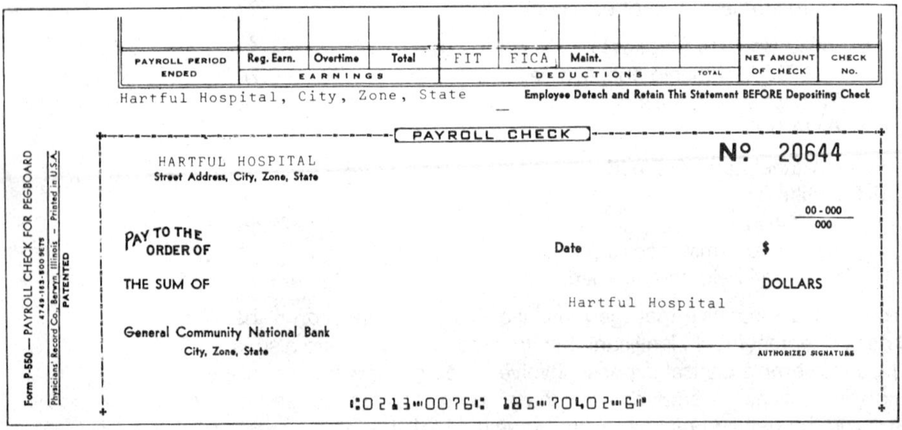

The individual time cards (or carbon copies of the payroll checks), sorted by department, are now summarized to obtain departmental totals for gross pay, deductions, and net pay. These totals then are entered in the payroll journal as indicated in figure 64. (An alternative procedure would be to list each employee in the journal individually, but this may not be feasible.) The illustrative entry includes figures for the nursing service administrative office only, with FIT and FICA withholdings assumed to be 20% and 6%, respectively. We also assume, for simplicity, that Hartful Hospital pays all of its employees once each month. The column totals shown in the journal therefore are totals for May 1977. If the hospital paid its employees every 2 weeks or twice each month, a separate journal would be prepared for each pay period.

As indicated in the payroll journal, May payroll withholdings were $48,400 for federal income taxes and $16,520 for FICA taxes. The hospital's matching share of FICA taxes for the month is recorded in the general journal by the following entry on May 31, 1977:

Employee Benefits—FICA	8710.0	$16,520	
FICA Withheld and Accrued	2036.0		$16,520
To accrue hospital's share of FICA taxes on May payroll.			

In the next chapter you will see the entries that are made by Hartful Hospital to voucher and pay the payroll taxes withheld and accrued.

Notice that the May net payroll of $227,080 is not credited to cash (even though the payroll checks have already been written) but to the accrued payroll liability account (account 2031.0). As you will see in the next chapter, a single voucher is prepared in this amount and is entered in the hospital's voucher register as follows:

Accrued Payroll	2031.0	$227,080	
Accounts Payable	2020.0		$227,080
To record payroll voucher.			

Immediately following this, a check for $227,080 is drawn against the hospital's general checking account and is entered in the cash disbursements journal as shown below:

Accounts Payable	2020.0	$227,080	
Cash	1011.0		$227,080
To record issuance of check for May payroll.			

This check is deposited in the hospital's payroll checking account but no entry is made in the payroll checking account to record the deposit. The individual payroll checks, you remember, were drawn on the payroll checking account but no entry was made to that account for those checks. When the payroll checks are cashed by employees, the payroll checking account automatically clears to the zero or imprest balance maintained in the account. This procedure removes a large volume of paychecks from general checking and simplifies reconciliation of the payroll checking account.

Each departmental total in the gross pay column is posted at the end of the month to the general ledger salaries and wages expense accounts indicated. Other postings to the general ledger are of column totals. In addition to those in the general ledger, postings also must be made to the employees' individual earnings records which often take the form illustrated in figure 65. This detailed record, which is required by tax laws and regulations, is in effect a subsidiary ledger supporting the departmental salaries and wages expense accounts. (In some systems, the payroll subsidiary ledger

Figure 64
Payroll Journal

1977 Date		Department	Check Numbers	Gross Payroll Account Numbers	Gross Payroll Amount Dr.	Deductions from Payroll Credits: FIT Withheld	FICA Withheld	Other	Total	Accrued Payroll Cr.
5	31	Nursing Services:								
		Administrative Office	231-233	6010.1	2,750	550	165		715	2,035
		Nursing Units		6021.1	161,400					
		Operating Rooms		6210.1	8,200					
		Emergency Rooms		6230.1	6,400					
		Central Supply		6250.1	7,700					
		Other Professional Services:								
		Administrative Office		7010.1	3,800					
		Laboratory		7011.1	8,200					
		Radiology		7040.1	7,700					
		Pharmacy		7070.1	4,900					
		Anesthesia		7080.1	5,500					
		Medical Staff		8030.1	12,000					
		General Services:								
		Administrative Office		8040.1	2,000					
		Dietary		8050.1	9,400					
		Plant O. & M.		8060.1	6,200					
		Housekeeping		8090.1	7,500					
		Laundry		8110.1	6,800					
		Fiscal Services:								
		Administrative Office		8211.1	4,100					
		Accounting		8212.1	6,700					
		Admitting		8241.1	5,300					
		Administrator's Office		8310.1	5,250					
		Administrative Services:								
		Administrative Office		8311.1	2,200					
		Purchasing		8331.1	3,900					
		Personnel		8371.1	4,100					
		Totals			292,000	48,400	16,520		64,920	227,080
					Debit	Credit	Credit	Credit	Credit	Credit
						2035.0	2036.0			2031.0

Figure 65
Employees' Individual Earnings Record

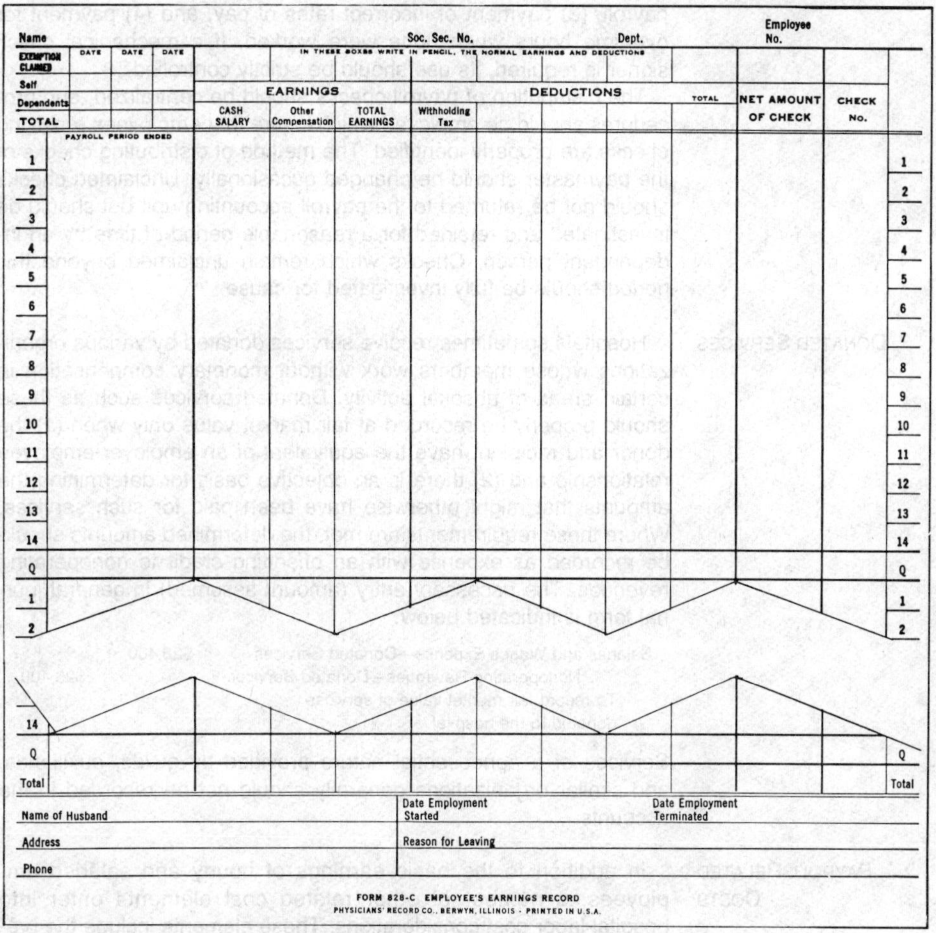

Name | Soc. Sec. No. | Dept. | Employee No.

EXEMPTION CLAIMED | DATE | DATE | DATE | IN THESE BOXES WRITE IN PENCIL, THE NORMAL EARNINGS AND DEDUCTIONS

Self

Dependents

TOTAL

PAYROLL PERIOD ENDED	EARNINGS			DEDUCTIONS					NET AMOUNT OF CHECK	CHECK No.
	CASH SALARY	Other Compensation	TOTAL EARNINGS	Withholding Tax				TOTAL		
1										1
2										2
3										3
4										4
5										5
6										6
7										7
8										8
9										9
10										10
11										11
12										12
13										13
14										14
Q										Q
1										1
2										2
14										
Q										Q
Total										Total

Name of Husband | Date Employment Started | Date Employment Terminated

Address | Reason for Leaving

Phone

FORM 828-C EMPLOYEE'S EARNINGS RECORD
PHYSICIANS' RECORD CO., BERWYN, ILLINOIS · PRINTED IN U.S.A.

consists of individual files for each employee containing either the time cards or copies of the payroll checks.) The information in this subsidiary ledger is needed in the preparation of various quarterly and annual tax reports and forms.

The employees responsible for compilation of payrolls should neither sign nor distribute payroll checks. Once prepared, the unsigned checks should be examined by the disbursing authority who should be satisfied, insofar as feasible, as to their accuracy and authenticity. This may involve a check of certain computations on a sample basis and a comparison of payees and pay rates with independently controlled personnel records. (In many instances, these procedures are performed by the hospital's internal auditors.)

Care particularly must be given to (1) inclusion of nonexistent persons on the payroll of a department, (2) issuance of any checks to former employees whose names have not been removed from the payroll, (3) payment of incorrect rates of pay, and (4) payment for overtime hours when none were worked. If a mechanical check signer is required, its use should be strictly controlled.

The distribution of payroll checks should be centralized, and procedures should be employed which insure that employees receiving checks are properly identified. The method of distributing checks or the paymaster should be changed occasionally. Unclaimed checks should not be returned to the payroll accounting unit but should be investigated and retained for a reasonable period of time by an independent person. Checks which remain unclaimed beyond this period should be fully investigated for cause.

Donated Services

Hospitals sometimes receive services donated by various organizations whose members work without monetary compensation in certain areas of hospital activity. Donated services such as these should properly be recorded at fair market value only when (1) the donor and recipient have the equivalent of an employer-employee relationship and (2) there is an objective basis for determining the amounts that might otherwise have been paid for such services. Where these requirements are met, the determined amounts should be recorded as expense with an offsetting credit to nonoperating revenues. The necessary entry (amount assumed) in general journal form is indicated below:

Salaries and Wages Expense—Donated Services	$28,400	
Nonoperating Revenues—Donated Services		$28,400
To record fair market value of services donated to the hospital.		

Services of a nonessential nature provided by guilds, auxiliaries, and similar organizations generally should not be recorded in the accounts.

Payroll-Related Costs

In addition to the basic earnings of hourly and salaried employees, a number of other related cost elements enter into hospital-labor cost considerations. These elements include the previously discussed overtime earnings, vacation, holiday, and sick pay, and the FICA taxes imposed on hospitals. Some other elements are unemployment taxes, workmen's compensation insurance, life and hospitalization insurance premiums paid for employees by the hospital, and pension plan costs. The total of these and other employee benefits constitutes a substantial cost to the hospital—often 25% or more of total employee compensation.

Vacation Pay

After a specified period of employment, hospital employees generally are entitled to an annual vacation with full pay. Assuming a 2-week vacation each year, employees in effect are paid for 50 weeks of work over a 52-week period. The reality of the situation is that the vacation pay is earned by employees, and is incurred as a cost by the hospital, during the 50 working weeks. It is incorrect, therefore, to defer recognition of vacation pay as an expense until it is actually paid. Instead, vacation pay should be charged to expense in the periods during which it is earned by employees.

To illustrate the necessary entries, let us assume that a hospital has 200 employees, each of whom earns $250 per week and is entitled to a 2-week vacation each year. The proper weekly payroll entry for this group (disregarding withholdings) is as follows:

Salaries and Wages Expense*	$52,000	
Cash		$50,000
Accrued Vacation Pay Liability		2,000
To record weekly payroll, including accrual for vacation pay.		

*Classified by departmental expense centers.

In other words, each employee earns $500 (i.e., $250 × 2 weeks) of vacation pay over the 50 weeks of work, or $10 per week. This means that $2,000 (i.e., $10 × 200 employees) should be charged to expense weekly with a corresponding accrual of the vacation-pay liability. When vacations are taken, the liability account is debited and cash is credited.

UNEMPLOYMENT TAXES

In addition to FICA taxes, hospitals may also be subject to federal and state tax laws dealing with unemployment compensation. The federal unemployment (FUTA) tax is at this writing 3.2% of the first $4,200 of taxable wages paid to each employee during a given year, but a 2.7% credit may be allowed for participation in a state unemployment tax (SUTA) program. Thus, the federal tax in effect is 0.5 percent. State tax laws vary, but we will assume a 2.7% rate.

In any event, the hospital must accrue these taxes for each payroll by making an entry such as the following (assuming a $50,000 payroll):

Employee Benefits—FUTA (0.5% × $50,000)	$ 250	
Employee Benefits—SUTA (2.7% × $50,000)	1,350	
FUTA Taxes Payable		$ 250
SUTA Taxes Payable		1,350
To record payroll tax expenses.		

Notice that these taxes are charged to the employee benefits account under the unassigned expense classification rather than to departmental expense centers. To charge these expenses to departments as a part of the normal accounting routine is troublesome and of little month-to-month value. These expenses are, however, allocated to departmental expense centers in the cost-finding procedure at the end of the year.

Observe that the unemployment taxes are paid by the hospital; these taxes are not withheld from employees' wages. Periodically, as required by law, the hospital must submit unemployment tax reports and remit the taxes to the appropriate governmental agency.

OTHER COST ELEMENTS

States have workmen's compensation laws which provide various benefits to disabled workers. In some cases, a tax is imposed on the employer, but more often the state laws establish standard benefits and allow hospitals to provide for such benefits through the purchase of appropriate insurance from a commercial insurance company. The premiums paid by the hospital are charged to expense (employee benefits); a minor portion, if any, of the cost is deducted from employees' pay.

Life, health, accident, disability, dental, and hospitalization insurance plans on a group basis often are established by hospitals in behalf of their employees. Participation in these group programs generally is voluntary, but the hospital frequently pays a substantial portion of the premiums as an employee benefit. Such payments by the hospital naturally are chargeable to expense in the employee benefits classification.

Increasing attention has been given in recent years to the establishment of pension and retirement plans for hospital employees. All or most of the costs of such programs often are paid by the hospital. A discussion of the rather complex accounting procedures involved is beyond the scope of this text.

This concludes the discussion of payroll accounting. Having studied this and the materials on revenues and cash receipts in the preceding chapter, we can now begin our examination of Hartful Hospital's procedures for nonlabor expenses, accounts payable, and cash disbursements.

QUESTIONS

1. Give 4 reasons to explain why employee compensation generally comprises two-thirds or more of total operating expenses in hospitals.

2. An employee of Grant Hospital is paid $2.80 per hour for a regular workweek of 40 hours. During a given week, this employee worked a total of 50 hours. Compute the employee's earnings for the week.

3. What is the current FICA tax rate? What is the maximum annual amount of FICA tax charged per employee?

4. An employee of Lincoln Hospital earns a salary of $1,450 per month, payable on the first day of the following month. Assume that federal income tax withholding is 20% and that the FICA tax is 5.85%. With respect to this one employee, make the necessary entries to

   a. Record the employee's earnings, tax deductions, and accrued payroll liability for January 1978
   b. Accrue the hospital's share of FICA taxes at January 31, 1978
   c. Record issuance of the paycheck on February 1, 1978
   d. Record remittance of January payroll taxes to the government

5. Other than taxes, list 5 types of withholdings that often are made from hospital employees' paychecks.

6. Describe briefly the general procedures involved in the compilation of gross payroll in a hospital for a given pay period.

7. How should donated services be accounted for by hospitals?

8. The fair market value of donated services received by Washington Hospital during April 1978, was $31,400. Make the necessary entry at April 30, 1978, to record these donated services.

9. Describe briefly the basic features of a good internal control system with respect to the hospital payroll.

10. Wilson Hospital has 450 employees, each of whom earns $300 per week and is entitled to a 2-week vacation each year. Disregarding withholdings, make the proper weekly payroll entry for this group of employees. Twenty of these employees take their vacations during the first 2 weeks of June. Make the necessary entry to record the paychecks issued to these 20 employees for the 2-week vacation period.

11. Kennedy Hospital's gross payroll for January 1978 is $250,000. Assuming a 0.5% federal unemployment tax rate and a 2.7% state unemployment tax rate, make the necessary entry to accrue the hospital's unemployment tax expense for January 1978.

12. As a part of the regular accounting routine, should unemployment taxes and the hospital's share of FICA taxes be charged to departmental cost center accounts? Explain.

13. Explain briefly how state workmen's compensation laws affect hospital payroll accounting.

14. Describe briefly the operation of an imprest payroll checking account. What are the advantages of such a system?

15. An employee of Jefferson Hospital is paid $2.80 per hour for a regular work-week of 40 hours. During a particular week, this employee worked 48 hours. Assume that the FICA tax is 6% and that 18% of the employee's gross pay is to be withheld for federal income taxes. Assume also that the federal unemployment tax is 0.5% and that the state unemployment tax is 2.5%. Make all necessary entries relating to this situation. (Disregard any consideration of vacation pay accrual.)

16. Madison Hospital's payroll for the month ended May 31, 1978, is summarized below:

Gross payroll, $462,000
FIT withheld, 5.85%
FICA withheld, 20%
FUTA rate, 0.5%
SUTA rate, 2.5%

Indicate how the May payroll would be entered in the journal *and* ledger systems described in chapter 13.

17. What information would you expect to find on an employee's individual earnings record? Be specific.

18. An employee of Madison Hospital earns a salary of $800 per month, payable on the first day of the following month. Assume the following tax rates:

FIT	18.0%
FICA	6.0
FUTA	0.5
SUTA	2.0

With respect to this one employee, make all necessary entries to record the March 1978 payroll and related matters. Indicate the journal in which each entry should be made.

14
Expenses, Payables, and Cash Disbursements

In accounting for hospital expenses, considerable attention naturally is given to salaries, wages, and employee benefits because these costs added together typically represent more than 60% of total operating expenses. The remaining expenses, however, must never be regarded lightly. Very substantial amounts are expended each year for supplies, utilities and other kinds of purchased services, insurance, interest, and other items. Effective management of these nonlabor costs means using sound accounting procedures.

So, in this chapter we shall examine Hartful Hospital's accounting system as it relates to these expenses, along with the corresponding liabilities and cash disbursements. We shall touch briefly on the purchasing and receiving functions, describe the voucher system, and illustrate the use of the voucher register and the cash disbursements journal. In the last part of this chapter, you also will see a summary of postings from all of Hartful Hospital's journals to the general ledger accounts. This is provided in an effort to tie together the materials of chapters 10 through 14.

Purchasing

The purchasing of supplies and services is a function of major importance in the hospital. It cuts across all departmental lines and accounts for a significant percentage of the hospital's annual expenditures. The purchasing responsibility consists basically of acquiring required supplies and services of the appropriate quality, in the proper quantity, at the times needed, and at reasonable costs. Ideally the purchasing function should be centralized and performed by an organized purchasing department headed by an experienced purchasing agent. This tends to minimize waste and duplication through standardization of buying and use of the many supply items required in the provision of hospital services. Limited authority to purchase certain products and services, however, sometimes must be given to selected department heads. In smaller hospitals, administrative personnel may do the buying personally or will carefully supervise and coordinate it.

To set the wheels of purchasing in motion, the purchasing department must be made aware of the need to purchase. This may be accomplished through the preparation of a *purchase requisition* form such as the one illustrated in figure 66. The form is generally executed by a department head or inventory storekeeper. A copy of the purchase requisition is sent to the purchasing department to inform that department of the items to be purchased; a duplicate copy is retained in a file as evidence that the request was made.

Figure 66
Purchase Requisition

HARTFUL HOSPITAL

PURCHASE REQUISITION PURCHASE ORDER NO. ____________

DEPARTMENT ____________ DATE ____________ 19 ____

FLOOR OR DIVISION ____________ DATE REQUIRED ____________ 19 ____

TO ELIMINATE DELAY KINDLY FURNISH COMPLETE DESCRIPTION OF ARTICLE.

QUANTITY	UNIT	DESCRIPTION OF ARTICLE	(State Fully what Item is to be used for)	UNIT PRICE

REQUESTED BY ____________ APPROVED BY ____________

SEND ORIGINAL TO PURCHASING AGENT. DUPLICATE IS RETAINED BY STORE ROOM CLERK OR DEPARTMENT HEAD.

The purchasing department, noting that the purchase requisition is properly authorized, makes appropriate choices of quantity, price, and vendor, in accordance with prescribed administrative policies. A *purchase order*, one form of which is presented in figure 67, is then prepared to acquire the supplies or services desired. The purchase order generally is a multipart form with copies:

1. One copy of the purchase order is sent to the accounting department for subsequent use in invoice audit and approval for payment. The information may also be useful in the forecasting of cash disbursements.
2. A second copy is sent to the requisitioning department or storekeeper as notification that the order has been placed.

The originator of the purchase will match this copy with its retained copy of the purchase requisition.

3. Two copies are sent to the vendor company. One of these copies is for the vendor's own use; the other is signed and returned to the hospital's purchasing department as an acknowledgement of the order and the vendor's agreement to fill it.
4. In some systems, another copy of the purchase order is routed to the hospital's receiving department (or to the inventory storeroom where the storekeeper performs the receiving function). This copy, however, generally should not provide information as to quantitites ordered.
5. A final copy is retained by the purchasing department in an unfilled orders file which is carefully monitored to avoid delays in the acquisition of desired items.

Figure 67
Purchase Order

PURCHASE ORDER

HARTFUL HOSPITAL
ADDRESS
CITY – STATE – ZIP CODE

Nº 49793
THIS ORDER NUMBER MUST APPEAR ON ALL CORRESPONDENCE, INVOICES, PACKAGES AND SHIPPING PAPERS

DATE ______ 19__
DEPT. ______
SHIP VIA ______
F.O.B. ______
TERMS ______
DELIVERY REQUIRED ______

TO

QUANTITY	DESCRIPTION	PRICE	PER UNIT	AMOUNT

FORM P-432 – PHYSICIANS' RECORD CO., BERWYN, ILLINOIS • PRINTED IN U.S.A.

BY ______

1

When the vendor returns the acknowledgment copy of the purchase order to indicate his acceptance of the order on the terms specified, the purchasing department will match this document with the copy of the purchase order in the unfilled-orders file. The documents will be retained in this file and monitored until the purchasing department is notified of the receipt of the items purchased. A purchase order constitutes a contract with a supplier, and so all required information (including quantities, adequate description, price, and terms) must be carefully indicated.

Figure 68
Receiving Report

HARTFUL HOSPITAL
RECEIVING REPORT

NO.__________

DATE________________19____

RECEIVED FROM______________________________

ADDRESS______________________________

PURCHASE ORDER NO.__________

QUANTITY	UNIT	DESCRIPTION OF ARTICLE

RECEIVED O. K.______________________________

RECEIVING

Upon receipt of purchased goods from suppliers, the hospital's receiving department or agent has the responsibility for counting, weighing, or otherwise measuring the quantities of goods received. The quality and condition of the goods is also checked. As a result of this process, a *receiving report* such as the one shown in figure

68 may be prepared. (In some systems, the packing slip, bill of lading, or a copy of the purchase order may serve this purpose.) After the incoming shipment has been examined in this way, the goods are moved into the hospital storerooms or else directed to the appropriate department. They remain there, under the storekeeper's control, until issued from the inventory for use in various departments of the hospital.

Thus, the receiving report is prepared as a record of the quantity of goods actually received. A copy of the receiving report is sent to the purchasing department where it is used to clear the related purchase order from the unfilled-orders file. A second copy is routed to the accounting department to be used in subsequent invoice processing and approval for payment. Another copy follows the goods into the storeroom, and a final copy may be retained by the receiving department as a work record.

Figure 69
Voucher Package

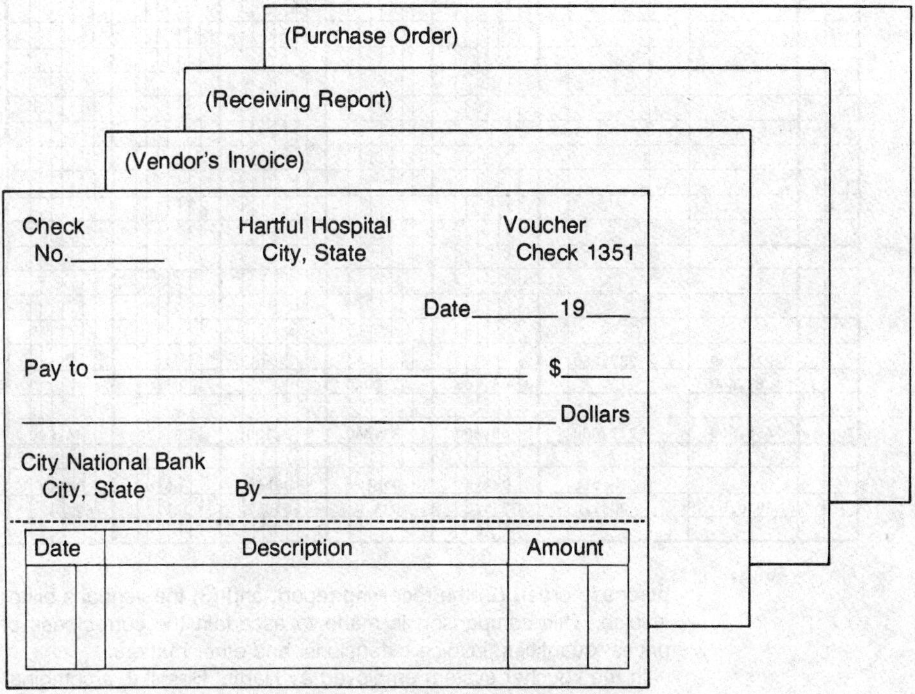

RECORDING PURCHASES

In due course, the vendor will bill the hospital for the items purchased. The vendor's invoice, when it arrives in the incoming mail, should be sent directly from the mailroom to the accounting department. In the accounting department, the 3 documents relating to the purchase are then matched. These documents are (1) the

Figure 70
Voucher Register

1977		Accounts		Payroll Related Debits			Nursing Service Expense		
Date		Payable Cr.	(✓)	Accrued Payroll	FIT Withheld	FICA W/H & Accrued	Adm. Office	Nursing Units	Operating Rooms
5	1	450	✓						
	2	4,690	✓					1,060	
	10	16,000	✓						
	31	227,080	✓	227,080					
	31	81,440	✓		48,400	33,040			
Totals		458,600		227,080	48,400	33,040	2,100	23,120	4,600
		Credit 2020.0		Debit 2031.0	Debit 2035.0	Debit 2036.0	Debit 6010.2	Debit 6021.2	Debit 6210.2

purchase order, (2) the receiving report, and (3) the vendor's bill or invoice. This comparison is made to ascertain the correctness of prices, quantities, invoice extensions, and other matters.

In the voucher system employed by Hartful Hospital, a combination voucher/check is now prepared in duplicate and is attached to the other three documents to form what is called a *voucher package* as illustrated in figure 69. The package is turned over to the accounting employee responsible for maintaining the hospital's *voucher register*. On the basis of the information contained in the approved voucher packages, the transactions are entered as dem-

Debits		Other Professional Service Expense Debits					Medical Staff Expense
Emergency Rooms	Central Supply	Adm. Office	Laboratory	Radiology	Pharmacy	Anesthesia	
					450		
			1,820	1,400			
3,900	9,800	1,700	4,100	4,700	7,460	2,200	1,748
Debit 6230.2	Debit 6250.2	Debit 7010.2	Debit 7011.2	Debit 7040.2	Debit 7070.2	Debit 7080.2	Debit 8030.2

onstrated in figure 70 in the voucher register. Once these entries are made, the voucher packages are placed in a file for unpaid vouchers where they are retained until their respective due dates. This file functions as the accounts payable subsidiary ledger in some accounting systems; in other systems, postings are made to individual vendor or supplier accounts in much the same manner as described earlier for accounts receivable. In any case, the subsidiary record for accounts payable should be reconciled regularly with the control account for accounts payable in the general ledger.

Examine the illustrative entries in the voucher register. On May 1,

(Figure 70 continued)
Voucher Register

General Services Expense Debits					Fiscal Services Expense Debits		
Adm. Office	Dietary	Plant O. & M.	House-keeping	Laundry	Adm. Office	Accounting	Admitting
	410						
1,300	21,500	14,124	3,800	4,300	2,400	7,008	6,100
Debit	Debit	Debit	Debit	Debit	Debit	Debit	Debit
8040.2	8050.2	8060.2	8090.2	8110.2	8211.2	8212.2	8241.2

1977, for example, you see the entry to record a $450 voucher for the purchase of certain drugs and pharmaceuticals. This required a debit to the pharmacy supplies and other expense account (account 7070.2) and a credit to accounts payable (account 2020.0). The entry indicates how individual vouchers might be journalized in the register. As an alternative, all the vouchers issued on a given day may be summarized and entered on a single line of the register, as illustrated by the entry of May 2, 1977. The sample entry of May 10, 1977, relates to the purchase of an item of depreciable equipment. This entry demonstrates the use of the sundry debit and credit col-

Administrative Services Expense Debits					Sundry Debits and Credits		
Administrator's Off.	Adm. Office	Governing Board	Purchasing	Personnel	Account Numbers	Dr.	Cr.
					1170.0	16,000	
3,800	1,100	1,000	1,020	1,200		16,000	
Debit	Debit	Debit	Debit	Debit			
8310.2	8311.2	8312.2	8331.2	8371.2			

umns, and emphasizes the fact that all disbursements (no matter what the purpose) must be vouchered through accounts payable.

Notice also the voucher register entries of May 31, 1977.

Payroll Journal

Salaries and Wages Expense	*	$292,000	
FIT Withheld	2035.0		$ 48,400
FICA Withheld and Accrued	2036.0		16,520
Accrued Payroll	2031.0		227,080

To record May payroll.

*Various departmental account numbers.

General Journal

Employee Benefits—FICA	8710.0	$ 16,520	
FICA Withheld and Accrued	2036.0		$ 16,520
To record hospital's share of FICA taxes on May payroll.			

The vouchering of the May payroll requires the preparation of (1) a voucher in the amount of $227,080 to record the amount to be transferred from the hospital's general checking account to its payroll checking account and (2) a voucher for $81,440 to record the hospital's liability to the government for payroll taxes withheld and accrued. You will shortly see entries in the cash disbursements journal to record the payment of these vouchers.

Recording Cash Disbursements

Just prior to their due dates, the approved voucher packages are removed from the file for unpaid vouchers and are sent to the hospital's treasurer or other disbursing authority. These voucher packages, with the unsigned check included, may be examined by the disbursing officer if he wishes to satisfy himself as to the propriety of the disbursements proposed. When satisfied, the disbursing officer signs the checks and mails them directly to the vendor. (Signed checks should not be returned to the accounting department for mailing.) All documents in the voucher packages then are indelibly stamped or perforated *PAID* to prevent their reuse in support of another disbursement. The packages then are returned to the accounting department to the person responsible for the cash disbursements journal. This employee now records the paid vouchers in this journal as illustrated in figure 71. After these entries are made, the voucher packages marked as paid are placed in a file for paid vouchers; here they are kept for the period specified by the hospital's record retention policies.

Observe the illustrative entries in the journal. Check number 2275, for example, was issued on May 9, 1977, in payment of the $450 voucher seen earlier in the voucher register. As a 2% discount was taken and credited to the purchases discounts account, the check was written for only $441. On May 31, 1977, check number 2690 was issued to transfer the amount of the net payroll for May from the hospital's general checking account to its payroll checking account. Check number 2691 was written to the government to remit the May payroll taxes withheld and accrued. (All checks issued on a given day may be summarized and entered on a single line of the journal, rather than journalizing checks individually.)

Summing Up

To summarize the Hartful Hospital illustration that has been pursued in the last five chapters, let us examine the general ledger postings from all journals and present the hospital's financial statements for the 5 months ended May 31, 1977. The revenue and cash receipts journals were shown in chapter 12, the payroll journal was illustrated in chapter 13, and the voucher register and cash disbursements journal were provided in this chapter. Now, in figure 72, Hartful Hospital's general journal for May is reproduced to indicate the adjusting entries that were necessary at the end of the month.

Figure 71
Cash Disbursements Journal

1977 Date	Description	Check Numbers	Cash Cr.	Purchases Discounts Cr.	Accounts Payable Dr.	Dr.	Sundry Debits and Credits: Account Numbers	Dr.	Cr.
5 9	Central Pharmaceutical Co.	2275	441	9	450				
31	Payroll Checking Account	2690	227,080		227,080				
31	Internal Revenue Service	2691	81,440		81,440				
	Totals		451,295	2,309	453,604				
			Credit 1011.0	Credit 5171.0	Debit 2020.0	Debit			

Figure 72
General Journal

1977 Date		Accounts and Explanations	Account Numbers	Dr.	Cr.
5	31	Inpatient Receivables — Discharged	1032.0	412,975	
		Inpatient Receivables — Inhouse	1031.0		412,975
		To transfer unpaid account balances from inhouse to discharged receivables.			
	31	Accrued Interest Receivable	1029.0	1,350	
		Interest Income	9051.0		1,350
		To accrue interest earned in May.			
	31	Deductions from Revenues — Bad Debts	5510.0	3,700	
		Deductions from Revenues — Contractual Adjustments	5520.0	11,400	
		Deductions from Revenues — Charity Service	5540.0	6,600	
		Allowance for Uncollectible Accounts:			
		Bad Debts	1061.0		3,700
		Contractual Adjustments	1062.0		11,400
		Charity Service	1066.0		6,600
		To adjust allowance accounts to correct balances.			
	31	Insurance Expense	8610.0	1,800	
		Prepaid Expenses	1120.0		1,800
		To adjust for expiration of insurance premiums.			
	31	Depreciation Expense	8510.0	28,000	
		Accumulated Depreciation — Buildings	1250.0		13,000
		Accumulated Depreciation — Equipment	1270.0		15,000
		To record depreciation expense for May.			
	31	Employee Benefits	8710.0	16,520	
		FICA Withheld and Accrued	2036.0		16,520
		To accrue hospital's share of FICA taxes on May payroll.			
	31	Interest Expense	8690.0	14,700	
		Accrued Interest Payable	2051.0		14,700
		To accrue interest expense for May.			

It is suggested that you trace all the postings from each of Hartful Hospital's journals to the general ledger accounts provided in figure 73 at pages 246–250. The posting references are as follows:

Posting Reference	
BB	Balance, May 1, 1977 (assumed)
IRJ	Inpatient revenue journal (chapter 12, page 208)

1977 Date		Accounts and Explanations	Account Numbers	Dr.	Cr.
5	31	Deferred Rental Income	2113.0	1,800	
		Rental Income	5155.0		1,800
		To record rental income earned in May.			

Posting Reference

- ORJ Outpatient revenue journal (chapter 12, page 210)
- CRJ Cash receipts journal (chapter 12, pages 214–215)
- PJ Payroll journal (chapter 13, page 226)
- VR Voucher register (chapter 14, pages 238–239)
- CDJ Cash disbursements journal (chapter 14, page 243)
- GJ General journal (chapter 14, page 244)

Figure 73
General Ledger Accounts

Cash— General Checking 1011.0

BB	180,000	CDJ	451,295
CRJ	447,500		

Cash— Payroll Checking 1012.0

Petty Cash Fund 1014.0

BB	500		

Temporary Investments 1020.0

BB	150,000		

Accrued Interest Receivable 1029.0

BB	5,400		
GJ	1,350		

Inpatient Receivables— Inhouse 1031.0

BB	110,000	CRJ	43,020
IRJ	453,995	GJ	412,975

Inpatient Receivables— Discharged 1032.0

BB	800,000	CRJ	401,850
GJ	412,975		

Outpatient Receivables 1044.0

BB	16,000	CRJ	57,900
ORJ	64,800		

Allowance for UAs— Bad Debts 1061.0

		BB	11,000
		GJ	3,700

Allowance for UAs— Contractual Adjs. 1062.0

		BB	56,000
		GJ	11,400

Allowance for UAs— Charity Service 1066.0

		BB	28,000
		GJ	6,600

Inventories 1110.0

BB	96,000		

Prepaid Expenses 1120.0

BB	14,000	GJ	1,800

Land 1130.0

BB	175,000		

Buildings 1150.0

BB	5,000,000		

Equipment 1170.0

BB	3,000,000		
VR	16,000		

Accumulated Depreciation— Buildings 1250.0

		BB	1,200,000
		GJ	13,000

Accumulated Depreciation— Equipment 1270.0

		BB	900,000
		GJ	15,000

Notes Payable 2010.0

		BB	80,000

Accounts Payable 2020.0

CDJ	453,604	BB	65,000
		VR	458,600

Accrued Payroll 2031.0

VR	227,080	PJ	227,080

FIT Withheld 2035.0

VR	48,400	PJ	48,400

FICA Withheld and Accrued 2036.0

VR	33,040	PJ	16,520
		GJ	16,520

Accrued Interest Payable 2051.0

		BB	18,300
		GJ	14,700

Deferred Rental Income 2113.0

GJ	1,800	BB	9,600

Bonds Payable 2190.0

		BB	2,400,000

Hospital Equity 2210.0

		BB	4,559,240

Revenue and Expense Summary 2219.0

Nursing Services Revenues Nursing Units—IP 3021.1

		BB	896,500
		IRJ	187,500

Operating Rooms—IP Revenues 3210.1

		BB	104,400
		IRJ	26,100

Operating Rooms—OP Revenues 3210.2

		BB	15,600
		ORJ	3,900

Emergency Rooms—IP Revenues 3230.1

		BB	57,600
		IRJ	14,400

Emergency Rooms—OP Revenues 3230.2

		BB	36,100
		ORJ	9,000

Central Supply—IP Revenues 3250.1

		BB	136,400
		IRJ	34,100

Central Supply—OP Revenues 3250.2

		BB	22,800
		ORJ	5,700

Laboratory—IP Revenues 4011.1

		BB	225,680
		IRJ	56,420

Laboratory—OP Revenues 4011.2

		BB	68,160
		ORJ	17,040

Radiology—IP Revenues 4040.1

		BB	355,340
		IRJ	88,835

Radiology—OP Revenues 4040.2

		BB	86,520
		ORJ	21,630

Pharmacy—IP Revenues 4070.1

		BB	99,840
		IRJ	24,960

Pharmacy—OP Revenues 4070.2

		BB	23,520
		ORJ	5,880

Anesthesia—IP Revenues 4080.1

		BB	86,720
		IRJ	21,680

Anesthesia—OP Revenues 4080.2

		BB	6,600
		ORJ	1,650

Cafeteria Sales 5061.0

		BB	83,920
		CRJ	18,480

Rental Income 5155.0

		BB	4,800
		GJ	1,800

(Figure 73 continued)

Purchase Discounts	5171.0		
		BB	9,240
		CDJ	2,309

Deductions from Revenues—Bad Debts	5510.0		
BB	12,600		
GJ	3,700		

Deductions from Revenues—Contractual Adjs.	5520.0		
BB	126,400		
CRJ	31,600		
GJ	11,400		

Deductions from Revenues—Charity Service	5540.0		
BB	67,600		
CRJ	14,400		
GJ	6,600		

Nursing Services Adm. Office—S & W	6010.1		
BB	11,200		
PJ	2,750		

Nursing Services Adm. Office—S & E	6010.2		
BB	8,400		
VR	2,100		

Nursing Units S & W	6021.1		
BB	645,600		
PJ	161,400		

Nursing Units S & E	6021.2		
BB	92,480		
VR	23,120		

Operating Rooms S & W	6210.1		
BB	32,800		
PJ	8,200		

Operating Rooms S & E	6210.2		
BB	18,400		
VR	4,600		

Emergency Rooms S & W	6230.1		
BB	25,600		
PJ	6,400		

Emergency Rooms S & E	6230.2		
BB	15,600		
VR	3,900		

Central Supply S & W	6250.1		
BB	30,800		
PJ	7,700		

Central Supply S & E	6250.2		
BB	39,200		
VR	9,800		

Other Prof. Services Adm. Off.—S & W	7010.1		
BB	15,200		
PJ	3,800		

Other Prof. Services Adm. Off.—S & E	7010.2		
BB	6,800		
VR	1,700		

Laboratory S & W	7011.1		
BB	32,800		
PJ	8,200		

Laboratory S & E	7011.2		
BB	16,400		
VR	4,100		

Radiology S & W	7040.1		
BB	31,800		
PJ	7,700		

Radiology S & E	7040.2		
BB	17,800		
VR	4,700		

Pharmacy S & W	7070.1		
BB	19,600		
PJ	4,900		

Account	Account No.	Entry	Amount	Entry	Amount
Pharmacy S & E	7070.2	BB	29,800	VR	7,460
Anesthesia S & W	7080.1	BB	23,000	PJ	5,500
Anesthesia S & E	7080.2	BB	8,700	VR	2,200
Medical Staff S & W	8030.1	BB	49,000	PJ	12,000
Medical Staff S & E	8030.2	BB	6,800	VR	1,748
General Services Adm. Off.—S & W	8040.1	BB	7,900	PJ	2,000
General Services Adm. Off.—S & E	8040.2	BB	5,200	VR	1,300
Dietary S & W	8050.1	BB	37,600	PJ	9,400
Dietary S & E	8050.2	BB	86,000	VR	21,500
Plant O & M S & W	8060.1	BB	24,800	PJ	6,200
Plant O & M S & E	8060.2	BB	56,500	VR	14,124
Housekeeping S & W	8090.1	BB	29,100	PJ	7,500
Housekeeping S & E	8090.2	BB	15,200	VR	3,800
Laundry S & W	8110.1	BB	27,200	PJ	6,800
Laundry S & E	8110.2	BB	15,300	VR	4,300
Fiscal Services Adm. Off.—S & W	8211.1	BB	16,500	PJ	4,100
Fiscal Services Adm. Off.—S & E	8211.2	BB	9,600	VR	2,400
Accounting S & W	8212.1	BB	26,800	PJ	6,700
Accounting S & E	8212.2	BB	31,300	VR	7,008
Admitting S & W	8241.1	BB	21,200	PJ	5,300
Admitting S & E	8241.2	BB	24,500	VR	6,100

(Figure 73 continued)

Administrator's Office S & W 8310.1

BB	20,600		
PJ	5,250		

Administrator's Office S & E 8310.2

BB	15,700		
VR	3,800		

Administrative Services Adm. Off.—S & W 8311.1

BB	8,900		
PJ	2,200		

Governing Board S & E 8312.2

BB	3,700		
VR	1,000		

Purchasing S & W 8331.1

BB	15,600		
PJ	3,900		

Administrative Services Adm. Off.—S & E 8311.2

BB	4,600		
VR	1,100		

Personnel S & W 8371.1

BB	16,400		
PJ	4,100		

Personnel S & E 8371.2

BB	4,700		
VR	1,200		

Purchasing S & E 8331.2

BB	4,100		
VR	1,020		

Insurance Expense 8610.0

BB	5,900		
GJ	1,800		

Interest Expense 8690.0

BB	48,700		
GJ	14,700		

Depreciation Expense 8510.0

BB	112,000		
GJ	28,000		

General Contributions 9041.0

		BB	10,900
		CRJ	2,250

Interest Income 9051.0

		BB	5,400
		GJ	1,350

Employee Benefits 8710.0

BB	66,300		
GJ	16,520		

After all journals are posted, a trial balance (not illustrated here) was taken of the general ledger account balances at May 31, 1977. Let us assume that this trial balance indicated the necessary equality of debit and credit balances.

Using the May 31, 1977, general ledger balances, we present Hartful Hospital's income statement for the 5 months ended May 31, 1977, in figure 74. Notice that the totals contained in this statement are supported by a schedule of gross revenues from services to patients (figure 75) and a schedule of operating expenses (figure 76). Examine this statement and accompanying schedules to acquaint yourself with both their format and content. You may also find it useful to trace some of the statement figures back to the general ledger accounts.

Figure 77 presents Hartful Hospital's balance sheet at May 31, 1977. It is suggested that you also examine the format and content of this statement; you also should trace some of the balance sheet figures back to the general ledger accounts. It is very important that you have a good understanding of the flow of financial data from the journals, through the ledgers, and into the hospital's financial statements.

Figure 74
Hartful Hospital
Income Statement
Five Months Ended May 31, 1977

Gross Revenues from Services to Patients:		
Nursing Services		$1,550,100
Other Professional Services		1,190,475
Total (Schedule A)		2,740,575
Less Deductions from Revenues:		
Bad Debts	$ 16,300	
Contractual Adjustments	169,400	
Charity Service	88,600	
Total Deductions from Revenues		274,300
Net Revenues from Services to Patients		2,466,275
Other Operating Revenues:		
Cafeteria Sales	102,400	
Rental Income	6,600	
Purchases Discounts	11,549	
Total Other Operating Revenues		120,549
Total Operating Revenues		2,586,824
Less Operating Expenses:		
Nursing Services	1,150,050	
Other Professional Services	321,708	
General Services	381,724	
Fiscal Services	161,508	
Administrative Services (including $140,000 of depreciation and $63,400 of interest)	411,790	
Total Operating Expenses (Schedule B)		2,426,780
Operating Income		160,044
Add Nonoperating Revenues:		
General Contributions	13,150	
Interest Income	6,750	
Total Nonoperating Revenues		19,900
Net Income		$ 179,944

Figure 75
Hartful Hospital
Gross Revenues from Services to Patients — Schedule A
Five Months Ended May 31, 1977

	Inpatients	Outpatients	Total
Nursing Services:			
Nursing Units	$1,084,000		$1,084,000
Operating Rooms	130,500	$ 19,500	150,000
Emergency Rooms	72,000	45,100	117,100
Central Supply	170,500	28,500	199,000
Total Nursing Service Revenues	1,457,000	93,100	1,550,100
Other Professional Services:			
Laboratory	282,100	85,200	367,300
Radiology	444,175	108,150	552,325
Pharmacy	124,800	29,400	154,200
Anesthesia	108,400	8,250	116,650
Total Other Professional Service Revenues	959,475	231,000	1,190,475
Totals	$2,416,475	$ 324,100	$2,740,575

Figure 76
Hartful Hospital
Operating Expenses
Five Months Ended May 31, 1977

Schedule B

	Salaries and Wages	Supplies and Other Exp.	Total
Nursing Services:			
Administrative Office	$ 13,950	$ 10,500	$ 24,450
Nursing Units	807,000	115,600	922,600
Operating Rooms	41,000	23,000	64,000
Emergency Rooms	32,000	19,500	51,500
Central Supply	38,500	49,000	87,500
Total Nursing Services Expense	932,450	217,600	1,150,050
Other Professional Services:			
Administrative Office	19,000	8,500	27,500
Laboratory	41,000	20,500	61,500
Radiology	39,500	22,500	62,000
Pharmacy	24,500	37,260	61,760
Anesthesia	28,500	10,900	39,400
Medical Staff	61,000	8,548	69,548
Total Other Professional Services Expense	213,500	108,208	321,708
General Services:			
Administrative Office	9,900	6,500	16,400
Dietary	47,000	107,500	154,500
Plant Operation and Maintenance	31,000	70,624	101,624
Housekeeping	36,600	19,000	55,600
Laundry	34,000	19,600	53,600
Total General Services Expense	158,500	223,224	381,724
Fiscal Services:			
Administrative Office	20,600	12,000	32,600
Accounting	33,500	38,308	71,808
Admitting	26,500	30,600	57,100
Total Fiscal Services Expense	80,600	80,908	161,508
Administrative Services:			
Administrator's Office	25,850	19,500	45,350
Administrative Office	11,100	5,700	16,800
Governing Board		4,700	4,700
Purchasing	19,500	5,120	24,620
Personnel	20,500	5,900	26,400
Depreciation		140,000	140,000
Insurance		7,700	7,700
Interest		63,400	63,400
Employee Benefits		82,820	82,820
Total Administrative Services Expense	76,950	334,840	411,790
Total Operating Expenses	$1,462,000	$ 964,780	$2,426,780

Figure 77
Hartful Hospital
Balance Sheet
May 31, 1977

		Assets	
Current Assets:			
Cash In Bank		$ 176,205	
Petty Cash		500	
Temporary Investments		150,000	
Accrued Interest Receivable		6,750	
Receivables from Patients	$ 942,025		
Less Allowance for Uncollectibles	116,700	825,325	
Inventories		96,000	
Prepaid Expenses		12,200	
Total Current Assets			$1,266,980
Property, Plant, and Equipment:			
Land		175,000	
Buildings		5,000,000	
Equipment		3,016,000	
Total		8,191,000	
Less Accumulated Depreciation		2,128,000	
Net Property, Plant, and Equipment			6,063,000
Total Assets			$7,329,980
	Liabilities and Capital		
Current Liabilities:			
Notes Payable		$ 80,000	
Accounts Payable		69,996	
Accrued Interest Payable		33,000	
Deferred Rental Income		7,800	
Total Current Liabilities			$ 190,796
Bonds Payable			2,400,000
Total Liabilities			2,590,796
Hospital Equity, January 1, 1977		4,559,240	
Add Net Income for 5 Months Ended May 31, 1977		179,944	
Hospital Equity, May 31, 1977			4,739,184
Total Liabilities and Hospital Equity			$7,329,980

QUESTIONS

1. What is the purpose of a purchase requisition? Who prepares it? How many copies are usually made? To whom are the copies sent, and why?

2. What is the purpose of a purchase order? Who prepares it? How many copies are usually made? To whom are the copies sent, and why?

3. Describe briefly the purchasing function in hospitals.

4. Describe briefly the receiving function in hospitals.

5. What is the purpose of a receiving report? Who prepares it? How many copies are usually made? To whom are the copies sent, and why?

6. What documents generally are included in a voucher package?

7. Describe the voucher system as a means of internal control over cash disbursements by hospitals.

8. On September 6, 1978, Hoover Hospital purchased $2,500 of dietary supplies on account, terms 2/10, n/30. The invoice from the supplier is paid on September 15, 1978. Indicate, in detail, how these transactions would be recorded in the hospital's voucher register, cash disbursements journal, accounts payable subsidiary ledger, and general ledger.

9. How often should postings be made from (a) the voucher register and (b) the cash disbursements journal?

10. Jackson Hospital purchased a new item of equipment for $45,000 on May 27, 1978. The supplier's invoice was paid on June 10, 1978. Indicate how these transactions should be recorded in the hospital's voucher register, cash disbursements journal, and general ledger.

PROBLEMS

A. The following is the adjusted trial balance for Harding Hospital at May 31, 1978 (the fiscal year ends June 30):

		Dr.	Cr.
1011.0	Cash—general checking	$ 172,000	
1014.0	Petty cash fund	750	
1020.0	Temporary investments	160,000	
1029.0	Accrued interest receivable	6,200	
1031.0	Inpatient receivables—inhouse	97,400	
1032.0	Inpatient receivables—discharged	831,500	
1044.0	Outpatient receivables	18,100	
1061.0	Allowance for uncollectible accounts—bad debts		$ 12,300
1062.0	Allowance for uncollectible accounts—contractual adjustments		53,700
1066.0	Allowance for uncollectible accounts—charity service		29,800
1110.0	Inventories	89,000	
1120.0	Prepaid expenses	12,900	
1130.0	Land	155,000	
1150.0	Buildings	5,500,000	
1170.0	Equipment	2,800,000	
1250.0	Accumulated depreciation—buildings		1,075,000
1270.0	Accumulated depreciation—equipment		840,000
2010.0	Notes payable		90,000
2020.0	Accounts payable		73,400

		Dr.	Cr.
2031.0	Accrued payroll		–0–
2035.0	FIT withheld		–0–
2036.0	FICA withheld and accrued		–0–
2051.0	Accrued interest payable		$ 19,700
2113.0	Deferred rental income		7,800
2190.0	Bonds payable		2,500,000
2210.0	Hospital equity		4,934,350
2219.0	Revenue and expense summary		–0–
3021.1	Nursing service revenues—inpatient nursing units		901,300
3210.1	Operating rooms—inpatient revenues		98,200
3210.2	Operating rooms—outpatient revenues		14,400
3230.1	Emergency rooms—inpatient revenues		58,100
3230.2	Emergency rooms—outpatient revenues		37,900
3250.1	Central supply—inpatient revenues		140,500
3250.2	Central supply—outpatient revenues		21,300
4011.1	Laboratory—inpatient revenues		231,600
4011.2	Laboratory—outpatient revenues		77,700
4040.1	Radiology—inpatient revenues		341,600
4040.2	Radiology—outpatient revenues		84,800
4070.1	Pharmacy—inpatient revenues		100,900
4070.2	Pharmacy—outpatient revenues		22,600
4080.1	Anesthesia—inpatient revenues		87,500
4080.2	Anesthesia—outpatient revenues		5,900
5061.0	Cafeteria sales		91,500
5155.0	Rental income		5,200
5171.0	Purchase discounts		8,700
5510.0	Deductions from revenues—bad debts	$ 14,800	
5520.0	Deductions from revenues—contractual adjustments	131,300	
5540.0	Deductions from revenues—charity service	59,900	
6010.1	Nursing services administrative office—salaries and wages	12,300	
6010.2	Nursing services administrative office—supplies and expense	7,200	
6021.1	Nursing units—salaries and wages	656,600	
6021.2	Nursing units—supplies and expense	87,200	
6210.1	Operating rooms—salaries and wages	31,300	
6210.2	Operating rooms—supplies and expense	17,100	

		Dr.	Cr.
6230.1	Emergency rooms—salaries and wages	$26,600	
6230.2	Emergency rooms—supplies and expense	14,500	
6250.1	Central supply—salaries and wages	30,700	
6250.2	Central supply—supplies and expense	38,100	
7010.1	Other professional services administrative office—salaries and wages	14,900	
7010.2	Other professional services administrative office—supplies and expense	7,700	
7011.1	Laboratory—salaries and wages	33,100	
7011.2	Laboratory—supplies and expense	15,700	
7040.1	Radiology—salaries and wages	32,800	
7040.2	Radiology—supplies and expense	16,900	
7070.1	Pharmacy—salaries and wages	20,100	
7070.2	Pharmacy—supplies and expense	31,600	
7080.1	Anesthesia—salaries and wages	19,500	
7080.2	Anesthesia—supplies and expense	9,700	
8030.1	Medical staff—salaries and wages	52,900	
8030.2	Medical staff—supplies and expense	7,100	
8040.1	General services administrative office—salaries and wages	8,500	
8040.2	General services administrative office—supplies and expense	4,800	
8050.1	Dietary—salaries and wages	38,200	
8050.2	Dietary—supplies and expense	91,700	
8060.1	Plant operation and maintenance—salaries and wages	23,000	
8060.2	Plant operation and maintenance—supplies and expense	62,300	
8090.1	Housekeeping—salaries and wages	30,400	
8090.2	Housekeeping—supplies and expense	14,300	
8110.1	Laundry—salaries and wages	25,500	
8110.2	Laundry—supplies and expense	14,600	
8211.1	Fiscal services administrative office—salaries and wages	15,300	
8211.2	Fiscal services		

		Dr.	Cr.
	administrative office—supplies and expense	$ 8,200	
8212.1	Accounting—salaries and wages	25,900	
8212.2	Accounting—supplies and expense	19,400	
8241.1	Admitting—salaries and wages	22,800	
8241.2	Admitting—supplies and expense	17,500	
8310.1	Administrator's office—salaries and wages	24,700	
8310.2	Administrator's office—supplies and expense	7,400	
8311.1	Administrative services administrative office—salaries and wages	7,900	
8311.2	Administrative services administrative office—supplies and expense	3,700	
8312.2	Governing board—supplies and expense	2,900	
8331.1	Purchasing—salaries and wages	14,600	
8331.2	Purchasing—supplies and expense	5,400	
8371.1	Personnel—salaries and wages	17,300	
8371.2	Personnel—supplies and expense	3,800	
8510.0	Depreciation expense	115,600	
8610.0	Insurance expense	6,100	
8690.0	Interest expense	51,700	
8710.0	Employee benefits	67,500	
9041.0	General contributions		$ 11,400
9051.0	Interest income		6,300
		$11,983,450	$11,983,450

Required. (1) Prepare an income statement for the 11 months ended May 31, 1978. (2) Prepare a balance sheet at May 31, 1978. Support the income statement with separate schedules for gross revenues and operating expenses as illustrated in figures 75 and 76.

B. Refer to the May 31, 1978, trial balance provided in problem A. above, and assume the following column totals in Harding Hospital's *special journals* for June 1978:

1. *Inpatient revenue journal:*

		Dr.	Cr.
1031.0	Inpatient receivables—inhouse	$462,500	
3021.1	Nursing units—inpatient revenues		$188,900
3210.1	Operating rooms—inpatient revenues		27,200
3230.1	Emergency rooms—inpatient revenues		15,100

		Dr.	Cr.
3250.1	Central supply—inpatient revenues		$ 36,500
4011.1	Laboratory—inpatient revenues		57,300
4040.1	Radiology—inpatient revenues		89,600
4070.1	Pharmacy—inpatient revenues		25,700
4080.1	Anesthesia—inpatient revenues		22,200

2. *Outpatient revenue journal:*

		Dr.	Cr.
1044.0	Outpatient receivables	$ 70,300	
3210.2	Operating rooms		$ 4,200
3230.2	Emergency rooms		9,700
3250.2	Central supply		6,800
4011.2	Laboratory		18,300
4040.2	Radiology		23,100
4070.2	Pharmacy		6,400
4080.2	Anesthesia		1,800

3. *Cash receipts journal:*

		Dr.	Cr.
1011.0	Cash—general checking	$494,100	
5520.0	Deductions from revenues—contractual adjustments	29,700	
5540.0	Deductions from revenues—charity service	14,800	
1031.0	Inpatient receivables—inhouse		$ 44,600
1032.0	Inpatient receivables—discharged		413,300
1044.0	Outpatient receivables		58,400
5061.0	Cafeteria sales		19,700
5155.0	General contributions		2,600

4. *Payroll journal:*

		Dr.	Cr.
6010.1	Nursing service administrative office	$ 2,750	
6021.1	Nursing units	159,200	
6210.1	Operating rooms	7,900	
6230.1	Emergency rooms	6,600	
6250.1	Central supply	7,300	
7010.1	Other professional services—administrative office	3,900	
7011.1	Laboratory	8,400	
7040.1	Radiology	7,500	
7070.1	Pharmacy	5,100	
7080.1	Anesthesia	5,400	
8030.1	Medical staff	12,000	
8040.1	General services administrative office	2,000	
8050.1	Dietary	9,600	
8060.1	Plant operation and maintenance	6,100	
8090.1	Housekeeping	7,300	
8110.1	Laundry	7,100	
8211.1	Fiscal services administrative office	4,100	
9212.1	Accounting	6,800	
8241.1	Admitting	5,600	
8310.1	Administrator's office	5,250	

		Dr.	Cr.
8311.1	Administrative services administrative office	$ 2,200	
8331.1	Purchasing	3,900	
8371.1	Personnel	4,100	
2035.0	FIT withheld		$ 49,200
2036.0	FICA withheld		17,300
2031.0	Accrued payroll		223,600

5. *Voucher register:*

		Dr.	Cr.
2020.0	Accounts payable		$461,500
2031.0	Accrued payroll	$223,600	
2035.0	FIT withheld	49,200	
2036.0	FICA withheld and accrued	34,600	
6010.2	Nursing service administrative office	1,800	
6021.2	Nursing units	22,500	
6210.2	Operating rooms	4,700	
6230.2	Emergency rooms	4,100	
6250.2	Central supply	9,300	
7010.2	Other professional services—administrative office	1,400	
7011.2	Laboratory	4,500	
7040.2	Radiology	4,800	
7070.2	Pharmacy	7,600	
7080.2	Anesthesia	2,100	
8030.2	Medical staff	1,300	
8040.2	General services administrative office	1,100	
8050.2	Dietary	23,400	
8060.2	Plant operation and maintenance	12,200	
8090.2	Housekeeping	3,600	
8110.2	Laundry	4,200	
8211.2	Fiscal services administrative office	2,100	
8212.2	Accounting	6,300	
8241.2	Admitting	5,800	
8310.2	Administrator's office	2,300	
8311.2	Administrative services—administrative office	900	
8312.2	Governing board	1,000	
8331.2	Purchasing	800	
8371.2	Personnel	1,300	
1170.0	Equipment	25,000	

6. *Cash disbursements journal:*

		Dr.	Cr.
1011.0	Cash—general checking		$448,600
5171.0	Purchases discounts		2,700
2020.0	Accounts payable	$451,300	

In addition to the above special journal information, you are provided with the following *general journal* entries made by Harding Hospital during June 1978:

	Account Numbers	Dr.	Cr.
7. Inpatient receivables—discharged	1032.0	$410,600	
Inpatient receivables—inhouse	1031.0		$410,600
To transfer unpaid account balances from inhouse to discharged receivables.			
8. Accrued interest receivable	1029.0	1,400	
Interest income	9051.0		1,400
To accrue interest earned in May.			
9. Deductions from revenues:			
Bad debts	5510.0	3,900	
Contractual adjustments	5520.0	12,400	
Charity service	5540.0	7,300	
Allowance for uncollectible accounts:			
Bad debts	1061.0		3,900
Contractual adjustments	1062.0		12,400
Charity service	1066.0		7,300
To adjust allowance accounts to correct balances.			
10. Insurance expense	8610.0	1,600	
Prepaid expenses	1120.0		1,600
To adjust for expiration of insurance premiums.			
11. Depreciation expense	8510.0	31,400	
Accumulated depreciation—buildings	1250.0		14,300
Accumulated depreciation—equipment	1270.0		17,100
To record depreciation expense for June.			
12. Employee benefits	8710.0	17,300	
FICA withheld and accrued	2036.0		17,300
To accrue hospital's share of FICA taxes on June payroll.			
13. Interest expense	8690.0	15,800	
Accrued interest payable	2051.0		15,800
To accrue interest expense for June.			
14. Deferred rental income	2113.0	1,400	
Rental income	5155.0		1,400
To record rental income earned in June.			

Required. (1) Establish the May 31, 1978, balances in general ledger accounts. (2) Make all necessary postings from the special journals and the general journal to the general ledger accounts. (3) Prepare an adjusted trial balance at June 30, 1978. (4) Prepare an income statement for the year ended June 30, 1978. (5) Prepare a balance sheet at June 30, 1978.

15
Principles of Fund Accounting

In addition to the resources received from patients and third-party payers in payment for health care services provided by the hospital, some hospitals also receive contributions, donations, gifts, grants, and endowment resources. Certain of these resources might be available, at the discretion of the governing board, for the financing of the regular day-to-day operating activities of the hospital *if* the donor places no restrictions on the donated resources. Let us assume, for example, that an individual gives Hartful Hospital $25,000 in cash and says to the hospital, "Use this money however you wish!" There is no stipulation by the donor concerning any specific purpose for which the money is to be applied. In cases such as this, regardless of the amount involved, the resources are classified as *unrestricted resources*. While the receipt of such resources must be recorded by the hospital as nonoperating revenue (account 9041.0—general contributions), such resources may be used for capital or operating needs as determined by the governing board.

Other donated resources received by hospitals, however, may be restricted by donors to specific uses and purposes such as construction of new hospital buildings, purchase of new equipment, or the financing of hospital charity work, research, and educational activities. Such resources are not available for any purpose designated by the governing board or hospital managers. Let us assume, for example, that an individual gives Hartful Hospital $25,000 in cash, and says to the hospital, "Use this money to purchase new equipment for your radiology department." In all cases of this kind, regardless of the amount involved, the resources are classified as *restricted resources*. Such resources must be employed or expended by the hospital precisely as required by the donors. There is both a legal and a moral obligation on the part of the hospital to comply fully with donors' restrictions and stipulations. Failing to observe the stated wishes of donors, or not providing a proper accounting for the use or disposition of donor-restricted resources, may give rise to very serious legal penalties.

Aside from the legal obligation to fulfill donors' requirements, there is also an administrative or managerial need to maintain in the accounting records a careful distinction between unrestricted and restricted resources. A hospital's managers, in making financing and investing decisions, must have information regarding which resources are available for any general operating purpose and which resources are not so available but whose use is limited to particular donor-restricted purposes. Otherwise, unauthorized and even illegal use might be made of certain hospital resources. Furthermore, donors often require from the hospital a periodic accounting for the use of resources provided by them.

The system of fund accounting has evolved in response to these stewardship and accountability requirements. It is the objective of this chapter to give you an opportunity to learn the principles of that system of accounting. Since a majority of voluntary community hospitals employ fund accounting procedures, the materials in this chapter deserve your attention. The discussion, however, will be of an introductory character. A more advanced treatment of the subject may be found in the author's *Hospital Financial Accounting—Theory and Practice*.

Nature of Fund Accounting

Fund accounting may be defined as a system of accounting in which the resources (and related obligations) of a hospital are segregated in the accounting records into self-balancing sets of accounts regarded as independent accounting entities, called *funds*, for the purpose of carrying on specific activities and attaining particular objectives in accordance with legal and other restrictions or limitations. In view of this rather lengthy and complex definition, perhaps you would appreciate the nature of fund accounting more easily if we considered a simple example. Take a moment to examine figure 78, a condensed balance sheet (figures are shown in thousands of dollars) for an assumed Community Hospital.

Figure 78
Community Hospital
Balance Sheet
September 30, 1977

Assets	$8,500
Liabilities	$2,500
Hospital equity	6,000
Total liabilities and hospital equity	$8,500

This balance sheet could be quite misleading as to the financial position of Community Hospital, however, if there are legal restrictions on the hospital's use of certain of its assets. Assuming this to be the case, a revised balance sheet is presented in figure 79 as it would appear in accordance with the principles of fund accounting.

Clearly, this revised balance sheet provides a much different impression of Community Hospital's financial position. We see that, of the $8,500 of assets, only $4,000 are unrestricted and available for general operating purposes. These are the only assets which can be used to pay the $1,900 of liabilities reported in the unrestricted fund. The other $4,500 of hospital assets are restricted by donors to particular uses, whatever they may be. So, the total column in figure 79 really has no significance and should not be included in a fund accounting balance sheet. It is included here only to indicate the relationship between figures 78 and 79.

Figure 79
Community Hospital
Balance Sheet
September 30, 1977

	Unrestricted Fund	Restricted Funds			Total All Funds
		Fund A	Fund B	Fund C	
Assets	$4,000	$1,000	$2,000	$1,500	$8,500
Liabilities	$1,900	$ 200	$ 400	$ –0–	$2,500
Hospital equity	2,100	800	1,600	1,500	6,000
Total liabilities and equity	$4,000	$1,000	$2,000	$1,500	$8,500

Thus, in fund accounting, assets and related liabilities are segregated in the hospital's accounts and reports into unrestricted and restricted "funds," depending upon the absence or presence of donor restrictions. In this context the term *funds* does not mean "cash" but simply a self-balancing group of related accounts. Observe that each fund, unrestricted and restricted, consists of equal debits (assets) and credits (liabilities and equity). This equality is maintained throughout all operations in the accounting process.

Notice that Community Hospital has a single unrestricted fund. In fund accounting, there is one (and only one) unrestricted fund. On the other hand, the hospital has 3 restricted funds. Restricted resources, as you will shortly see, are classified according to the 3 major types of restrictions that are externally imposed on assets donated to the hospital.

An extremely important point to recognize here is that the term *restricted* should be used only to refer to resources that are *externally* restricted. That is, when we speak of restricted funds, we are referring to a self-balancing set of accounts containing assets whose use has been restricted by a person or other entity external to the hospital. A hospital's governing board, by its actions, can *designate* certain assets to certain uses, but the board does not have the power to *restrict* their use in terms of the hospital's legal relationships with its creditors.

The board can make whatever designations it wishes for internal management purposes, but, if donors do not restrict the use of resources they contribute to the hospital, the board cannot do it for them. Moreover, what the board can do, it can undo. So, let us not refer to "board-restricted funds." If the board wishes to earmark certain assets for a particular purpose, it may do so but the term *board-designated assets* should be used to describe the situation. Assets that are so designated, however, are unrestricted assets and must be reported as a part of the hospital's unrestricted fund. It might be noted, however, that some hospitals have begun to utilize separately incorporated foundations for receiving donations in order to obtain greater flexibility in restricting funds for special purposes.

Types of Funds

In fund accounting as employed by hospitals, there are 2 major categories of funds: unrestricted and restricted. There is only one unrestricted fund, but restricted funds are classified into 3 types: (1) specific purpose funds, (2) plant replacement and expansion funds, and (3) endowment funds. Let us now briefly describe the nature and content of the unrestricted fund and each of the three types of restricted funds.

Unrestricted Fund

An unrestricted fund is maintained by all hospitals using fund accounting. This fund includes all hospital resources, with related obligations, that are not restricted by such external authority as donors. All of the resources of this fund are available for general operating and capital activities at the discretion of the hospital's governing board. In addition, the accounts of the unrestricted fund include all the revenues and expenses to be reported in the hospital's income statement. Think back to the extended Hartful Hospital illustration of the last 5 chapters; all the accounts included there were unrestricted fund accounts. The chart of accounts presented in chapter 10 is, except for a few accounts to be added in this chapter, a chart of accounts for Hartful Hospital's unrestricted fund.

Restricted Funds

Some hospitals receive substantial amounts of resources by donation. If no strings are attached by donors, such resources are recorded in the unrestricted fund regardless of any action that might be taken by the hospital's governing board. It must be presumed that if the donor wished to restrict the use of the resources, the donor would do so at the time of contribution. If no such restrictions are made by the donors, the governing board cannot do it for them because such board actions would not be proper or legally binding.

A majority of donated resources, however, generally are restricted in some way by donors. These resources are of 3 types: (1) resources restricted for specific operating purposes, (2) resources restricted for acquisition of plant assets, and (3) resources restricted as endowments. A chart of accounts for each of these 3 types of restricted funds (and some additional unrestricted fund accounts) is presented in figure 80. The account numbering system closely conforms to the system prescribed in the AHA's *Chart of Accounts for Hospitals* manual. Account numbers are constructed according to a system.

1. The first digit of account numbers for restricted funds is either *1* or *2*, with the following designations:

First Digit		
1	=	Asset accounts
2	=	Liability and equity accounts

Notice that all accounts of restricted funds are either asset, liability, or equity accounts; there are no revenue or expense accounts in the restricted funds, although the use of such accounts would be logical and useful.

2. The second digit of account numbers for restricted funds is either *5*, *6*, or *7*, with the following designations:

Second Digit		
5	=	Plant replacement and expansion fund accounts
6	=	Specific purpose fund accounts
7	=	Endowment fund accounts

Thus, the second digit of these account numbers identifies the type of restricted fund to which the account is related.

3. The third and fourth digits are employed to provide a primary subclassification of the accounts by specific type of asset, liability, or equity.

The AHA manual also provides for the use of fifth and sixth digits where needed by individual hospitals. We will limit restricted fund account numbers, for our present purposes, to 5 digits as shown in figure 80.

• ***Specific Purpose Fund.*** Resources restricted by donors for purposes other than plant asset acquisitions or endowments are recorded in the specific purpose fund. Assume, for example, that Hartful Hospital receives $25,000 in cash from a donor who restricts the use of the money to a specific purpose such as charity service, research activities, working capital, or educational programs conducted by the hospital. The specific purpose fund entry is

Cash	1611.0	$25,000	
Donated Resources Received	2613.1		$25,000
To record receipt of donated resources restricted to specific purposes.			

Once recorded as specific purpose funds, these resources remain restricted funds until such time as the specified purposes are completed by appropriate activity in the unrestricted fund, such as provision of charity service to patients, conduct of research, inclusion in working capital, or carrying on of educational programs.

As expenditures are made for these specific purposes by the unrestricted fund, periodic transfers of the previously restricted resources are made to the unrestricted fund from the specific purpose fund. Assuming that the above $25,000 is transferred to the unrestricted fund to finance educational programs, the necessary entries are as follows:

Specific Purpose Fund

Transfers to Unrestricted Fund	2614.1	$25,000	
Cash	1611.0		$25,000
To record transfer of resources to the unrestricted fund to finance educational programs.			

Unrestricted Fund

Cash	1011.0	$25,000	
Transfers from Restricted Funds for Education	5021.0		$25,000
To record resources received from specific purpose fund to finance educational programs.			

Notice that the account (5021.0) credited in the unrestricted fund is a *revenue* account in the "other operating revenues" classification. Since expenditures for the educational programs are recorded as unrestricted fund expenses, this credit accomplishes an appropriate matching of revenues and expenses. Similar procedures would be followed for transfers related to charity work and research activities.

Until transfers such as the above are made, however, the resources carried in the specific purpose fund should be prudently invested. Income and gains on these temporary investments should be credited to the appropriate specific purpose fund accounts (for example, accounts 2613.2 and 2613.3). At the end of each fiscal year these accounts (as well as accounts 2612.4, 2613.1, and 2614.1) should be closed to the specific purpose fund balance (account 2611.0).

• ***Plant Replacement and Expansion Fund.*** Cash and other assets received by the hospital from donors and other external authorities who restrict the use of those resources to the acquisition of plant assets are included in the plant replacement and expansion fund. Assume, for example, that a donor gives the hospital $80,000 for the purchase of a new item of equipment for the radiology department. The entry to be made in the plant replacement and expansion fund is the following:

Cash	1511.0	$80,000	
Donated Resources Received	2513.1		$80,000
To record receipt of donated resources restricted to purchase of plant assets.			

Until the equipment is purchased by the unrestricted fund, this $80,000 remains in the plant replacement and expansion fund. The $80,000 usually is placed in some form of income-producing investment. Income and gains on such investments should be credited to accounts 2513.2 and 2513.3. At the end of the year, these accounts (along with accounts 2512.1, 2512.4, 2513.1, and 2514.1) are closed to the plant replacement and expansion fund balance account (account 2511.0).

When the equipment is purchased by the unrestricted fund, the $80,000 (plus any net investment income) is transferred to the unrestricted fund. Entries to record the transfer are shown on page 270.

Plant Replacement and Expansion Fund

	Account	Debit	Credit
Transfers to Unrestricted Fund	2514.1	$80,000	
Cash	1511.0		$80,000
To record transfer of resources to unrestricted fund to finance purchase of equipment for radiology.			

Unrestricted Fund

	Account	Debit	Credit
Cash	1011.0	$80,000	
Transfers from Plant Replacement and Expansion Fund	2212.2		$80,000
To record receipt of resources from plant replacement and expansion fund to finance purchase of equipment.			

The credit in the unrestricted fund is made to an unrestricted fund balance account, *not* a revenue account; plant assets, including those with previously restricted resources, are *not* recorded in the plant replacement and expansion fund but the unrestricted fund.

Figure 80
Hartful Hospital
Chart of Accounts—Restricted Funds*

	Account Numbers			
	Plant Replacement and Expansion Fund	Specific Purpose Fund	Endowment Fund	Unrestricted Fund
ASSETS:				
Cash—General Checking Account	1511.0	1611.0	1711.0	
Investments	1520.0	1620.0	1720.0	
Accrued Income Receivable	1529.0	1629.0	1729.0	
Pledges Receivable	1581.0	1681.0	1781.0	1081.0
Allowance for Uncollectible Pledges	1582.0	1682.0	1782.0	1082.0
Due from Unrestricted Fund	1591.0	1691.0	1791.0	
Due from Plant Replacement and Expansion Fund		1692.0	1792.0	1092.0
Due from Specific Purpose Fund	1593.0		1793.0	1093.0
Due from Endowment Fund	1594.0	1694.0		1094.0
Other Assets	1530.0	1630.0	1730.0	
LIABILITIES AND FUND BALANCES:				
Due to Unrestricted Fund	2581.0	2681.0	2781.0	
Due to Plant Replacement and Expansion Fund		2682.0	2782.0	2082.0
Due to Specific Purpose Fund	2583.0		2783.0	2083.0
Due to Endowment Fund	2584.0	2684.0		2084.0
Fund Balance	2511.0	2611.0	2711.0	
Transfers from Unrestricted Fund	2512.1			
Transfers from Plant Replacement and Expansion Fund				2212.2
Transfers from Specific Purpose Fund				**
Transfers from Endowment Fund	2512.4	1612.4		**
Donated Resources Received	2513.1	2613.1	2713.1	
Investment Income	2513.2	2613.2		
Investment Gains and Losses	2513.3	2613.3	2713.3	
Transfers to Unrestricted Fund	2514.1	2614.1		
Transfers to Plant Replacement and Expansion Fund				2214.2

*Including additional unrestricted fund accounts.
**See text discussion at pages 269 and 270.

In some instances, a hospital will receive pledges from donors to contribute money for future purchases of plant assets. The receipt of such pledges should be recorded in the plant replacement and expansion fund as follows:

Pledges Receivable	1581.0	$40,000	
Allowance for Uncollectible Pledges	1582.0		$ 4,000
Donated Resources Received	2513.1		36,000
To record receipt of pledges (estimated to be 90% collectible) restricted to the acquisition of plant assets.			

A similar procedure is followed for the receipt of pledges relating to other funds. Figure 80 has accounts provided in the other funds.

Another important point concerns the procedure to be followed when plant assets are donated in kind to a hospital. Assume, for example, that a donor gives the hospital an item of equipment having a fair market value of $80,000 (rather than giving the hospital $80,000 with which to purchase the equipment). Where this occurs, *no entry* is made in the plant replacement and expansion fund. Instead, the following entry is made in the unrestricted fund:

Equipment	1170.0	$80,000	
Value of Donated Plant Assets	2213.0		$80,000
To record receipt of donated equipment at fair market value.			

The account credited is not a revenue account but an unrestricted fund balance account. A donation of plant assets in kind is assumed to be a contribution to the permanent capital of the hospital and is not reported as revenue in the income statement.

• ***Endowment Fund.*** Endowments consist of contributed resources which, by donor restriction, are not to be expended but are to be held intact for the production of income. Let us assume, for example, that Hartful Hospital receives $100,000 from a donor who specifies that the money is to be invested in securities and held as an endowment of the hospital. The endowment fund entries are

Cash	1711.0	$100,000	
Donated Resources Received	2713.1		$100,000
To record receipt of resources to be held as an endowment.			
Investments	1720.0	$100,000	
Cash	1711.0		$100,000
To record the investment of endowment funds received.			

At the year's end, account 2713.1 (along with account 2713.3) is closed to the endowment fund balance account (2711.0).

Income from investments of endowment funds may be donor restricted or immediately available for general operating purposes. If the income is restricted by the donor to specific operating purposes, for example, this income should not be recorded in the endowment fund but should be recorded directly in the specific purpose fund as follows (amount assumed):

Cash	1611.0	$ 7,500	
Transfers from Endowment Fund	2612.4		$ 7,500
To record receipt of income earned on endowment fund investments and restricted to specific operating purposes.			

If the income is donor restricted to the acquisition of plant assets, the income should be recorded directly in the plant replacement

Figure 81
Hartful Hospital
Income Statement
Year Ended December 31, 1977

Gross Revenues from Services to Patients:		
Nursing Services		$3,565,282
Other Professional Services		2,738,130
Total		6,303,412
Less Deductions from Revenues:		
Bad Debts	$ 53,790	
Contractual Adjustments	389,620	
Charity Service (net of specific purpose gifts of $34,000)	194,920	
Total Deductions from Revenues		638,330
Net Revenues from Services to Patients		5,665,082
Other Operating Revenues:		
Cafeteria Sales	235,520	
Transfers from Restricted Funds for Research and Education	92,000	
Rental Income	14,680	
Purchase Discounts	23,169	
Total Other Operating Revenues		365,369
Total Operating Revenues		6,030,451
Less Operating Expenses:		
Nursing Services	2,499,194	
Other Professional Services	972,099	
General Services	763,448	
Fiscal Services	355,318	
Administrative Services (including $322,000 of depreciation and $145,820 of interest)	988,296	
Total Operating Expenses		5,578,355
Operating Income		452,096
Add Nonoperating Revenues:		
General Contributions	28,930	
Unrestricted Income from Endowment Fund	41,000	
Interest Income on Unrestricted Fund Investments	14,850	
Total Nonoperating Revenues		84,780
Net Income for the Year		$ 536,876

and expansion fund through accounts 1511.0 and 2512.4 in the manner illustrated above.

On the other hand, the income earned on endowment fund investments may not be donor restricted in any way. In these cases, the income should be recorded directly in the unrestricted fund as follows (amount assumed):

Cash	1011.0	$ 7,500	
Unrestricted Income from Endowment Fund	9055.0		$ 7,500
To record receipt of unrestricted income from endowment fund investments.			

Notice that the credit in the unrestricted fund is made to a revenue account to be reported as "nonoperating revenues" in the hospital's income statement.

Thus, investment income on endowment funds is directly recorded in a fund other than the endowment fund. It generally is not correct to record such income in the endowment fund initially and later to transfer it to another fund. Gains and losses on such investments, however, generally are recorded in the endowment fund (account 2713.3) on the theory that gains and losses follow the principal rather than the income of the fund.

Financial Statements

To illustrate the effect of fund accounting on the financial statements of the hospital, we will provide here an assumed set of statements for Hartful Hospital for the year ended December 31, 1977. In addition to the income statement and balance sheet, a new statement—the statement of changes in fund balances—is introduced to provide an analysis and summary of all changes which occurred in the fund balances during the year.

Income Statement

Hartful Hospital's income statement for 1977 is presented in figure 81 in condensed form. While this statement is virtually identical in format and content to the statement illustrated in chapter 14, we can see certain indications of the hospital's use of fund accounting. First, among the deductions from revenues, you will notice that the amount of charity service has been reduced by $34,000 which was transferred to the unrestricted fund from the specific purpose fund during 1977. In other words, the value of charity services provided in 1977 was $228,920, but the $34,000 received from the specific purpose fund was credited against it to produce the income statement figure of $194,920. Thus, amounts received from the specific purpose fund to finance the hospital's charity work are netted against the charity service figure rather than being shown in the statement as revenues.

Second, the other operating revenues include $92,000 transferred from the specific purpose fund to the unrestricted fund to finance a part of the hospital's research and educational activities. This is the accounting treatment that is recommended by the AHA *Chart of Accounts* manual for such transfers. It is generally not practical to attempt to credit such transfers to the related research and education expense accounts.

Finally, notice that $41,000 of unrestricted income earned on the investments of the endowment fund is included in the nonoperating revenues classification. If such income were restricted by donors, it would not be reported in the income statement. Instead, it would be recorded as an addition to the fund balance account of either the specific purpose fund or the plant replacement and expansion fund.

Figure 82
Hartful Hospital
Statement of Changes in Fund Balances
Year Ended December 31, 1977

Unrestricted Fund		
Fund Balance, January 1		$4,559,240
Net Income for the Year		536,876
Transfers from Plant Replacement and Expansion Fund for Plant Asset Acquisitions		150,000
Donated Medical Equipment		35,000
Fund Balance, December 31		$5,281,116
Restricted Funds		
Specific Purpose Fund:		
Fund Balance, January 1		$ 245,612
Donated Resources Received		142,000
Investment Income		18,248
Investment Gains (Net)		7,600
Transfers to Unrestricted Fund for		
Charity Service	$ (34,000)	
Research and Education	(92,000)	(126,000)
Fund Balance, December 31		$ 287,460
Plant Replacement and Expansion Fund:		
Fund Balance, January 1		$1,580,050
Donated Resources Received		196,330
Investment Income		112,477
Investment Gains (Net)		1,472
Transfer to Unrestricted Fund for Plant Asset Acquisitions		(150,000)
Fund Balance, December 31		$1,740,329
Endowment Fund:		
Fund Balance, January 1		$2,800,000
Donated Resources Received		100,000
Investment Gains (Net)		21,400
Fund Balance, December 31		$2,921,400

STATEMENT OF CHANGES IN FUND BALANCES

A statement of changes in fund balances for the year ended December 31, 1977, is provided in figure 82. The purpose of this statement is to summarize all of the changes which occurred in the fund balance accounts (all funds) during the year. It provides essential information that cannot be obtained from an examination of the income statement and balance sheet alone.

Observe that the statement begins with an analysis of the changes in the unrestricted fund balance. In addition to being increased by the year's net income, the fund balance was increased by a $150,000 transfer from the plant replacement and expansion fund to finance certain acquisitions of plant assets and by the fair market value ($35,000) of medical equipment contributed in kind to the hospital by a donor. You may recall from the preceding discussion that neither of these 2 items are ever to be recorded as revenue or included in the income statement. Receipts of plant assets in kind, or receipts of cash restricted by donors to the acquisition of plant assets, are considered contributions to the permanent capital of the hospital rather than revenues.

The analysis of changes in the specific purpose fund balance includes the amount ($142,000) of resources received by the hospital during 1977 which were restricted by donors to specific operating purposes (charity service, research, and education). Such resources, at the time received, are not treated as revenues of the unrestricted fund but, as indicated here, are recorded in the specific purpose fund. The balance of the specific purpose fund also was increased during 1977 by $18,248 of income and $7,600 of net gains on the investments of the fund. The fund balance was decreased by $126,000 of transfers to the unrestricted fund ($34,000 for charity work and $92,000 for research and education costs). As noted earlier, these 2 items are included in the hospital's income statement.

A similar analysis appears in the statement with respect to the changes in the fund balance accounts of the other 2 restricted funds. Two points might be emphasized here. First, the $150,000 reduction of the plant replacement and expansion fund balance is the same item shown as a direct addition to the unrestricted fund balance. Second, notice that investment income is not shown as an element of change in the endowment fund balance. All endowment fund investment income is recorded directly in one of the other funds as previously indicated at page 274. Transfers of resources from the endowment fund to other funds (or from other funds to the endowment fund) rarely occur.

BALANCE SHEET

The December 31, 1977, balance sheet of Hartful Hospital is presented in figure 83 in accordance with the principles of fund accounting. Notice that the assets, liabilities, and capital balances are segregated by funds. The total assets of each fund equal the total of each fund's liabilities and fund balance. Users of this balance sheet can readily see that $7,960,625 of resources are unrestricted and available for general operating purposes while other resources

Figure 83
Hartful Hospital
Balance Sheet
December 31, 1977

ASSETS

Unrestricted Fund

Current Assets:			
Cash		$ 192,068	
Temporary Investments		175,000	
Accrued Interest Receivable		8,124	
Receivables—Patients	$1,192,563		
Less Allowance for Uncollectibles	122,056	1,070,507	
Due from Other Funds		41,000	
Inventories		87,000	
Prepaid Expenses		9,260	
Total Current Assets			$1,582,959
Property, Plant, and Equipment:			
Land		175,000	
Buildings		5,000,000	
Equipment		3,505,345	
Total		8,680,345	
Less Accumulated Depreciation		2,302,679	
Net Property, Plant, and Equipment			6,377,666
Total Unrestricted Fund Assets			$7,960,625

Restricted Funds

Specific Purpose Fund:			
Cash		$ 10,300	
Investments		289,160	
Total Specific Purpose Fund Assets			$ 299,460
Plant Replacement and Expansion Fund:			
Cash		$ 9,267	
Pledges Receivable	$ 184,929		
Less Allowance for Uncollectibles	20,450	164,479	
Investments		1,591,583	
Total Plant Replacement and Expansion Fund Assets			$1,765,329
Endowment Fund:			
Cash		$ 1,371	
Investments		2,924,029	
Total Endowment Fund Assets			$2,925,400

LIABILITIES AND FUND BALANCES

Unrestricted Fund

Current Liabilities:		
Notes Payable	$ 125,000	
Accounts Payable	72,384	
Accrued Payroll	31,270	
Payroll Taxes Withheld and Accrued	9,242	
Accrued Interest Payable	40,163	
Deferred Rental Income	1,450	
Total Current Liabilities		$ 279,509
Bonds Payable		2,400,000
Total Liabilities		2,679,509
Unrestricted Fund Balance		5,281,116
Total Unrestricted Fund Liabilities and Fund Balance		$7,960,625

Restricted Funds

Specific Purpose Fund:		
Due to Unrestricted Fund	$ 12,000	
Fund Balance	287,460	
Total Specific Purpose Fund Liabilities and Fund Balance		$ 299,460
Plant Replacement and Expansion Fund:		
Due to Unrestricted Fund	$ 25,000	
Fund Balance	1,740,329	
Total Plant Replacement and Expansion Fund Liabilities and Fund Balance		$1,765,329
Endowment Fund:		
Due to Unrestricted Fund	$ 4,000	
Fund Balance	2,921,400	
Total Endowment Fund Liabilities and Fund Balance		$2,925,400

are restricted by donors or other external authorities to particular purposes. In other words, $299,460 of resources are restricted to specific operating purposes, $1,765,329 of resources are restricted to plant asset acquisitions, and a total of $2,925,400 of resources are restricted for endowment purposes. Similarly, the liabilities to be paid from the resources of each fund are classified by funds. Note also that the individual fund balance figures at December 31 are those previously seen in the statement of changes in fund balances (figure 82).

Among the current assets of the unrestricted fund is an item of $41,000 due from the restricted funds. This is balanced by the "due to unrestricted fund" liabilities shown in the restricted funds ($12,000 in the specific purpose fund, $25,000 in the plant replacement and expansion fund, and $4,000 in the endowment fund). Interfund receivables and payables of this sort may arise when interfund transfers are appropriate but resources are not currently available. Such receivables and payables may represent interfund borrowings, however. All such borrowings should be documented and formally approved by the hospital's governing board.

QUESTIONS

1. Distinguish between unrestricted and restricted resources.

2. Define *fund accounting*. Why is fund accounting a recommended system of accounting for hospitals?

3. What is a "board-designated fund"? Explain why the resources of funds of this kind are not classified as restricted resources.

4. Fort Hospital received donations of (a) an item of medical equipment having a fair market value of $100,000 and (b) $100,000 cash restricted by the donor to the purchase of medical equipment. How should each of these donations be accounted for when received? Explain why the treatment differs.

5. Finn Hospital received a $300,000 cash donation that is restricted by the donor. In what fund do you think this $300,000 should be recorded?

6. Finn Hospital received a $300,000 cash donation that was not restricted by the donor in any manner. The governing board of the hospital, however, voted to restrict this $300,000 to the purchase of plant assets. In what fund should this donation be recorded? Please explain.

7. When should resources be transferred from the specific purpose fund to the unrestricted fund?

8. When should resources be transferred from the plant replacement and expansion fund to the unrestricted fund of the hospital?

9. When, if ever, should resources be transferred from (a) the unrestricted fund to the plant replacement and expansion fund? (b) the endowment fund to the unrestricted fund?

10. If investments held in a restricted fund are sold at a gain, in what fund should the gain be recorded?

11. In what fund should unrestricted investment income earned on endowment fund investments be recorded?

12. In the context of "fund accounting," what does the word *fund* mean?

13. List, and describe briefly, each of the 4 types of funds generally employed in hospital accounting.

14. During 1978, Flair Hospital's unrestricted fund received $18,000 cash from its specific purpose fund. Of this total, $13,000 was for charity service and $5,000 for research activities. How should the $18,000 be recorded in the accounts of the unrestricted fund?

PROBLEMS

A. Fine Hospital employs an unrestricted fund, a specific purpose fund, a plant replacement and expansion fund, and an endowment fund. Certain of the transactions completed by the hospital during 1978 are indicated below:

1. The hospital received a $150,000 cash donation not restricted by donors in any manner.
2. The hospital received, as a donation, laboratory equipment having a fair market value of $40,000.
3. The hospital received a $40,000 cash donation restricted by donor to the purchase of new laboratory equipment. The equipment was subsequently purchased at a cost of $45,000.
4. The hospital received a $30,000 cash donation restricted by donor to the financing of charity service by the hospital. The specified charity service was subsequently provided by the hospital.
5. The hospital received a $14,000 cash donation restricted by donor to the financing of certain research activities by the hospital. The specified research activity was subsequently completed by the hospital.
6. The hospital received pledges in the amount of $90,000 from donors who wished to contribute to future purchases of plant assets. It is estimated that 85% of these pledges will prove to be collectible.
7. The hospital received a $500,000 cash donation restricted by donor as a permanent endowment of the hospital. Subsequently
   a. The $500,000 was invested in corporate securities.
   b. The $500,000 of investments earned $35,000 of dividends and interest during 1978. According to the provisions of the endowment, 60% of the investment income is restricted to the purchase of plant assets and the remaining 40% is unrestricted.
8. The unrestricted fund borrowed $75,000 from the specific purpose fund. The loan was subsequently repaid in full along with interest of $3,000.

Required. Prepare, in general journal form, the necessary entries to record all the above transactions. Be sure to specify the particular fund in which each entry should be made.

B. Faultless Hospital provides you with the following account balances at March 31, 1978:

Cash—endowment fund	$ 18,000
Inventories	27,000
Deferred revenue (current)	6,000
Accumulated depreciation	242,000

Investments—board-designated	$ 47,000
Notes payable to banks	11,000
Receivables—patients	57,000
Investments—specific purpose fund	92,000
Bonds payable	80,000
Prepaid expenses (current)	5,000
Investments—unrestricted fund (current)	14,000
Accrued expenses payable	13,000
Cash—board-designated	5,000
Investments—endowment fund	303,000
Accounts payable	41,000
Land	8,000
Allowance for uncollectible accounts	15,000
Mortgage payable (noncurrent)	135,000
Equipment	260,000
Cash—plant replacement and expansion fund	17,000
Cash—unrestricted fund (current)	14,000
Building	320,000
Current portion of long-term debt	10,000
Investments—plant replacement and expansion fund	174,000
Cash—specific purpose fund	3,000

Required. Prepare, in good form, an all-funds balance sheet for Faultless Hospital at March 31, 1978.

C. Frankly Hospital provides you with the following information taken from its accounting records at September 30, 1978, the end of its fiscal year:

Interest expense		$ 11,000
Transfer received from specific purpose fund for		
Charity service	$ 14,000	
Education	9,000	23,000
Transfer received from plant replacement and expansion fund for purchase of plant assets		52,000
Nursing service expense		134,000
Deductions from revenues		99,000
Income from board-designated investments		7,000
General services expense		108,000
Depreciation expense		12,000
Unrestricted gifts and bequests		36,000
Gross patient service revenues		422,000
Fiscal services expense		29,000
Unrestricted income from endowment fund		21,000
Other professional services expense		101,000
Other operating revenues		31,000
Administrative services expense		22,000
Unrestricted fund balance, October 1, 1977		325,000

Required. (1) Prepare an income statement for the year ended September 30, 1978. (2) Prepare a statement of changes in the unrestricted fund balance for the year ended September 30, 1978.

D. Fondly Hospital provides you with the following information which relates to the year ended June 30, 1978:

Cafeteria sales		$ 240,000
Transfer to unrestricted fund from plant replacement and expansion fund for plant-asset acquisitions		120,000
Cash—unrestricted fund (current)		190,000
Cash—endowment fund		1,000
Accrued salaries and wages payable		32,000
Nursing services expense		2,500,000
Gross revenues—nursing services		3,600,000
General contributions (unrestricted)		29,000
Donated medical equipment		40,000
Donated resources received—endowment fund		90,000
Land		166,000
Cash—plant replacement and expansion fund		9,300
Unrestricted fund balance, June 30, 1978		?
Deductions from revenues—bad debts		54,000
General services expense		770,000
Deferred rental income (current)		2,000
Due to unrestricted fund from		
Specific purpose fund	$ 15,000	
Plant replacement and expansion fund	34,000	
Endowment fund	6,000	55,000
Gross revenues—other professional services		2,800,000
Unrestricted income from endowment fund		28,000
Investment income—specific purpose fund		17,000
Endowment fund balance, June 30, 1978		?
Investment income—plant replacement and expansion fund		108,000
Temporary investments—unrestricted fund (current)		180,000
Equipment		3,500,000
Notes payable		80,000
Bonds payable		2,500,000
Cash—specific purpose fund		12,000
Accrued interest receivable		9,000
Accumulated depreciation		2,400,000
Deductions from revenue—charity service		201,000
Other professional services expense		987,000
Prepaid expenses (current)		8,000
Investments—endowment fund		3,000,000
Accounts payable		75,000
Specific purpose fund balance, June 30, 1978		?
Buildings		5,500,000
Inventories		110,000
Rental income		15,000
Fiscal services expense		354,000
Purchase discounts		26,000
Deductions from revenue—contractual adjustments		403,000
Payroll taxes withheld and accrued		7,000
Plant replacement and expansion fund balance, June 30, 1978		?

Accrued interest payable		41,000
Donated resources received—specific purpose fund		124,000
Investment gains		
Specific purpose fund	8,000	
Plant replacement and expansion fund	3,000	
Endowment fund	14,000	25,000
Administrative services expense		1,004,000
Donated resources received—plant replacement and expansion fund		230,000
Transfers from specific purpose fund to unrestricted fund for:		
Charity service	29,000	
Research	40,000	
Education	52,000	121,000
Receivables—patients		1,300,000
Investments—specific purpose fund		290,000
Allowance for uncollectible accounts		140,000
Investments—plant replacement and expansion fund		1,600,000
Income on unrestricted fund investments		13,000
Plant asset pledges receivable (net)		206,000

Required. Prepare in good form (1) an income statement for the year ended June 30, 1978, (2) a statement of changes in fund balances for the year ended June 30, 1978, and (3) a balance sheet at June 30, 1978.

IV
Selected Financial Accounting Topics

16
Quick Assets

The quick assets of a hospital consist of cash and those other assets which, relatively speaking, can be quickly and directly converted into cash, that is, temporary investments and receivables. This chapter provides a discussion of certain of the accounting problems and procedures related to such assets. Although cash, marketable securities, and receivables may appear in any fund, most of the materials of this chapter relate to the quick assets of the hospital's unrestricted fund. You should recognize, however, that the accounting methods and practices described here are largely applicable to the quick assets found in the restricted funds.

CASH

Cash may be defined as consisting of actual money and other immediately available resources or credit instruments generally accepted as media of exchange and used as money equivalents. This includes coin and paper currency, demand deposits in banks, checks, and money orders. Postage stamps, however, are supplies, not cash. Postdated checks and IOUs from employees are properly treated as receivables. The very essence of cash is its availability as a medium of exchange, its purchasing power.

Considerable attention is given to cash accounting because of its rather obvious value as the means of financing hospital activities. Cash also is the asset likely to be most susceptible to fraudulent misappropriation by employees and others. Finally, it should be recognized that, because of the large volume of cash transactions, the incidence of honest errors can be quite high unless appropriate accounting procedures and internal controls are observed.

BANK RECONCILIATIONS

The bank reconciliation should be regarded as one of the more important accounting and internal control procedures. It will aid in the prevention and detection of fraud, the discovery of any errors in accounting records, and the determination of the accuracy of the bank statement. Bank statements, of course, should be delivered unopened to the person who is to perform the reconciliation, and they should remain in that person's control until the reconciliation is completed. Reconciliations should be supervised by the hospital controller or his delegate and should be performed by someone who does not handle cash or cash records.

Figure 84
Homecity Hospital
Bank Reconciliation—General Checking Account
November 30, 1977

				Books		Bank	
				Dr.	Cr.	Dr.	Cr.
Balances, 11/30				182,062			168,934
Deposits in transit, 11/30:							
	Date		Amount				
	11/29		21,604				
	11/30		18,217				
Total							39,821
Checks outstanding, 11/30:							
	Date	Number	Amount				
	10/19	4259	1,361				
	10/27	4326	412				
	11/10	4533	89				
	}	}	}				
	11/30	4715	145				
Total						19,655	
Bank service charges for November					37		
NSF checks returned by bank:							
Robert M. Patient check dated 11/14; deposited 11/17			519				
William L. Patient check dated 11/20; deposited 11/21			909				
Total					1,428		
Collection of treasury bills by bank				25,000			
Bank errors:							
Deposit of 11/27 omitted from bank statement			16,400				
Check of Othercity Hospital erroneous charged against our account			187				
Total							16,587
Book errors:							
Check #4649 for $234, dated 11/15, erroneously journalized as $324				90			
Totals				207,152	1,465	19,655	225,342
Offsets				1,465			19,655
Adjusted balances, 11/30				205,687			205,687

A bank reconciliation is primarily a matter of adjusting two incorrect cash balances (the ledger balance and the bank balance) to a correct amount representing the actual amount of cash over which the hospital has control, that is, the cash balance to be reported in the balance sheet. Ordinarily, the book balance will be incorrect for 2 reasons: (1) items may have been subtracted from the bank statement balance but not from the book balance (for example, bank service charges and patients' checks deposited by the hospital which prove uncollectible) and (2) items may have been added to the bank balance but not to the book balance (for example, collections of items by the bank for the hospital). On the other hand, the bank statement balance normally will be incorrect because (1) items may have been added to the book balance but not to the bank balance (for example, hospital deposits in transit at the bank statement date) and (2) items may have been subtracted from the book balance but not from the bank balance (for example, checks issued and outstanding at the bank statement date). In addition, the book and bank balances may be incorrect because of errors made by either the hospital or the bank (banks *do* make errors).

To illustrate the bank reconciliation procedure, assume that the general checking account of Homecity Hospital has a November 30, 1977, general ledger balance of $182,062. Within a few days after the end of the month, the hospital receives the November bank statement which reports a November 30, 1977, balance of only $168,934! Neither of these figures should be reported as the cash balance in the hospital's month-end balance sheet. The 2 figures must be reconciled to an adjusted (correct) balance. This is accomplished through a reconciliation of the book and bank balances in the manner illustrated in figure 84.

The reconciliation begins with the entry of the November 30 balances in the respective book and bank columns. The $182,062 book balance is obtained from the general ledger account (1011.0); the $168,934 bank balance is found on the November bank statement. Typically, it is to be hoped, the book balance is a debit balance while the bank balance normally is a credit balance (from the bank's point of view, the hospital's balance is a liability of the bank). If the account is overdrawn, of course, the book balance will be a credit, and the bank balance will be a debit.

The next step is to list the deposits in transit at November 30. A deposit in transit is a deposit made by the hospital (usually on the last day or so of the month) which does not appear on the bank statement for that month. At some banks there may be a lag or delay of a day or so in recording customer's deposits, particularly where the customer makes deposits after banking hours through night depository systems. Deposits in transit may be identified by a comparison of deposits as shown on the bank statement with entries in the cash receipts journal. If the hospital deposits all receipts daily and intact (as it should), daily debits to cash in the journal will be the same amounts as the daily bank deposits. If a deposit was listed as in transit on the prior month's reconciliation, the person making the reconciliation also should ascertain that the deposit appears on the current month's bank statement. (Note that deposits are debits on the hospital's books but appear as credits on the bank statement since, from the bank's point of view, the hospital's balance is a liability.)

Notice that Homecity Hospital has 2 deposits in transit at November 30 which total $39,821. This amount has been included in the hospital's November receipts per books but does not appear as deposits on the November bank statement. To reconcile, therefore, the $39,821 is credited (added) to the bank balance in the reconciliation. As a part of the December 31, 1977, reconciliation process, the person preparing it should make sure that this $39,821 appears as deposits on the December bank statement.

Next, the checks outstanding at November 30 are listed by date, number, and amount on the reconciliation. When the November bank statement is received, the checks included with the statement are arranged in numerical order and are compared (1) with the listing of checks outstanding on the prior month's (October) reconciliation and (2) with the hospital's cash disbursements journal and payroll journal entries of the current month. An investigation should be made of checks that remain outstanding from the prior month's reconciliation to determine if payment should be stopped on such checks. And, perhaps on a sample basis, the endorsements on cancelled checks might be examined for possible irregularities.

At November 30, Homecity Hospital has a total of $19,655 of outstanding checks. These are checks which have been written and included in the hospital's disbursements but which have not yet been presented to the hospital's bank for payment. The bank has no knowledge of this "float" and consequently has not reduced the hospital's checking account balance for those checks. This situation arises because payees sometimes hold the hospital's checks for a few days before cashing them, because of delays in the postal system, and because of the time it takes for checks to clear the banking system. In any event, the outstanding checks are debited to (deducted from) the bank balance in the reconciliation since the hospital no longer has control of the amount of money represented by such items. The person who prepares the December 31 reconciliation should determine whether or not these $19,655 of outstanding checks clear the bank in December.

The November bank statement includes a number of debit and credit memos which specify certain special items which have been charged or credited by the bank to the hospital's account. One of the debit memos indicates that the bank service charge for November was $37. This has been deducted by the bank in arriving at the hospital's November 30 balance but the $37 has not yet been recorded in the hospital's November disbursements. The bank service charges are credited to the books column of the reconciliation.

Two other debit memos are for NSF (not sufficient funds) checks that were received from patients, recorded as cash receipts, and deposited by the hospital during November. Unfortunately, those patients did not have sufficient funds in their checking accounts to cover these checks. These checks appeared as deposits (November 17 and 21) on the bank statement but, when their NSF status was determined, the bank subsequently charged them back against the hospital's account. So, to reconcile, the $1,428 of bad checks must be credited to the book balance in the reconciliation. These defaulting patients should immediately be contacted to work out an agreement as to when and how they plan to make these checks good. The writing of bad checks is a serious matter, and steps should be taken by the hospital to recover such amounts.

The November bank statement also includes a credit memo representing the collection by the bank of $25,000 of treasury bills for the hospital. These bills, which are issued by the U.S. Treasury Department, were being held as temporary investments by the hospital. They matured late in November and were turned over to the bank for collection from the government. (A part of the November service charge relates to the fee charged by the bank for this collection service.) The $25,000 appearing on the bank statement as a deposit must be debited to the books column of the reconciliation.

Comparisons made of the bank statement with the hospital's cash records uncovered certain errors made by the bank during November as well as an error made by the hospital's accounting personnel during the month. One of the bank errors was an omission from the bank statement of a $16,400 deposit which was made by the hospital on November 27. Apparently, the bank credited this deposit in error to another customer's account. In order to reconcile, the omitted deposit must be credited to the bank columns of the reconciliation. The bank also made an error in charging one of Othercity Hospital's checks for $187 against Homecity Hospital's account. This is reconciled by a credit to the bank columns.

The error made by Homecity Hospital was in journalizing check number 4649, written for $234 in payment of an account payable, in the incorrect amount of $324. This caused an understatement of $90 (i.e., $324 − $234) in the month-end ledger cash balance. To reconcile, the $90 must be added back to the book balance.

After all necessary adjustments have been determined, each of the columns of the reconciliation is totaled. Then, the ledger credit column total is offset against the ledger debit column total, and the bank debit column total is offset against the bank credit column total. This provides the adjusted (correct) cash balance at November 30, or $205,687. This is the cash balance which should be reported in Homecity Hospital's balance sheet at November 30, 1977. But, since the general ledger account has a $182,062 balance, an adjusting entry is required in the hospital's general journal.

Cash—General Checking Account	$ 23,625	
Accounts Receivable—Patients	1,428	
Fiscal Services—Supplies and Expense	37	
Temporary Investments		$ 25,000
Accounts Payable		90
To adjust accounts per November 30, 1977, bank reconciliation.		

The debit of $23,625 increases the general ledger cash balance to $205,687, the debit of $1,428 charges the bad checks back to the patients' accounts, and the $37 debit records the bank service charges as November expenses. The credit of $25,000 eliminates the treasury bills from the temporary investments account, and the credit of $90 corrects the error in accounts payable (when check number 4649 was entered in the cash disbursements journal, $90 too much was debited to the accounts payable account). Notice that no entry is necessary for deposits in transit, outstanding checks, or bank errors. The deposits in transit and the outstanding checks have already been recorded in the hospital's accounts; the bank errors will be called to the bank's attention so that they may be corrected by the bank in its December statement.

The bank reconciliation is an important document; it should not be destroyed. All reconciliations should be retained in appropriate files for review by the hospital's internal and external auditors.

Sometimes bank reconciliations are accomplished by adjusting the bank balance into agreement with the ledger balance (previously adjusted to a correct figure). While this method will produce a reconciliation and is employed by most auditors, the procedure illustrated in figure 84 is described here for pedagogical reasons and because it always produces the proper balance sheet figure for cash and organizes all the necessary adjustments in one place, and that is in the ledger debit and credit columns. Other reconciliation methods may not necessarily provide these two advantages.

As noted in chapter 14, the use of a special payroll checking account will greatly facilitate the bank reconciliation process. The special payroll account allows the large volume of payroll checks to be removed from the general checking account reconciliation. The payroll checking account ordinarily will require no reconciliation as it tends to reconcile itself to a zero or imprest balance. This is true because the deposit of the net payroll amount in the account is exactly offset by the total of the individual payroll checks clearing the account. Should employees not cash their payroll checks promptly so as to accomplish this result within a reasonable time period, payroll checks may be printed to read "void if not presented for payment within 30 days." Other special checking accounts may be established, if useful, for other frequently recurring disbursements such as payroll taxes, equipment purchases, and interest payments on the hospital's long-term debt (bonds payable, for example).

IMPREST CASH FUNDS

A hospital should not keep cash on hand unnecessarily. All cash receipts should be deposited daily and intact: disbursements should never be made directly from cash receipts. Disbursements, as a general rule, should be made only by checks, properly authorized and supported by appropriate vouchers. Any violations of these basic control principles are open invitations to confusion, error, and fraud.

As a practical matter, however, provision usually must be made for the keeping of cash funds in limited amounts from which cash disbursements can be made for items for which the writing of checks is not feasible. Hospitals, for this reason, often must maintain several so-called petty cash funds, change funds, and check cashing funds. The need for such funds should be evaluated regularly so that their number and size will be neither excessive nor inadequate. All such funds should be accounted for on an *imprest* basis: that is, each fund should be established in a fixed amount which is replenished periodically when that amount has been exhausted. Responsibility for each imprest fund should be assigned to a specific employee who, as the fund custodian, has sole control over it.

• ***Petty Cash Funds***. To illustrate the accounting procedures for petty cash funds, assume that Homecity Hospital decides to establish such a fund in the imprest amount of $750. Accordingly, a check for this amount is drawn payable to the appointed petty cash custodian who cashes the check and places the money for safekeeping in a locked petty cash drawer or box. The entries are as follows:

Voucher Register

Petty Cash Fund	$ 750	
Accounts Payable		$ 750
To record voucher to establish imprest petty cash fund of $750.		

Cash Disbursements Journal

Accounts Payable	$ 750	
Cash—General Checking Account		$ 750
To record check issued to establish imprest petty cash fund of $750.		

Disbursements from the fund are made only by the petty cash custodian and then only in return for signed receipts, petty cash slips or vouchers, and other supporting documents. A typical petty cash disbursement form is illustrated in figure 85. As cash is paid out of the fund, these forms are completed and retained in the petty cash drawer or box.

When the fund is found to be nearly exhausted or routinely at the end of each month, a reimbursement check can be drawn to replenish the fund to its imprest amount. Assume that the contents of the petty cash box at this time are as follows:

Coin and currency	$ 87
Petty cash disbursement slips	635
IOU from employee	25
Total	$747

The coin and currency in the box, of course, were determined by actual count. The disbursement slips are removed from the box, totaled, and summarized according to the accounts to be debited for the expenditures. This summary analysis can be entered on the back of specially printed petty cash envelopes such as shown in figure 86. When the summary is completed, the cash disbursement slips are placed in the envelope which becomes a part of the voucher package for the check to be drawn to replenish the petty cash fund.

Figure 85
Petty Cash Disbursement Slip

PETTY CASH DISBURSEMENT

No.__________________ Date____________________19____

$____________

TO____

Amount____________________________________DOLLARS

For____

____

Account Number__________________________________

Approved By____________________ Received Payment____________________

FORM P-171 - P-W SYSTEM PHYSICIANS' RECORD CO., BERWYN, ILLINOIS PRINTED IN U.S.A.

For simplicity, let us assume that the petty cash disbursements of $635 are chargeable only to the accounting department ($415) and the laboratory department ($220). The necessary entries to replenish the fund are as follows:

Voucher Register

Accounting—Supplies and Expense	$415	
Laboratory—Supplies and Expense	220	
Accounts Receivable—Employees	25	
Cash Over and Short	3	
Accounts Payable		$663
To record voucher for check to replenish petty cash fund.		

Cash Disbursements Journal

Accounts Payable	$663	
Cash—General Checking Account		$663
To record check issued to replenish the petty cash fund.		

Notice that the employee's $25 IOU is debited to accounts receivable—employees. This represents an improper use of the petty cash fund, and the custodian should be instructed not to allow employees to borrow from the fund. Note also that the $3 shortage in the fund is debited to a special cash over and short account which is treated as either a miscellaneous expense or miscellaneous income account, depending upon its balance at the end of the reporting period.

The $663 check is drawn payable to the petty cash custodian who cashes it and places the money in the petty cash box. This $663 plus the $87, which was remaining in the fund at the time of reimbursement, brings the petty cash drawer up to a total of $750 again. These replenishments are made as often as the fund is depleted, or at least at the end of each monthly accounting period for control purposes.

Figure 86
Petty Cash Disbursements Summary

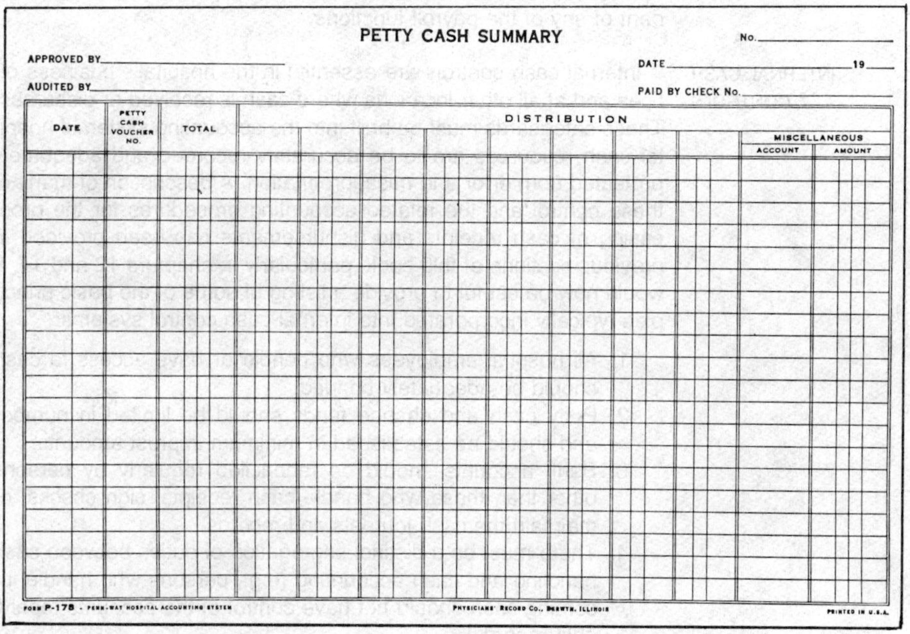
PETTY CASH SUMMARY

No. ______

APPROVED BY ______ DATE ______ 19 ___

AUDITED BY ______ PAID BY CHECK No. ______

DATE	PETTY CASH VOUCHER NO.	TOTAL	DISTRIBUTION							MISCELLANEOUS	
										ACCOUNT	AMOUNT

FORM P-178 - PENN-WAY HOSPITAL ACCOUNTING SYSTEM PHYSICIANS' RECORD CO., BERWYN, ILLINOIS PRINTED IN U.S.A.

It should be recognized that nowhere in the reimbursement process is the petty cash account debited or credited. This is done only when the imprest amount of the fund is increased or decreased. If reimbursements are required so often as to be bothersome, the imprest amount of the fund might be considered inadequate. Assume, for example, that it is decided to increase the above fund to $1,000. A check therefore is drawn for $250 and is debited to the petty cash account. On the other hand, if reimbursements are infrequent, this may be an indication that the imprest amount is excessive. Suppose, for example, that a decision is made to reduce the $750 fund to an imprest amount of $400. In this case, one would remove $350 of currency from the petty cash box and deposit it in the hospital's general checking account, crediting the petty cash account.

• ***Other Imprest Funds***. Hospitals often establish change funds in relatively nominal amounts at cash receiving locations for the purpose of providing change to patients, employees, and visitors. These funds should be balanced daily to the total of recorded cash receipts plus the imprest amount of the change fund. In depositing cash receipts, over and short variations are considered to be in the day's receipts and not in the change fund which is retained in its imprest amount.

While hospital policy ordinarily should be that of not cashing any personal or payroll checks for anyone, check-cashing funds often are established as a convenience to employees. Where such check-cashing funds are necessary, they should be maintained on an imprest basis. The custodian of such funds should be independent of any of the payroll functions.

INTERNAL CASH CONTROLS

Internal cash controls are essential in the hospital's business offices and at all other locations where cash is received or disbursed. These safeguards must be built into the accounting system if hospital cash resources are to be accurately recorded and adequately protected from error and misappropriation. A description of many of these control and the related accounting procedures for the processing of cash receipts and disbursements has been provided in previous sections of this book, particularly in chapters 12 and 14. It would now be useful to provide a listing of some of the basic principles typically incorporated into internal cash control systems:

1. All hospital employees who handle or have access to cash should be adequately bonded.
2. Petty cash and change funds should be limited in number and should be established in minimum imprest amounts.
3. Bank accounts should be reconciled regularly by persons other than those who handle cash receipts, sign checks, or maintain the cash journals and records.
4. There must be a distinct segregation of duties between cash handling and cash accounting (e.g., persons who handle incoming cash should not have control of the accounts receivable records).
5. All cash record forms, such as checks, bank deposit tickets, cash receipt slips, and petty cash vouchers, should be prenumbered and accounted for by numerical sequence whenever this is feasible.
6. Definite responsibility for cash-handling functions and for custody of cash funds should be assigned to specific employees.
7. A minimum number of employees should be given access to cash.

Figure 87
Entries for Temporary Investments

Voucher Register

Date	Account / Explanation		Debit	Credit
10/1	Temporary Investments		$40,065	
	Accrued Interest Receivable		1,000	
	Accounts Payable			$41,065
	To record voucher for purchase of temporary investments as follows:			
	Purchase price (face value)	$40,000		
	Acquisition costs	65		
	Total cost	$40,065		
	Accrued interest:			
	$40,000 × .06 × 5/12	1,000		
	Total disbursement	$41,065		

Cash Disbursements Journal

Date	Account / Explanation	Debit	Credit
10/1	Accounts Payable	$41,065	
	Cash—General Checking Account		$41,065
	To record check issued for purchase of temporary investments.		

General Journal

Date	Account / Explanation	Debit	Credit
10/31	Accrued Interest Receivable	$ 200	
	Interest Income		$ 200
	To accrue interest income earned on temporary investments in October: $40,000 × .06 × 1/12.		

Cash Receipts Journal

Date	Account / Explanation	Debit	Credit
11/1	Cash—General Checking Account	$ 1,200	
	Accrued Interest Receivable		$ 1,200
	To record receipt of semiannual interest on temporary investments: $40,000 × .06 × 6/12.		

General Journal

Date	Account / Explanation	Debit	Credit
11/30	Accrued Interest Receivable	$ 200	
	Interest Income		$ 200
	To accrue interest income earned on temporary investments in November.		

General Journal

Date	Account / Explanation	Debit	Credit
12/31	Accrued Interest Receivable	$ 200	
	Interest Income		$ 200
	To accrue interest income earned on temporary investments in December.		

8. The work of business office personnel should be made complementary so that an error by one automatically will be discovered by another.
9. Physical protection should be provided through the use of vaults, bank facilities, cashiers' cages, locked cash drawers, and similar devices.
10. Definite procedures should be established in writing for the handling of all cash transactions.
11. Office procedures should be so arranged that misappropriations are unlikely to go undetected without the collusion of 2 or more employees.
12. Internal audits and surprise cash counts should be made by a responsible employee at irregular intervals.

While the above listing is not by any means complete, it is indicative of some of the principles and procedures to be observed in a sound internal control system. A more thorough treatment of the subject appears in the author's *Hospital Financial Accounting–Theory and Practice.*

TEMPORARY INVESTMENTS

Temporarily excessive cash balances should always be invested by the hospital in bank savings accounts, certificates of deposit, U.S. treasury bills, or in some other type of securities. The investment objective should be safety and a reasonable investment income. These temporary or short-term investments could appear in the hospital's restricted funds as well as in the unrestricted fund, although long-term investments are more commonly found in the endowment fund and in the plant replacement and expansion fund.

To illustrate the accounting procedures for temporary investments, at times referred to as marketable securities, let us assume that Homecity Hospital's cash budget indicates that $40,000 of cash will be available for investment for about 4 months. Accordingly, on October 1, 1977, the hospital purchases $40,000 of U.S. government bonds at face value. These 6% (per year) bonds pay interest semi-annually on November 1 and May 1 (3% each interest payment date). Assuming this to be an investment of the hospital's unrestricted fund, the entries for 1977 would be those illustrated in figure 87.

The voucher register entry records the investment at *cost* which is the quoted price paid for the securities plus brokerage fees and other acquisition costs. It is assumed here that the quoted price was 100% of face, or par, value and that acquisition costs totaled $65. For accounting purposes, then, the cost of this investment was $40,065. Had these securities been quoted at, say, 98, the price paid for them would have been $39,200 (i.e., 98% of $40,000), and the cost of the investment would have been recorded as $39,265 (i.e., $39,200 + $65).

Because these bonds were acquired between interest payment dates, the seller must be paid the accrued interest on the bonds since the last interest payment date, from May 1 to October 1, or 5 months' interest. This $1,000 is not charged to expense but to accrued interest receivable because it will be recovered by the hospital on November 1, when the issuer of the bonds pays 6 months' interest to bondholders. Accrued interest settlements always are made in this manner between investors who trade in bonds. It would not be convenient for the bond issuer to attempt to make these adjustments. Instead, the issuer always pays 6 months' interest on each interest payment date regardless of the length of time the investor has held the bonds.

On October 31, and at the end of each subsequent monthly reporting period so long as Homecity Hospital holds these bonds, a general journal adjusting entry is required to record the accrued interest income on the investment. The amount of this entry is an approximation of interest for one month; precise computations to exact days or cents can be made but are not really necessary in recording most accruals of this type. Note that the October 31 entry increases the balance of the accrued interest receivable account to $1,200 which is the amount of the semi-annual interest received the following day (November 1).

At December 31, the interest income account has a balance of $600, which is reported in Homecity Hospital's 1977 income statement as nonoperating revenue. The $400 of accrued interest receivable will be reported in the hospital's year-end balance sheet as a current asset. The December 31, 1977, balance sheet also will report the investment at its cost of $40,065. Suppose, however, that the December 31 quoted market price of these bonds has risen to 102 ($40,800), or has fallen to 97 ($38,800). Should the carrying value of the investment be adjusted (written up or down) to current market value? Under current generally accepted accounting principles, temporary investments in bonds usually are carried in the accounts and in the balance sheet at their original acquisition cost with market value indicated parenthetically or by footnote. Some accountants argue, however, that such investments should be valued at the *lower* of cost or market value; others believe that such investments should be reported at market value, whether this is higher or lower than cost. We will use the cost valuation.

To complete this illustration, let us assume that these investments are sold by the hospital at 102½ and accrue interest on January 1, 1978, with brokerage fees and other expenses of sale amounting to $76. The necessary cash receipts journal entry is

Cash—General Checking Account		$41,324	
Accrued Interest Receivable			$ 400
Temporary Investments			40,065
Gain on Sale of Temporary Investments			859
To record sale of temporary investment in bonds as follows:			
Sale price ($40,000 @ 102½)	$41,000		
Less brokerage and other expenses of sale	76		
Net	$40,924		
Accrued interest $40,000 × .06 × 2/12	400		
Total cash received	$41,324		

The credit to accrued interest receivable is necessary to eliminate the balance of that account as established by the income accruals at the end of November and December. A gain of $859 is realized on the sale; it is computed as the difference between the net proceeds ($40,924) and the cost of the investment ($40,065). This gain will be reported in the 1978 income statement of the hospital among the nonoperating revenues.

Similar procedures are followed in accounting for temporary investments in the hospital's restricted funds. The accounting procedures for long-term investments, however, is somewhat different. This matter will be pursued at length in chapter 19.

RECEIVABLES

The term *receivables*, as employed in hospital accounting, refers to the realizable cash value of the hospital's legal claim against its patients, third-party payers, and others. Such receivables arise primarily from the provision of health care services to patients on a credit basis. In effect, the hospital exchanges its services, including goods and supplies, for the patient's and/or the third party's promise to pay for such services in the future. It is an economic exchange measured in terms of the hospital's full established rates irrespective of expectations as to eventual collectibility. The resulting revenues and related receivables are recorded on the accrual basis in the time period in which the associated health care services are rendered. And, because there is usually a considerable time-lag between the rendering of services and the receipt of payment for those services, this gives rise to substantial amounts of accounts and notes receivable in hospital balance sheets.

Receivables may also exist in relatively small amounts from transactions that are only indirectly related to the provision of services to patients. Included in this category are accruals for various miscellaneous items such as interest and rental income earned but not yet received in cash, advances to employees, tuition charges receivable from students, and donors' pledges receivable. Full and separate disclosure should be made in the hospital balance sheet of all material amounts of these miscellaneous receivables.

Much of the accounting procedure relating to receivables has already been dealt with in earlier chapters. Here in chapter 16, the discussion will be confined to the balance sheet valuation of receivables, accounting for notes receivable, and internal controls.

VALUATION OF RECEIVABLES

Receivables should be reported in the hospital balance sheet at their net realizable or cash value. In other words, the gross amount of receivables recorded at full service rates in the accounts should be reduced to the net amount that can be reasonably estimated to be actually collectible in cash. Appropriate estimates, as described below, should be made of the amounts uncollectible due to bad debts, contractual adjustments, charity service, and other items. Such estimates should be treated as reductions of gross receivables in the balance sheet by the use of suitable "allowance" accounts. These amounts should also be included as "revenue deductions" in the income statement of the period in which the receivables arose. This procedure is required to secure a proper balance sheet valuation of the receivables as well as to obtain a proper matching of revenues and revenue deductions on an accrual basis.

• ***Bad Debts***. It is reasonable to expect that a certain amount of receivables arising from services provided to self-responsible patients will prove to be uncollectible. Uncollectible amounts also may arise from the uninsured portion of the accounts of patients covered by Blue Cross or other third-party payers. At the time of admission, or as soon thereafter as practicable, the financial status of each patient should be determined so that uncollectible amounts can be properly classified and distinguished as arising from (1) bad debts, (2) contractual adjustments, or (3) charity service. After adequate collection efforts have been expended to the point at which additional expenditures cannot be justified on the basis of prospective benefits, amounts remaining uncollected from self-responsible, noncharity patients should be considered bad debts.

At the end of each reporting period, an estimate must be made of the amount of receivables which ultimately will prove to be bad debts. This is necessary to prevent an overstatement of assets (receivables) in the balance sheet and to provide for a proper matching of revenues and revenue deductions in the income statement of the period in which the receivables originated. It is a procedure required under the accrual basis of accounting.

To illustrate, let us assume that 1977 is the initial year of operations for Homecity Hospital. During this year, the hospital provided $3,600,000 of services to patients and collected $3,000,000 of this amount. At the end of the year, then, accounts receivable total $600,000. Also assume that operating expenses for the year are $3,500,000 and that there were no charity patients or contractual adjustments. If nothing is done with respect to the possibility of bad debts, the hospital's year-end balance sheet will include $600,000 of accounts receivable among the assets, and the 1977 income statement will report a net income of $100,000 (in other words, $3,600,000 − $3,500,000).

In the first several months of the following year, $564,000 of the 1977 accounts receivable are collected. The remaining sum of $36,000, after diligent efforts to collect it, is deemed to be uncollectible accounts, or bad debts. Accordingly, an entry is made to write off these receivables and charge the $36,000 to the 1978 revenue deductions account. Observe, however, that the receivables and the related revenues were recorded in 1977.

This procedure obviously places the bad debt losses in the wrong year! The $36,000 of bad debts should have been given accounting recognition as deductions from revenues in 1977, the year in which the related revenue was recorded. This means that the net income for 1977 was overstated by $36,000. In addition, there was a $36,000 overstatement of assets (accounts receivable) in the December 31, 1977, balance sheet. The receivables should have been stated in that balance sheet at net realizable cash value, or $564,000.

The difficulty, of course, is that it is impossible to predict precisely which individual accounts will prove to be bad debts. It also is impossible to determine precisely the total dollar amount of accounts that will prove to be uncollectible in the future. We do not have perfect foresight. Nevertheless, a reasonable estimate can, and should be, made so that the degree of misstatement in the financial statements will be minimized. There are 3 methods by which bad debts may be estimated for accrual basis accounting purposes:

1. Application of a percentage, based on past experience, to the balance of accounts receivable at the end of the accounting period
2. Application of a percentage, based on past experience, to the total of charges to patients' accounts during the accounting period
3. Determination through an analysis of individual accounts in the patients' ledger, taking into account the length of time each account has remained unpaid (this method is called *aging* the accounts receivable)

As a matter of actual practice, hospitals generally employ all 3 methods, comparing the results of each so as to arrive at the most accurate estimate possible of probable bad debts.

The percentage used in these methods often is an average percentage based upon several prior years' experience and tempered by expectations of conditions that might exist in the subsequent collection period. Computations of such percentages, of course, should be based only on the self-responsible portions of patients' accounts receivable, since billings to third parties are generally collectible in full. In the following example, we will assume (1) that an average of 50% of the hospital's charges are 100% billed to third parties on assignment by patients, leaving 50% payable by patients themselves, and (2) that 40% of the year-end receivables have been billed to third-party payers on behalf of patients.

Let us return to the end of 1977 and attempt to estimate the amount of bad debts likely to arise in 1978 from the $600,000 of accounts receivable at Homecity Hospital. If we use the first method and assume that the appropriate bad debts percentage is 9%, bad debts will be estimated at $30,000 as follows:

Accounts receivable, 12/31/77	$600,000
Less third-party portion (40%)	240,000
Self-responsible portion	$360,000
Percentage of bad debts	9%
Estimated bad debts	$ 32,400

On the other hand, if we use the second method and assume that the appropiate bad debts percentage is 2.5% of revenues, bad debts will be estimated at $45,000 as follows:

1977 charges to patients	$3,600,000
Less third-party portion (50%)	1,800,000
Self-responsible portion	$1,800,000
Percentage of bad debts	2.5%
Estimated bad debts	$ 45,000

You should not assume from this example that the second method will always provide a larger estimate than the first method. It can be said that method 2 may be statistically superior to method 1 because of the larger base (charges rather than receivables) the second method employs. But, under either method, the critical factor is the soundness of assumptions and judgments underlying the determination of the bad debts percentage.

The aging procedure (method 3) is likely to provide the most accurate estimate of bad debts. It also is the most managerially useful method in that it requires a detailed, account-by-account examination of patients' receivables. The procedure involves the classification of account balances into "age" groups, depending upon the number of days that have elapsed since the date of discharge, as illustrated in figure 88. (In some cases, the aging may be made on the basis of time elapsed since the date of the last payment received on the account. Our illustration merely provides a "DLP"—date of last payment—column to indicate this information when it is desired.)

As you can see in the aging schedule, a total is obtained for each age group: for example, $160,000 of receivables are 1–30 days "old," $43,000 are in the 31–60-day group, and so on. Appropriate percentages based on past experience are then applied to these totals to obtain an estimate of probable bad debts. As you might expect, the percentage that is applied increases with the age of the accounts. The older the account, the less likely it is to be collected.

Using the bad debt estimate provided by the aging schedule, the required adjusting entry at the end of 1977 is as follows:

Deductions from Revenue—Bad Debts	$37,800	
Allowance for Uncollectible Accounts—Bad Debts		$37,800
To record required provision for bad debts per accounts receivable aging schedule.		

Thus, the 1977 income statement will include the $37,800 of estimated bad debts as a deduction from the patient service revenues of the year. And, the balance sheet at December 31, 1977, will show the allowance account as follows:

Accounts Receivable	$600,000	
Less Allowance for Uncollectible Accounts—Bad Debts	37,800	$562,200

In this way, the accounts receivable are reduced to net realizable value for balance sheet presentation purposes.

Let us now assume that, during 1978, $564,000 of these accounts are collected by the hospital. The hospital credit manager

Figure 88
Accounts Receivable Aging Schedule
December 31, 1977

Patient Name	Account Balance	Third-Party Portion	Self-		
			Total	Inhouse	1-30
Able, Marcus C.	1,420	690	730	730	
Active, James R.	2,466	1,314	1,152		1,152
Adams, Mary P.	608		608		
Agar, Thomas J.	1,190		1,190		
Akron, Louise M.	782		782		
Allen, Richard Q.	532		532		
Ammons, Peter C.	808	355	453	453	
Etc.					
Totals	600,000	240,000	360,000	90,000	160,000
Bad debt percentages				.02	.05
Estimated bad debts			37,800	1,800	9,000

concludes that the remaining $36,000 of accounts are definitely uncollectible. The summary entries are the following:

Cash Receipts Journal

Cash—General Checking Account	$564,000	
Accounts Receivable		$564,000
To record collections on 1977 accounts receivable during 1978.		

Responsible Portion						
Elapsed Days Since Discharge						
31-60	61-90	91-180	Over 180	DLP	Remarks	
			608			
	1,190					
782						
		532				
43,000	30,000	22,000	15,000			
.10	.20	.35	.60			
4,300	6,000	7,700	9,000			

General Journal

Allowance for Uncollectible Accounts—Bad Debts	$ 36,000	
Accounts Receivable		$ 36,000
To record the write-off of accounts deemed to be bad debts.		

The specific accounts written off at this time are removed or otherwise eliminated from the active section of the patients' subsidiary ledger. These records are placed in an inactive file and are retained under the control of a responsible employee who does not have access to incoming cash receipts. This is designed to prevent the theft of subsequent cash collections, if any, on previously written-off accounts. Where such recoveries are made, the credit should be made to the allowance account or to a special account designated "recovery of accounts written off."

To complete this illustration, assume that Homecity Hospital's accounts receivable at the end of 1978 total $685,000. Bad debts are estimated at $41,000, determined in the manner previously described for the end of 1977. The required adjusting entry for bad debts at December 31, 1978, is the following:

General Journal

Deductions from Revenues—Bad Debts		$ 39,200	
Allowance for Uncollectible Accounts—Bad Debts			$ 39,200
To record required provision for bad debts as follows:			
Required allowance account balance (credit)	$41,000		
Present allowance account balance (credit)	1,800		
Required adjustment	$39,200		

Recall that bad debts were estimated in the amount of $37,800 at the end of 1977, but actual write-offs during 1978 were only $36,000. This means that the allowance account is left with a $1,800 credit balance at December 31, 1978. Since a credit balance of $41,000 is required (based on an aging schedule or one of the other methods of estimation), the adjustment need be made for only $39,200. On the other hand, if 1978 write-offs had been (say) $38,000, the allowance account would have had a December 31, 1978, *debit* balance of $200. And, in that case, the above entry would have been made for $41,200 in order to obtain the desired $41,000 credit balance in the allowance account.

• ***Contractual Adjustments***. Under contractual agreements with third-party payers, hospitals often receive less than their full rates and are sometimes prohibited by the terms of the contract from recovering the difference from the patients that are covered by the contract. In such cases, the amount of these uncollectible differences—called contractual adjustments—included in year-end accounts receivable must be determined. This may be done by a direct analysis of individual accounts or on a percentage basis developed either from a sample of the accounts or from past experience. The procedure is similar to that for estimating bad debts.

To illustrate, recall (from figure 88) that the third-party portion of Homecity Hospital's December 31, 1977, receivables was $240,000, measured in terms of the hospital's full service rates. Earlier, it was assumed that the third-party payers paid 100% of such rates; now let us assume that the hospital is reimbursed on the average at only 95% of such rates. If this 5% difference is not billable to the patients involved, the following adjusting entry is required at December 31, 1977:

General Journal

Deductions from Revenues—Contractual Adjustments	$ 12,000	
Allowance for Uncollectible Accounts— Contractual Adjustments		$ 12,000
To record required provision for estimated contractual adjustments included in year-end accounts receivable.		

Including the previously determined estimate of bad debts, the December 31, 1977, balance sheet presentation of receivables might be as follows:

Accounts Receivable	$600,000	
Less Allowance for Uncollectible Accounts (Estimated Bad Debts, $37,800, and Contractual Adjustments, $12,000)	49,800	$550,200

The 1977 income statement, of course, will include the $12,000 of estimated contractual adjustments as a deduction from the patient service revenues of the year. Where the precise amounts of contractual adjustments can be determined, they may be credited directly to accounts receivable rather than to the allowance account.

Assume now that payments received on these accounts from third-party payers in 1978 amount to $229,400. The necessary entries are summarized below in a single cash receipts journal entry:

Cash Receipts Journal

Cash—General Checking Account	$229,400	
Deductions from Revenues—Contractual Adjustments	10,600	
Accounts Receivable		$240,000
To record receipt of payments for third-party portion of 12/31/77 receivables.		

Notice that the $10,600 debit is made here to the revenue deductions account and not to the allowance account because of the assumed design of the cash receipts journal (see the cash receipts journal illustrated in figure 61 at pages 214-215).

So, at the end of 1978, the allowance for uncollectible accounts for contractual adjustments remains with the $12,000 credit balance established at the end of 1977. If the amount of contractual adjustments at December 31, 1978, is estimated at (say) $14,500, the required adjusting entry is as follows:

General Journal

Deductions from Revenues—Contractual Adjustments	$ 2,500	
Allowance for Uncollectible Accounts— Contractual Adjustments		$ 2,500
To record required provision for contractual adjustments at 12/31/78 as follows:		

Required allowance	$14,500
Present balance of allowance account	12,000
Required adjustment	$ 2,500

On the other hand, if the $10,600 were debited to the allowance account in the above cash receipts journal entry, the December 31, 1978, adjustment would be made in the amount of $13,100 ($14,500 minus the remaining $1,400 balance of the allowance account). Either procedure is satisfactory.

The above illustrations for bad debts and contractual adjustments were presented in annual terms for ease of exposition. You *must* understand, however, that these adjustments are made in actual practice on a monthly basis. This is necessary in order to make the monthly financial statements more accurate and useful for internal management purposes.

• ***Charity Service***. As indicated in previous chapters, particularly in chapter 7 at pages 119-120, uncollectible receivables arising from the provision of charity service to patients may be accounted for through the use of an allowance account such as that described above for contractual adjustments. This method may be used where the amount of charity service in receivables is determined by estimate rather than by specific identification. In many cases, however, such amounts are readily determinable, and the use of the allowance account method is not necessary. Instead, charity service is recorded by direct credits to the receivables account.

ACCOUNTING FOR NOTES RECEIVABLE

It is not uncommon for hospitals to accept interest-bearing promissory notes from patients who, faced with a substantial hospital bill, require an extended period of time to accumulate the resources with which to pay their accounts. Although hospital managements historically have regarded the charging of interest with some disfavor, the use of interest-bearing notes receivable by hospitals is increasingly being viewed as both necessary and justifiable.

To illustrate the accounting procedures, assume that a patient gives Homecity Hospital an 8%, 90-day promissory note on March 1, 1978, in settlement of his $9,000 account with the hospital. The total interest on this note is $180 (i.e., $9,000 × .08 × 90/360), or $2 per day. It should be recognized as earned income by the hospital through monthly accruals as shown in figure 89. Elapsed days between any 2 dates are computed by counting the first day or the last day, but not both; in other words, the number of days between March 1 and March 31 is 30. It is assumed here that the note in question is a *term* note receivable—that is, that the face amount of the note and all interest is payable in a single sum on the maturity date of the note (May 30, 1978). Accounting for *installment* notes receivable, where the principal amount and interest is payable in periodic installments, is discussed fully in the author's *Hospital Financial Accounting—Theory and Practice*.

Should the patient fail to pay the note at maturity, the debit of $9,180 is made to dishonored notes receivable rather than to cash. The failure of the patient to honor the note, however, in no way changes the fact that interest income of $180 was earned. If further collection efforts are unsuccessful, the $9,180 may be written off as a bad debt.

To illustrate how patients' notes receivable may be used as a

Figure 89
Accounting for Notes Receivable

General Journal

3/1	Notes Receivable	$9,000	
	Accounts Receivable		$9,000
	To record receipt of 8%, 90-day note receivable for $9,000.		
3/31	Accrued Interest Receivable	$ 60	
	Interest Income		$ 60
	To record interest earned in March: $9,000 × .08 × 30/360.		
4/30	Accrued Interest Receivable	$ 60	
	Interest Income		$ 60
	To record interest earned in April: $9,000 × .08 × 30/360.		

Cash Receipts Journal

5/30	Cash—General Checking Account	$9,180	
	Interest Income		$ 60
	Accrued Interest Receivable		120
	Notes Receivable		9,000
	To record collection of note and accrued interest.		

source of funds by the hospital, let us backtrack to March 31. Assume that the first 2 entries in figure 89 have already been made, and that the hospital *discounts* the note receivable at a local bank. Assuming that the bank discount rate is 12%, the entry to record the discounting of the note is as follows:

Cash Receipts Journal

3/31 Cash—General Checking Account	$8,996	
Interest Expense	64	
Accrued Interest Receivable		$ 60
Notes Receivable Discounted		9,000
To record the discounting of a $9,000 note receivable at 12% at local bank.		

The maturity value of this note is $9,180, and there are 60 days remaining before that maturity date. The discount charged by the bank (rounded to the nearest dollar) therefore is $184 (i.e., $9,180 × .12 × 60/360). The proceeds of the note to the hospital are $8,996 (i.e., $9,180 − $184); that is, on March 31 the bank gives the hospital $8,996 for the patient's note. The hospital gives up the right to receive the $9,180 maturity value of the note. This will be collected by the bank.

Notice the above credit to notes receivable discounted. This is called a *contingent liability* account; so, assuming that the note was discounted "with recourse" (as is usual), the hospital is obligated to pay the bank $9,180 at the maturity date of the note if the patient does not. This account is presented in the hospital's balance sheet as a direct deduction from notes receivable in the asset section.

No other entries related to this note are made by the hospital until the May 30 maturity date. Following are the entries to be made on May 30 by the hospital, assuming (1) that the patient pays the bank and (2) that the patient does not pay the bank:

(1) *General Journal*

Notes Receivable Discounted	$9,000	
Notes Receivable		$9,000
To record payment by patient of discounted note receivable.		

(2) *Voucher Register*

Notes Receivable Discounted	$9,000	
Notes Receivable Dishonored	9,195	
Notes Receivable		$9,000
Accounts Payable		9,195
To record voucher for payment of discounted note receivable dishonored by patient.		

Cash Disbursements Journal

Accounts Payable	$9,195	
Cash—General Checking Account		$9,195
To record check issued to pay bank for dishonored note receivable discounted.		

When a discounted note is dishonored, the bank generally will make a charge often called a "protest fee." In this case, the fee was $15, making the total payment to the bank $9,195 (i.e., $9,000 + $180 + $15). Notice that the face amount of the note, the interest, and the protest fee is charged back to the patient by the debit to notes receivable dishonored. If collection efforts are not fruitful, the $9,195 may be written off as a bad debt.

INTERNAL CONTROL

Various internal control principles and procedures have been discussed in earlier chapters, particularly in chapter 12 where you observed that the control of receivables and the control of revenues is closely linked; so, let us limit this discussion to a few general observations about the internal control of hospital receivables.

Receivables control begins in the admitting process, where complete and accurate information must be secured so that an initial determination can be made of each patient's financial status and unnecessary delays may be avoided in subsequent billing and collection efforts. Once patients are admitted, the system should be such as to provide a high degree of assurance that *all* billable services rendered are promptly and accurately charged to patients' accounts. Unrecorded revenues are unlikely to be charged; if not charged, they will not be billed; and, if not billed, they will not be collected. Having complete and accurate charges to patients' accounts, the objective becomes that of maximum collection of such charges at the earliest practicable time.

The billing function usually should be performed by someone other than those who maintain the patients' subsidiary ledger records or the cashiers. Sound procedures should be followed (as described in chapter 12) as collections are received to assure that patients' accounts are promptly and accurately credited. Noncash credits made to accounts receivable deserve particular attention, as such credits may be used to hide errors and defalcations. Finally, the regular reconciliation of subsidiary ledgers with receivables control accounts must be recognized as an essential internal control practice.

QUESTIONS

1. What are "quick assets"?

2. Define *cash*. Are postage stamps, postdated checks, and employee IOUs properly includable in "cash"? If not, how should such items be classified in the balance sheet?

3. For what reasons are bank reconciliations prepared? By whom should bank reconciliations be prepared?

4. Explain how you would determine the appropriate imprest amount in which to establish a petty cash fund.

5. Under what circumstances is the petty cash account debited or credited?

6. List 10 of the most important basic principles typically incorporated into internal cash control systems.

7. Name 3 methods by which bad debts may be estimated for accrual basis accounting purposes. Which method is best?

8. Describe briefly some of the procedures which should be observed in maintaining effective internal control over hospital receivables.

9. Identify and explain the nature of 3 deductions that may be made in arriving at a balance sheet valuation for accounts receivable.

10. Define the term *temporary investments*. List some common types of temporary investments available to hospitals.

11. Hearty Hospital's general ledger cash in bank account shows a balance of $213,597 at November 30. The November bank statement, however, shows a balance of $244,129 at the same date. List 4 types of factors which may cause such a difference, and give an example of each.

12. Briefly describe the imprest system for operating a petty cash fund and state the principal advantages of the imprest system from the standpoint of internal control.

PROBLEMS

A. On June 1, Marshall Hospital established a petty cash fund in the imprest amount of $500. On June 14, the contents of the petty cash fund were as follows and the fund was reimbursed:

Coin and currency	$221
Petty cash expense vouchers	216
IOU from employee	10
Check of another employee made payable to Marshall Hospital	50

On June 16 the imprest amount of the petty cash fund was reduced to $300.

Required. (1) Prepare the necessary entries in general journal form at June 1, 14, and 16. (2) Why do you think the imprest amount of the petty cash fund was reduced on June 16?

B. Midway Hospital decided to establish a petty cash fund on May 1 in the imprest amount of $750. The following transactions relating to the fund took place during May:

1. The fund was established on May 1.
2. The fund was replenished on May 15 at a time when the contents of the fund were as follows.

Currency and coin	$ 42
Expense vouchers	681
Employee IOU	25

3. On May 16 it was decided to increase the imprest amount of the fund to $1,000.
4. The fund was replenished on May 31 at a time when the contents of the fund were as follows.

Currency and coin	$173
Expense vouchers	837

Required. (1) Prepare general journal entries to record all the petty cash transactions for May. (2) Assuming that the petty cash fund was *not* reimbursed on May 31, prepare the necessary May 31 adjusting entry.

C. Mason Hospital's general ledger cash in bank account shows a balance of $346,920 at October 31. An examination of the October bank statement in comparison with the cash records of the hospital, however, discloses the following information:

1. The October 31 balance per bank statement was $465,900.
2. A deposit in transit at October 31 was for $12,800.
3. Checks outstanding at October 31 totaled $89,300.
4. A patient's NSF $5,100 check was returned by the bank with its October statement.
5. Bank service charges for October were $120.
6. The bank inadvertently credited another of its depositors for the Mason Hospital's October 26 bank deposit of $10,600.
7. Matured temporary investments of $50,000, plus interest of $2,000, were cashed and credited by the bank to the hospital's checking account on October 29.
8. A hospital employee journalized a properly drawn check for $700 as $7,000 on October 11 in settlement of an account payable.

Required. Prepare (1) a bank reconciliation at October 31 for Mason Hospital (2) the necessary adjusting entry at October 31.

D. Mature Hospital's comparison of its cash records with its March bank statement provides the following information:

	Per Books	Per Bank
1. Balances, February 28	$14,755	$15,862
Receipts	15,431	17,495
Disbursements	13,744	16,087
Balances, March 31	16,442	17,270

2. Deposits in transit totaled $1,375 at February 28 and $946 at March 31. Checks outstanding were $2,482 at February 28 and $1,949 at March 31.
3. Bank service charges on the March bank statement were $16.
4. An NSF $479 check of a Mature Hospital patient was returned by the bank with the March statement.
5. On March 30 the bank collected a Mature Hospital patient's note to the hospital of $2,000 plus $40 interest. The bank credited the hospital for collection of the note and debited the hospital $7 for the service provided.
6. A hospital bookkeeper on March 12 journalized a $487 deposit as $847. This money represented a collection on a patient's account.
7. On March 22 the bank charged the hospital's account with a $388 check of another of the bank's depositors. The bank indicated that this mistake would be corrected on the April bank statement.
8. On March 27 one of the hospital's bookkeepers journalized a $10 check as $100. This check was issued in settlement of an account payable.
9. On March 29 the bank failed to give the hospital credit for a $1,055 deposit of that date. When notified of the error on April 4, the bank made the correction to appear on the April bank statement.

Required. (1) Prepare a bank reconciliation at February 28. (2) Prepare a bank reconciliation at March 31. (3) Prepare the necessary March 31 adjusting entry.

E. According to its books, Mainstay Hospital has a cash balance of $438,104 at June 30. The June bank statement, however, shows a June 30 balance of $486,681. An investigation produces the following information:

1. The bank credited, in error, Mainway Hospital for a deposit of $28,417 made by Mainstay Hospital on June 22.
2. Bank service charges for June amounted to $27.
3. Outstanding checks at June 30 were $107,092.
4. A deposit of $39,865 was in transit at June 30.
5. The June bank statement shows a credit of $10,600 (including $600 interest) representing the proceeds of a patient's note collected for the hospital by the bank.
6. The bank returned patients' checks marked "not sufficient funds" in the amount of $2,606.
7. Check number 1791 issued in payment of an account payable of $200 was recorded in error by a hospital bookkeeper as $2,000 even though the check was drawn in the correct $200 amount.

Required. (1) Prepare a bank reconciliation at June 30. (2) Prepare the necessary adjusting journal entry at June 30.

F. Hammil Hospital purchased $60,000 of U.S. government bonds at face value and accrued interest on September 1, 1977. These 8% bonds pay interest semiannually on April 1 and October 1. Brokerage and other acquisition costs totaled $94. The bonds mature on April 1, 1982, but the hospital intends to hold these securities as a short-term investment in its unrestricted fund. On

January 1, 1978, these bonds are sold by the hospital at 103 and accrued interest, with brokerage fees and other expenses of sale amounting to $105. Hammil Hospital closes its books annually on December 31.

Required. (1) Prepare, in general journal form, all necessary entries for 1977 in connection with this investment. (2) Indicate how all matters relating to this investment should be presented in the hospital's 1977 financial statements. (3) Prepare the necessary entry, in general journal form, to record the sale of the bonds on January 1, 1978.

G. Holden Hospital purchased $75,000 of corporate bonds at face value and accrued interest on August 1, 1977, with brokerage and other acquisition costs amounting to $88. These 6% bonds pay interest semiannually on June 1 and December 1, and mature on June 1, 1979. The hospital intends to hold these bonds as a temporary investment of its unrestricted fund. On January 1, 1978, these bonds are sold by the hospital at 98 and accrued interest, with brokerage fees and other expenses of sale amounting to $73. Holden Hospital closes its books annually on December 31.

Required. (1) Prepare, in general journal form, all necessary entries for 1977 with respect to this investment. (2) Indicate how all matters relating to this investment should be presented in the hospital's 1977 financial statements. (3) Prepare the necessary entry, in general journal form, to record the sale of the bonds on January 1, 1978.

H. A patient gave Happy Hospital a 9%, 90-day promissory note on November 1, 1977, in settlement of his $12,000 account with the hospital. Happy Hospital closes its books annually on December 31.

Required. (1) Prepare, in general journal form, all necessary entries with respect to this note for 1977 and 1978. (2) Indicate how all matters relating to this note should be presented in the hospital's 1977 financial statements.

I. A patient gave Harkrader Hospital a 6%, 180-day promissory note on October 1, 1977, in settlement of his $8,000 account with the hospital. The hospital discounted this note on November 1, 1977, at a local bank whose discount rate is 9%. Harkrader Hospital closes its books annually on December 31.

Required. (1) Prepare, in general journal form, all necessary entries with respect to this note for 1977 and 1978. (2) Indicate how all matters relating to this note should be presented in the hospital's 1977 financial statements. (3) Prepare, in general journal form, the necessary entry at the maturity date of the note, assuming that the note is dishonored by the patient and the bank makes a protest fee charge of $22.

J. Hadley Hospital has $760,000 of accounts receivable at December 31, 1977. An aging schedule is prepared which indicates that bad debts should be estimated in the amount of $58,000. Before adjustment, however, the allowance for bad debts account has a December 31, 1977, credit balance of $3,700.

During 1978, $64,800 of the 1977 accounts receivable are written off as bad debts; the remainder of the accounts are collected.

At December 31, 1978, Hadley Hospital has $827,000 of accounts receivable, and an aging schedule is prepared which indicates that bad debts should be estimated in the amount of $71,000.

Required. (1) Make the necessary entry at December 31, 1977, to record the required provision for bad debts. (2) Make the necessary summary entry to record the write-off of uncollectible accounts in 1978. (3) Make the necessary entry at December 31, 1978, to record the required provision for bad debts. (4) Indicate the presentation of receivables in the hospital's December 31, 1978, balance sheet.

K. During 1977, Hamlet Hospital charged patients' accounts for a total of $3,500,000. Its general ledger at December 31, 1977 (the end of the fiscal year), shows the following balances:

Patients' accounts receivable	$425,000 Dr.
Allowance for uncollectible accounts—bad debts	4,300 Cr.

Required. Prepare the necessary adjusting entries for estimated bad debts under each of the following assumptions: (1) bad debts are estimated at 1% of charges, (2) bad debts are estimated at 6% of receivables, and (3) bad debts, based upon an aging of the receivables, are estimated at $31,900.

L. Haven Hospital's adjusted trial balance at December 31, 1977, included the following accounts:

Accounts receivable—patients	$500,000 Dr.
Allowance for uncollectible accounts	
Bad debts	40,000 Cr.
Contractual adjustments	50,000 Cr.
Charity service	20,000 Cr.

In 1978, with respect to the 1977 accounts receivable, write-offs were made as follows: bad debts $37,400, contractual adjustments $51,700, charity service $19,200. The remainder of the 1977 receivables were collected.

Haven Hospital's accounts receivable at December 31, 1978, totaled $600,000. Estimated uncollectibles at that date were bad debts 9%, contractual adjustments 11%, charity service 1%.

Required. Prepare the receivables section of Haven Hospital's balance sheet at December 31, 1978. Show all necessary computations to support the figures included in the presentation.

17
Inventories and Current Liabilities

The first part of this chapter is concerned with accounting procedures pertaining to the acquisition, usage, and valuation of hospital inventories. In a hospital, inventories include, besides drugs and pharmaceuticals shelved in the pharmacy, the foodstuffs located in dietary storerooms and numerous other items ranging from the cleaning supplies used in housekeeping to laboratory chemicals and radiological film. While the inventory asset of the hospital may not be of substantial size relative to other assets, the annual usage of supplies is a significant element of cost. As much as 12–15 % of total operating expense may be represented by the cost of supplies. And, like cash, the inventory of the hospital is highly susceptible to theft. It also should be recognized that the cost of maintaining an inventory—purchasing, receiving, storing, issuing, and insuring—is rather sizeable. Finally, it is necessary for accounting purposes that proper determinations be made of the costs of supplies used and of the costs of supplies remaining unused in the hospital inventory. Let us therefore not underestimate the importance of adequate accounting and internal control procedures with respect to inventories.

In the second part of this chapter, we want to pull together some of the previously discussed materials dealing with current liabilities. Certain other related matters not covered before will also be introduced in this section from a balance sheet point of view. The balance sheet classification of current liabilities, as you know, includes a wide variety of debts representing goods and services purchased on account, borrowings from banks, accruals for payrolls, payroll-related obligations, interest, and other expenses. In fact, all cash disbursements made by the hospital ordinarily must pass through current liability accounts of one kind or another. These accounts consequently deserve a considerable amount of accounting and managerial attention.

INVENTORIES

The operations of a hospital enterprise require the purchase and use of a stock of goods and supplies. A discussion of the purchasing and receiving functions was presented in chapter 14, and now we must turn to the problems of determining (1) the costs of supplies used (the debits to supplies expense accounts) and (2) the costs of supplies unused and on hand (the valuation of the inventory) for balance sheet purposes. These determinations require an inventory accounting system and the adoption of an inventory valuation method.

INVENTORY ACCOUNTING SYSTEMS

Most hospitals will employ 2 different inventory accounting systems concurrently. Certain types of supplies may be accounted for by the periodic inventory system, while concurrently others are maintained on a perpetual inventory basis. To illustrate the 2 systems, let us assume that we have the following information with respect to a particular supply item which we will refer to as *Item X*:

	Units	Unit Cost
Inventory, April 1	100	$6
Purchase, April 15	400	$6
Usage, April 20	350	$6

The month begins with $600 (i.e., 100 @ $6) in the inventory account. What entry is made on April 15 when 400 additional units are purchased? What entry should be made on April 20 to record the usage of 350 units? By what procedure is the inventory at April 30 determined? The latter 2 questions would be complicated somewhat if the April 15 purchase was made at a unit cost other than $6, but we will defer this complication to a later point.

• ***Periodic Inventory System***. Under the periodic inventory system, no day-to-day record of supplies in inventory is maintained in the accounting records. As supplies are purchased, they may be charged either to inventory or directly to expense. Assuming the latter, this would be the April 15 entry:

Supplies Expense	$2,400	
Accounts Payable		$2,400
To record purchase of supplies (400 units @ $6 per unit).		

Generally, the debit is made to a supplies expense account only if the department that will use the supplies is known. Otherwise, the debit must be made to an inventory account.

Whether the above debit is made to supplies expense or to inventory, no entry is made on April 20 when 350 units of these supplies are used in departmental activities. At the end of April, then, the accounts would appear as follows:

Inventory		Supplies Expense	
$600		$2,400	

The inventory account shows the inventory balance at April 1, not

April 30. The supplies expense account indicates the cost of supplies purchased, not the cost of supplies used. Both account balances are incorrect.

So, at April 30, either (1) a physical inventory (actual count) must be taken or (2) an estimate must be made of the number of units in the month-end inventory. In the absence of error or theft, this quantity will be found to be 150 units. Cost prices then are assigned to these units, and the account balances are adjusted accordingly:

Inventory	$ 300	
Supplies Expense		$ 300
To record increase in inventory and corresponding reduction in departmental supplies expense.		

This entry adjusts the inventory to the proper April 30 balance of $900 (i.e., 150 units @ $6) and reduces the supplies expense account balance to $2,100 (the 350 units used which cost $6 each).

If we assume that the April 15 purchase of 400 units was debited to inventory rather than to supplies expense, the necessary April 30 adjusting entry is the following:

Supplies Expense	$2,100	
Inventory		$2,100
To record the cost of supplies used during April (350 units at $6 each).		

So, regardless of the debit made in the April 15 entry, we end April with $900 in inventory and $2,100 in supplies expense.

The periodic inventory system has the advantage of simplicity; it is clerically inexpensive. Because monthly physical inventory counts usually are not practical (and accurate monthly inventory estimates may not be available), however, the account balances may be somewhat distorted until actual counts and appropriate adjustments can be made. The degree of misstatement usually is not serious for interim reporting purposes, but physical inventories should be taken at least once each year, generally at the end of the fiscal period. The major disadvantage of the periodic inventory system is that the accounting records do not provide a means for control. The physical inventory indicates what the inventory is, of course, but the accounting records do not indicate what the inventory should be. Significant shortages may go undetected.

• ***Perpetual Inventory System***. Under the perpetual inventory system, records are maintained to provide a continuous record of supplies purchased, used, and on hand. Supplies accounted for on this basis are always charged to inventory accounts when purchased. The necessary April 15 entry is as follows:

Inventory	$2,400	
Accounts Payable		$2,400
To record purchase of 400 units of supplies at $6 per unit.		

An entry is also made in subsidiary inventory ledger records to reflect this inventory addition, raising the inventory balance to 500

Figure 90
Perpetual Inventory Ledger Card

LOCATION ______ ITEM ______ STOCK NO. ______

DESCRIPTION   UNIT

VENDOR		VENDOR		DATE	MAXIMUM	MINIMUM
1		3				
2		4				

ORDERED				RECEIVED					ISSUED					BALANCE ON HAND		
DATE 19__	ORDER NO.	VENDOR NO.	QUANTITY	DATE 19__	ORDER NO.	QUANTITY	PRICE	AMOUNT	DATE 19__	REQ. NO.	QUANTITY	PRICE	AMOUNT	QUANTITY	PRICE	AMOUNT

(P-477 BACK)

units having a total cost of $3,000 (the April 1 inventory of 100 units at $6 each plus the April 15 purchase of 400 units at $6 each). Perpetual inventory ledger cards such as the one illustrated in figure 90 may be used for this purpose, or the subsidiary records may be maintained by electromechanical equipment. Whatever the means employed, a continuous record is maintained of the units (with unit costs) received, issued, and remaining on hand.

As the supplies are required by departments for use in day-to-day operations, stores requisition forms (see figure 91) are executed. The forms provide a record of the quantities and costs of supplies used by the various departments of the hospital. Copies of these forms are routed to the accounting department where they serve as the basis for entries to debit the supplies expense accounts and to credit the inventory accounts. The April 20 entry, for example, would be this:

Supplies Expense	$2,100	
Inventory		$2,100
To record the requisition from inventory of 350 units of supplies which cost $6 per unit.		

An entry also is made in the subsidiary ledger records to reflect a reduction of 350 units in the inventory, thus lowering the inventory balance to 150 units of this supply item. These subsidiary ledger records may be kept in terms of quantities only, unit costs only, or in both quantities and costs as illustrated in figure 90. At least once each year, a physical inventory is taken and the perpetual records are adjusted, if necessary, to reflect the actual count. The main point to be made here is that the perpetual quantity records, in the absence of accounting errors, indicate precisely what the inventory *should be* at any time.

The choice of inventory system depends mainly upon the characteristics of particular supply items. If the dollar value of annual usage is substantial, if the supplies have a high unit cost and are susceptible to theft, or if the supplies are directly billable to patients, the perpetual inventory system is often desirable. The perpetual system provides a continuous control over the inventory in that information is immediately available as to inventory levels. Purchasing is facilitated, the adequacy of supplies on hand is more assured, and shortages are readily identified. Perpetual records also are useful for purposes of maintaining adequate insurance coverage and for documentation of losses. Because it is a costly system, however, careful studies should be made to determine that the value of the benefits to be derived from perpetual records exceed the costs of installing and maintaining them.

Figure 91
Stores Requisition Form

STORES REQUISITION REQUISITION NO.________

DEPARTMENT________ DATE________19____

FLOOR OR DIVISION________ DATE REQUIRED________19____

QUANTITY		DESCRIPTION OF SUPPLIES NEEDED	TO BE USED IF PERPETUAL INVENTORIES ARE KEPT			
WANTED	DELIVERED		PRICE	PER	AMOUNT	ACCT. NO.

REQUESTED BY	APPROVED BY

SEND ORIGINAL TO STORE ROOM CLERK. DUPLICATE IS RETAINED BY DEPARTMENT HEAD.

INVENTORY VALUATION METHODS

The preceding example assumed a single unit cost of supplies. In actual practice, however, supplies typically are purchased during a given time period at different unit costs. A problem therefore arises in determining which unit costs relate to the supply items that have been used during the period and which apply to the units remaining in inventory at the end of the period. These determinations are important because of their direct effect upon the hospital's reported operating expenses and net income as well as upon the balance sheet valuation of the end-of-period inventory.

As a basis for subsequent illustrations, let us assume the following data with respect to a particular item of supplies:

1978 Date		Units	Costs Unit	Costs Total
May 1	Inventory	200	$ 2.00	$ 400
5	Purchase	400	2.50	1,000
10	Usage	300		
15	Purchase	500	3.00	1,500
20	Usage	600		
25	Purchase	100	3.50	350
				$ 3,250

The month begins with an inventory of 200 units which cost $2.00 each. During the month of May, a total of 1,000 more units were purchased at steadily increasing prices; and, because 900 units were used during the month, the May 30 inventory consists of 300 units. In this illustration, the total cost of the opening inventory and purchases is $3,250. What part of this total cost is the cost of supplies used during the month? What part should be assigned to the 300 units remaining in the month-end inventory? There are several different possible answers to these questions, depending upon the inventory valuation method that is adopted by the hospital.

• ***Specific Identification***. It may be possible to make a specific identification of unit purchase costs with individual units of inventory. If the inventory items are packaged or are in containers of some kind, the packages or cartons may be crayon-marked or tagged in some manner to show actual unit costs. Then, as items are removed from the inventory for issuance to departments, the stores requisition forms can be made to show these specifically identified unit costs. When the annual physical inventory is taken, the marked containers will provide the necessary unit cost figures for the pricing of the units in the inventory. Figure 92 provides an illustration of the type of form sometimes used in the taking of the physical inventory and in assigning costs to the units counted.

The specific identification method, however, is generally impracticable, if not impossible, to apply. This is true because of the multiplicity of products in hospital inventories and because the marking of unit costs on each item is either not feasible or too costly. It therefore is necessary to turn to some *assumed* flow of inventory units or costs. Some such generally accepted assumptions of flow are (1) average, (2) first in–first out, and (3) last in–first out. Different assumptions may be made for different classifications of inventory; the same assumption need not be applied to the inventory in its entirety.

Figure 92
Physical Inventory Record

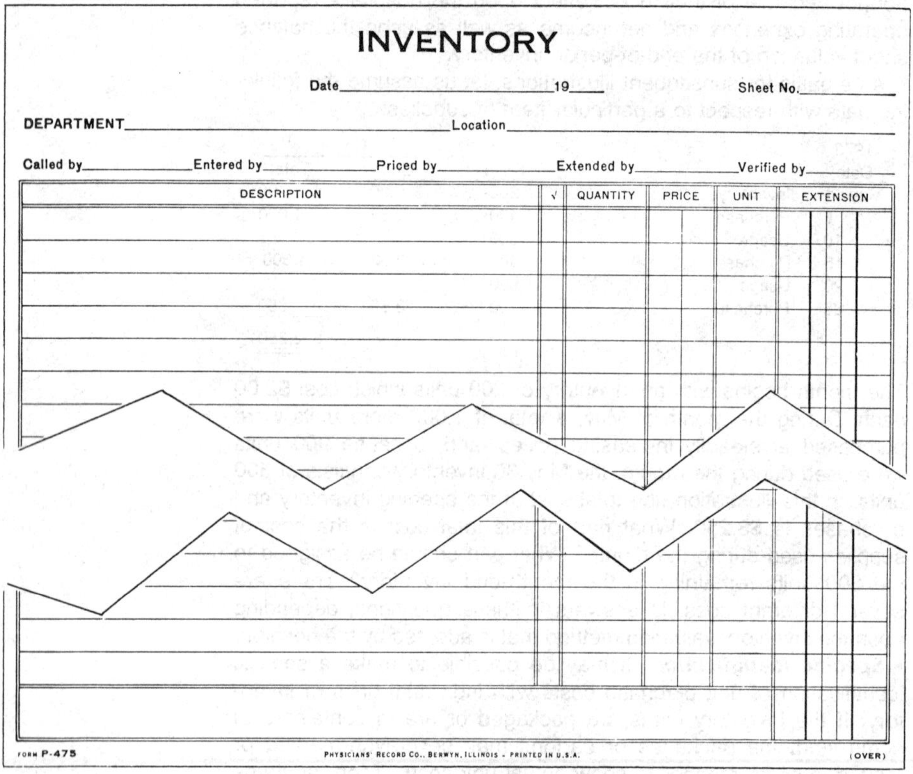

INVENTORY

Date____________ 19____ Sheet No.________

DEPARTMENT________________ Location________________

Called by________ Entered by________ Priced by________ Extended by________ Verified by________

DESCRIPTION	√	QUANTITY	PRICE	UNIT	EXTENSION

FORM P-475 PHYSICIANS' RECORD CO., BERWYN, ILLINOIS - PRINTED IN U.S.A. (OVER)

• ***Weighted-Average Costing***. Under weighted-average costing, the assumption is that the units issued from inventory are drawn more or less equally from each acquisition of supplies. It is not necessary, however, that the physical flow of the units in inventory be such as to correspond actually with the assumption.

If the *periodic inventory system* is employed, a weighted-average cost for the month of May would be computed as indicated in figure 93. This computation, which is made at the end of the month, indicates that the weighted-average cost per unit was $2.71 (rounded to the nearest cent). The May 31 inventory is therefore valued at $813 (300 units @ $2.71). This leaves $2,437 ($3,250 – $813) as the cost of supplies used during the month.

The necessary May 31 journal entry, assuming that the month's purchases were debited to the inventory account, is as follows:

Supplies Expense	$2,437	
Inventory		$2,437
To record cost of supplies used during May under weighted-average cost method, periodic inventory system.		

The credit in this entry reduces the inventory account balance from $3,250 (i.e., $400 + $1,000 + $1,500 + $350) to $813. Had purchases been debited to supplies expense, the month-end adjustment would have been a debit to inventory and a credit to supplies expense for $413.

Figure 93
Computation of Weighted-Average Cost
Periodic Inventory System

May 1	Inventory	200	units	@	$2.00	=	$ 400
5	Purchase	400	units	@	$2.50	=	1,000
15	Purchase	500	units	@	$3.00	=	1,500
25	Purchase	100	units	@	$3.50	=	350
		1,200					$3,250

Weighted = average cost ($3,250/1,200) = $2.71

If the *perpetual inventory system* is employed but the cost of units issued is recorded only at the end of each month or other convenient period, the computation of the weighted-average cost can be the same as shown above. On the other hand, it may be desirable to compute and record costs as supplies are issued from the inventory. This requires the computation of a new weighted-average cost after each purchase of supplies at a unit cost different from the current-average cost of the inventory. In other words, a "moving" weighted-average cost is computed as shown in figure 94 as it might appear on an inventory ledger card.

Figure 94
Computation of Weighted-Average Cost
Perpetual Inventory System

	Purchases			Issues			Balance		
		Cost			Cost			Cost	
Date	Units	Unit	Total	Units	Unit	Total	Units	Unit	Total
May 1							200	$2.00	$ 400
5	400	$2.50	$1,000				600	2.33	1,400
10				300	$2.33	$ 700	300	2.33	700
15	500	3.00	1,500				800	2.75	2,200
20				600	2.75	1,650	200	2.75	550
25	100	3.50	350				300	3.00	900
		Cost of supplies used				$2,350			

Thus, a new weighted-average cost is determined after each additional purchase. After the purchase of May 5, for instance, the recomputed average cost is $2.33, determined by a division of $1,400 by 600 units. As a result, the cost of supplies used is computed to be $2,350 (compared to $2,437 under the periodic inventory system), and the ending inventory is $900 (compared to $813).

• ***First-In–First-Out (FIFO) Costing***. The first-in–first-out (FIFO) costing method is based on the assumption that the supplies issued from inventory are obtained from the oldest stock. This means that the remaining units in inventory are stated in terms of the most recently incurred costs. The assumption appears logical in that some effort ordinarily is made to use up the oldest stock first. Nevertheless, the actual physical flow of the units need not conform exactly with the underlying FIFO assumption for this method to be acceptable.

If the *periodic inventory system* is used, the 300-unit inventory at May 31 would be valued as follows:

100 units @ $3.50 =	$ 350	(most recent purchase)
200 units @ $3.00 =	600	(from next most recent purchase)
300 units	$ 950	May 31 inventory valuation

Since the ending inventory is composed of the most recently incurred costs, the cost assigned to supplies used during the month is $2,300 (i.e., $3,250 – $900), the "oldest" costs.

If the *perpetual inventory system* is used in conjunction with FIFO costing, the same answers as above are obtained. The procedure is illustrated in figure 95 as it might appear on a subsidiary inventory ledger card. This allows the costs of supplies used to be determined at the time of issuance from inventory rather than at the end of the month only.

Figure 95
Computation of FIFO Cost
Perpetual Inventory System

	Purchases			Issues			Balance		
		Cost			Cost			Cost	
Date	Units	Unit	Total	Units	Unit	Total	Units	Unit	Total
May 1							200	$2.00	$ 400
5	400	$2.50	$1,000				200	2.00	400
							400	2.50	1,000
10				200	$2.00	$ 400			
				100	2.50	250	300	2.50	750
15	500	3.00	1,500				300	2.50	750
							500	3.00	1,500
20				300	2.50	750			
				300	3.00	900	200	3.00	600
25	100	3.50	350				200	3.00	600
							100	3.50	350
			Cost of supplies used			$2,300			

Figure 96
Computation of LIFO Cost
Perpetual Inventory System

	Purchases			Issues			Balance		
		Cost			Cost			Cost	
Date	Units	Unit	Total	Units	Unit	Total	Units	Unit	Total
May 1							200	$2.00	$ 400
5	400	$2.50	$1,000				200	2.00	400
							400	2.50	1,000
10				300	$2.50	$ 750	200	2.00	400
							100	2.50	250
15	500	3.00	1,500				200	2.00	400
							100	2.50	250
							500	3.00	1,500
20				500	3.00	1,500			
				100	2.50	250	200	2.00	400
25	100	3.50	350				200	2.00	400
							100	3.50	350
				Cost of supplies used		$2,500			

• ***Last-In–First-Out (LIFO) Costing***. The last-in–first-out (LIFO) method is based on the assumption that the supplies issued from inventory are drawn from the most recently purchased stock; the units are charged out of the inventory at the most recently incurred costs. This means that the ending inventory will be stated in terms of the earliest (oldest) costs experienced. It is somewhat difficult to imagine a hospital supplies situation in which there would actually be a LIFO flow of physical units, but you must remember that the physical flow need not conform to the LIFO assumption for the use of the method to be acceptable. The LIFO procedure is really based on an assumed flow of costs rather than of units.

If the *periodic inventory system* is used, the physical inventory of 300 units at May 31 would have a cost computed as follows:

200 units @ $2.00 =	$ 400	(earliest costs; May 1 inventory)
100 units @ $2.50 =	250	(next earliest costs; May 5 purchase)
300	$ 650	May 31 inventory valuation

Since the May 31 inventory is composed of the earliest costs incurred, the cost of supplies issued during the month consists of the most recently incurred costs, or $2,600 (i.e., $3,250 – $650). Let us again emphasize the point that, while it is unlikely that the oldest physical units comprise the inventory at May 31, the LIFO method's validity does not depend upon the actual physical flow of the units of inventory.

If the *perpetual inventory system* is employed in conjunction with the LIFO method, the required procedure is illustrated in figure 96 as it might appear on a subsidiary inventory ledger card. As indicated, the perpetual LIFO cost of supplies used is $2,500 and the

May 31 inventory $750 (i.e., $400 + $350), while the periodic LIFO figures were $2,600 and $650. It should be noted that the periodic and perpetual inventory systems ordinarily do not produce the same results when the LIFO method is employed; they do produce the same results, however, when the FIFO method is used.

• ***Summary***. The hospital has a choice of the above inventory costing methods in most instances. Which method should be adopted? The method that is chosen should, of course, be theoretically sound and clerically feasible. Consideration also should be given to the probable effect of the method on the reported results of operations and financial position. The implications of each method with respect to third-party cost reimbursement contracts is also important.

Figure 97 summarizes the results obtained by the use of FIFO, average, and LIFO costing (the 3 most widely used methods) in conjunction with the perpetual inventory system. It can be seen from this illustration that, in a period of rising prices, the LIFO method produces the highest operating expenses (reimbursable costs) and the lowest inventory valuation. FIFO produces the opposite results. Weighted-average costing will provide results somewhere between those obtained from FIFO and LIFO.

Figure 97
Summary of Inventory Costing Methods
Perpetual Inventory System

	Costing Method		
	FIFO	Average	LIFO
Inventory, May 1	$ 400	$ 400	$ 400
Purchases	2,850	2,850	2,850
Total	$3,250	$3,250	$3,250
Less inventory, May 31	950	900	750
Cost of supplies used in May	$2,300	$2,350	$2,500

INTERNAL CONTROL

Matters pertaining to internal controls over the purchase and receipt of supplies for inventory were discussed in chapter 14. Once supplies are acquired, the initial internal control objective is largely that of protecting the inventory items from theft, damage, waste, and obsolescence, as they remain in storage and then are consumed in hospital operations. A major requirement is the assignment of responsibility to specific employees for inventories at each location in the hospital. The number of such locations should be minimized so that centralized control may be better achieved. The storage areas should be kept clean, adequately lighted, and locked, with access limited strictly to authorized employees. Supplies should be released from the storerooms only upon presentation of properly executed stores requisition forms. Listings of approved authorization signatures should be issued by administration and reviewed periodically. Maximum-minimum controls should be devised which permit inventories to be maintained in amounts which are neither inadequate nor excessive. Where perpetual inventory records are kept, these records should be reconciled with physical inventories taken at least on an annual basis.

CURRENT LIABILITIES

The traditional working definition of current liabilities commonly employed identifies them as those obligations which mature and normally will be paid within approximately one year from the balance sheet date. Included in the current liability classification are notes payable, accounts payable, current maturities of long-term debt, accrued liabilities for expenses and other items, and deferred revenues.

Figure 98
Accounting for Notes Payable
Interest Not Prepaid

	Cash Receipts Journal		
8/1	Cash—General Checking Account	$36,000	
	Notes Payable		$36,000
	To record issuance of 90-day, 10% note to local bank for a short-term loan of $36,000.		
	General Journal		
8/31	Interest Expense	$ 300	
	Accrued Interest Payable		$ 300
	To accrue interest expense on note for month of August: ($36,000 × .10 × 30/360).		
	General Journal		
9/30	Interest Expense	$ 300	
	Accrued Interest Payable		$ 300
	To accrue interest expense on note for month of September.		
	Voucher Register		
10/30	Interest Expense	$ 300	
	Accrued Interest Payable	600	
	Notes Payable	36,000	
	Accounts Payable		$36,900
	To record issuance of voucher for payment of note and interest to maturity date.		
	Cash Disbursements Journal		
10/30	Accounts Payable	$36,900	
	Cash—General Checking Account		$36,900
	To record issuance of check in payment of note and interest.		

Figure 99
Accounting for Notes Payable
Interest Prepaid

	Cash Receipts Journal		
8/1	Cash—General Checking Account	$35,100	
	Prepaid Interest Expense	900	
	Notes Payable		$36,000
	To record issuance of 90-day, 10% note to local bank for a short-term loan of $36,000 with interest deducted in advance.		
	General Journal		
8/31	Interest Expense	$ 300	
	Prepaid Interest Expense		$ 300
	To record expiration of prepaid interest on note for month of August ($900 × 1/3).		
	General Journal		
9/30	Interest Expense	$ 300	
	Prepaid Interest Expense		$ 300
	To record expiration of prepaid interest on note for month of September.		
	Voucher Register		
10/30	Interest Expense	$ 300	
	Notes Payable	36,000	
	Prepaid Interest Expense		$ 300
	Accounts Payable		36,000
	To record issuance of voucher for payment of note and to record expiration of prepaid interest for month of October.		
	Cash Disbursements Journal		
10/30	Accounts Payable	$36,000	
	Cash—General Checking Account		$36,000
	To record issuance of check in payment of note.		

NOTES PAYABLE

Notes payable are obligations in the form of promissory notes issued to trade creditors for the purchase of goods and services, to banks for loans of a short-term character, and to other organizations. Whereas trade accounts payable generally fall due within a month, notes may be outstanding for periods of 90, 180, or more days from the balance sheet date. This requires, for interim reporting purposes, the accrual of interest expense on a monthly basis.

To illustrate the accounting procedure involved, let us assume that a hospital issues its 90-day, 10% note to a local bank for a short-term loan of $36,000 on August 1, 1978. The interest on this note will be $900 (i.e., $36,000 × 10% × 90/360), or $10 per day. The maturity date of the note is October 30, 1978, which is 90 days from August 1. All necessary entries for this 90-day period are summarized in figure 98.

In some instances, local banking practices may dictate that interest on loans be deducted in advance from the loan proceeds. This, in effect, means that the hospital is prepaying the interest expense. If that were the case with respect to the above loan, the proceeds would be $35,100 (i.e., $36,000 - $900), and the $900 would be accounted for as prepaid interest expense as illustrated in figure 99. It should be noted here that the hospital is paying $900 interest for the use of $35,100 for 90 days; so the effective (actual) rate of interest is higher than the 10% rate quoted by the bank.

ACCOUNTS PAYABLE

Trade accounts payable originate from the purchase of supplies and services on account. In many such purchases, a cash discount is allowed to the hospital if the related invoices are paid within a specified period of time. It is important, therefore, that the accounting system provide assurance that invoices are paid, whenever possible, within the discount period. It can be a costly omission to fail to take these discounts. (It should be noted that *trade discounts*, which may be offered to the hospital by a supplier in the case of large-volume buying, or use of a bidding process in purchasing, are always considered a reduction in cost. Only the net cost of the supplies should be recorded in the hospital's accounts.)

To illustrate, assume that the hospital purchases $5,000 of supplies on account, with terms of 2/10, n/30, on October 31. This means that, if the invoice is paid within 10 days (by November 10), a 2% cash discount can be taken by the hospital. The discount would amount to $100 (i.e., 2% of $5,000), and a payment of only $4,900 (i.e., $5,000 – $100) would be required. If the hospital does not pay the invoice within ten days, however, the supplier must be paid the full $5,000 within 30 days. So, if the hospital waits until November 30 to pay the invoice, it is in effect paying an additional $100 (or 2%) for delaying its payment for 20 days. Since there are roughly 18 periods of 20 days in a year, missing the discount would be paying 36% interest (i.e., 18 × 2%) per year on purchases!

The procedure described in earlier chapters is indicated by the following journal entries for the above example:

Voucher Register

10/31	Supplies Expense	$5,000	
	Accounts Payable		$5,000
	To record voucher for purchase of supplies on account.		

Cash Disbursements Journal

11/10	Accounts Payable	$5,000	
	Purchases Discounts		$ 100
	Cash—General Checking Account		4,900
	To record check issued in payment of voucher.		

Notice here that purchase discounts are recorded only when taken, and they are treated as other operating income. If we can assume that all available discount opportunities will be taken, this procedure has a number of weaknesses. First, the voucher register entry overstates both the cost of the supplies and the amount of the liability. Second, income is not earned by purchasing. Last, if the discount is missed, no recognition is given to the discount lost in the accounting records. That is, the cash disbursements journal entry would be simply a debit to accounts payable and a credit to cash for $5,000.

An alternative procedure designed to overcome the weaknesses of the above system is indicated by the entries below:

Voucher Register

10/31	Supplies Expense	$4,900	
	Accounts Payable		$4,900
	To record voucher (net of discount) for purchase of supplies on account.		

Cash Disbursements Journal

11/10	Accounts Payable	$4,900	
	Cash—General Checking Account		$4,900
	To record check issued in payment of voucher.		

In this way, the supplies and the related liability are recorded at the amount which the hospital should pay; no discount earned is recorded if the invoice is paid on time. If the discount is missed, however, the payment entry will be as follows:

Cash Disbursements Journal

11/10	Accounts Payable	$4,900	
	Purchase Discounts Lost	100	
	Cash—General Checking Account		$5,000
	To record check issued in payment of voucher after discount period has elapsed.		

Here, the use of the purchase discounts lost account (which is treated as a financial expense) points up an inefficiency in the hospital's processing of its accounts payable. Thus, management's attention is drawn to a situation which requires corrective action. Management should be more interested in the amount of purchase discounts lost than in the amount of discounts taken.

CURRENT MATURITIES OF LONG-TERM LIABILITIES

Mortgages, bonds, and other long-term obligations of the hospital should be reported as current liabilities to the extent that they are to be paid within one year from resources classified as current assets. In many instances, such as with mortgage notes and bonds that mature in annual installments, a portion of the total obligation is presented as a current liability, and the balance of the debt remains in the long-term liability classification. Assume, for example, that a hospital issues $5,000,000 of bonds on January 1, 1978, and that $500,000 of this bond issue matures each year for 10 years, beginning January 1, 1979. The December 31, 1978, balance sheet therefore should report $500,000 among the current liabilities and $4,500,000 as long-term debt.

ACCRUED LIABILITIES

Accrued liabilities consist of obligations that arise as a result of past operations usually involving contractual commitments and tax legislation. Included in this balance sheet classification are accrued salaries and wages payable, payroll withholdings and tax accruals, and various expense items such as interest and rent. Because of their materiality, accrued payroll and payroll-related liabilities typically are reported separately from other accrued liabilities. Accounting procedures for these liabilities were discussed in several earlier chapters, particularly chapters 5 and 13.

DEFERRED REVENUES

Hospitals sometimes receive cash advances from patients, third-party payers, and others for services that are to be provided in the future. Prepayments of this kind—including patients' admission deposits; advances from third-party reimbursement agencies; and tuition, rent, and interest received in advance—are recorded as liabilities when they are received. If the provision of such future services will involve significant costs or be financed from the hospital's current resources, these advances are properly classified as current liabilities. It sometimes has been the practice to report all deferred revenues in a balance sheet classification located separately between current liabilities and long-term liabilities. This practice, however, should be avoided. Deferred revenues should be identified as either current or long-term liabilities and should be reported in the balance sheet accordingly.

INTERNAL CONTROL

The key to effective internal control over liabilities lies in (1) the approval of purchase, borrowing, payroll, or other transactions giving rise to liabilities and (2) the proper determination of the amounts in which such liabilities are recorded. The voucher system employed should require that authorizations and approvals be fully evidenced in writing before any liabilities are recorded and before disbursements are made to discharge them. Appropriate subsidiary ledger records should be maintained by employees who are independent of the general ledger accounting function. These detailed records should be reconciled with the related general ledger control accounts on a regular basis.

QUESTIONS

1. Indicate some of the major requirements for a good system of internal control over hospital inventories.

2. Distinguish between the periodic inventory system and the perpetual inventory system. What are the advantages and disadvantages of each system? Which system should be used by hospitals?

3. Indicate the reasons that a considerable amount of importance should be assigned to inventory accounting and management in a hospital.

4. Distinguish between the FIFO and LIFO inventory costing

methods. In a period of rising prices, which method would tend to result in the recording of the highest costs for supplies used? In a period of rising prices, which method would tend to result in the highest end-of-period inventory?

5. Potter Hospital had a 1977 net income of $164,000. Cost of supplies used during the year totaled $713,000. The hospital's inventory of supplies increased by $27,000, and accounts payable to suppliers increased by $39,400 during the 1977 year. What was the amount of cash paid to suppliers during 1977?

6. Because of an error, Paxton Hospital's December 31, 1977, inventory was understated by $19,000. What is the effect of this error on the hospital's reported net income for 1977 and its financial position at December 31, 1977? What effect, if any, will this error have on the hospital's 1978 net income?

7. Define *current liabilities*. Give 6 examples of accounts that are shown in the current liability section of the hospital's balance sheet.

8. What are the financial consequences of a continued failure to take advantage of cash discount opportunities in the payment of accounts payable?

9. Payton Hospital purchased supplies on account and paid the related invoice within the specified discount period. The following entries were made:

Supplies Expense	$3,000	
Accounts Payable		$3,000
Accounts Payable	$3,000	
Purchase Discounts		$ 60
Cash—General Checking Account		2,940

From a theoretical and practical point of view, what is "wrong" with these entries? Briefly explain the alternative "discounts lost" procedure.

10. What are some of the major features of a satisfactory system of internal control over hospital liabilities?

PROBLEMS

A. Pitter Hospital provides you with the following information with respect to a single supply item purchased and used in its radiology department:

May 1	Inventory	400 units	@	$7
8	Usage	300 units		
15	Purchase	200 units	@	$8
22	Purchase	200 units	@	$9
27	Usage	200 units		

Required. Compute the cost of supplies used in May, assuming (1) periodical LIFO costing, (2) perpetual LIFO costing, (3) periodical FIFO costing, and (4) periodical weighted average costing.

B. Given the following data relating to a single billable supply item purchased and sold by Patter Hospital:

	Units	Cost Per Unit	Cost Total
Inventory, October 1	200	$1,000	$ 200
Purchases			
October 5	200	2.00	400
October 15	400	3.00	1,200
October 25	200	4.50	900
Sales			
October 10	300		
October 20	400		

Required. Compute the cost of supplies sold to patients during October and the inventory valuation at October 31, assuming the following:

1. Periodic inventory system
   a. Weighted average costing
   b. FIFO costing
   c. LIFO costing
2. Perpetual inventory system
   a. Weighted average costing
   b. FIFO costing
   c. LIFO costing

G. Putter Hospital began operating a new department on April 1. This department purchased and issued a single supply item as follows:

April	1	Purchased 500 units @ $5
	5	Issued 300 units
	10	Purchased 200 units @ $6
	15	Purchased 300 units @ $7
	25	Issued 400 units

Required. Assuming that this supply item is billed to patients at $10 per unit, compute the gross profit made by this department during April if the costing methods used are (1) the perpetual FIFO and (2) the perpetual LIFO.

D. Pender Hospital issues its 90-day, 10% note to a local bank for a short-term loan of $48,000 on September 1, 1977. Interest on the note was *not* deducted in advance. The hospital's fiscal year ends on September 30.

Required. Prepare, in general journal form, all necessary entries for 1977 in connection with this note.

E. Pinson Hospital issues its 120-day, 12% note to a local bank for a short-term loan of $75,000 on October 1, 1977. Interest on the note *was* deducted in advance. The hospital's fiscal year ends on December 31.

Required. Prepare, in general journal form, all necessary entries for 1977 and 1978 in connection with this note.

F. Parkway Hospital provides you with the following information about the purchase and usage of one of its billable supply items:

1978				Costs	
Date			Units	Unit	Total
June	1	Inventory	300	$4.00	$1,200
	5	Purchase	500	4.60	2,300
	10	Usage	400		
	15	Purchase	450	5.20	2,340
	20	Usage	550		
	27	Purchase	200	5.50	1,100

This supply item is billed to patients at $8.00 per unit.

Required. Assume that Parkway Hospital employs the perpetual LIFO system of accounting for this supply item. (1) Prepare an inventory ledger card for the month of June, 1978. (2) Prepare, in general journal form, all necessary entries for the month of June, 1978. (3) Assume that the physical inventory at June 30, 1978, indicates that 480 units are on hand in the inventory. What adjusting entry, if any, would you suggest?

18
Plant Assets and Depreciation

A hospital's *plant assets* consist of land, land improvements, buildings, and equipment. Other descriptive terms such as *fixed assets, capital assets,* and *tangible assets* also are often used as synonyms for this classification of resources. In any event, these assets are not intended for sale in the normal course of business but are held for use over a period of years in the provision of hospital services. Except for land, plant assets deteriorate with use and the passage of time; they eventually wear out. This "wearing out" process, as you already know, is recognized in accounting through a procedure called *depreciation*, the rational and systematic allocation of the cost of plant assets to expense over their useful lives.

In previous chapters, only a necessary minimum of attention has been given to the problems of accounting for plant assets and depreciation. We should now explore in some detail the accounting concepts and procedures employed by hospitals in recording the acquisition, depreciation, and disposal of plant properties. These are matters of considerable significance because it is not at all unusual to find 60 or 70% of a hospital's assets invested in land, buildings, and equipment. Developing and maintaining adequate records of these long-lived assets clearly must be one of the imperatives of hospital accounting.

Acquisition of Plant Assets

Hospitals generally acquire plant assets either by purchase or donation. A purchase of plant assets should result only from a budgetary process and a carefully constructed program of capital expenditures. The amounts which can be spent for this purpose will be limited, and the available funds must be allocated in the most effective manner consistent with the long-range objectives of the hospital. This program should also include an ongoing effort to secure plant assets by donation so that donors are encouraged to contribute in a form and manner best suited to the hospital's real needs. All plant asset acquisitions, whether by purchase or by donation, should also require the approval of the governing board of the hospital.

As plant assets are acquired, appropriate accounting records should be established. This requires a proper account classification of the assets and an accurate determination of their "cost." In addition to the general ledger record, a suitable subsidiary ledger record also must be made for accounting and internal control purposes.

CLASSIFICATION OF PLANT ASSETS

Hospital plant assets, with the related accumulated depreciation accounts, traditionally have been classified in the following manner:

AHA Account Numbers	
1130	Land
1140	Land Improvements
1240	Accumulated Depreciation—Land Improvements
1150	Buildings
1250	Accumulated Depreciation—Buildings
1170	Fixed Equipment
1270	Accumulated Depreciation—Fixed Equipment
1180	Major Movable Equipment
1280	Accumulated Depreciation—Major Movable Equipment
1190	Minor Equipment
1290	Accumulated Depreciation—Minor Equipment

This classification, or some variation of it, probably is employed by a majority of hospitals. Let us briefly examine the nature and content of each of the 6 primary asset accounts.

- ***Land***. The land account includes the cost of earth surface owned by the hospital and used in the ordinary course of hospital operations. It includes all land used for building sites, yards and grounds, and parking areas. Land acquired for future expansion, and not currently in use, should not be included in the land account but should be reported among the long-term investments in the hospital's balance sheet. Since land does not deteriorate with use or the passage of time, it is not subject to depreciation.
- ***Land Improvements***. Land improvements consist of the cost of on-site water and sewer systems, fencing and walls, sidewalks, shrubbery and trees, and paving of roadways and parking lots. These costs are depreciable and therefore should be separately recorded in the accounts so as to distinguish them from land costs which are not depreciable.
- ***Buildings***. This account should reflect the cost of all buildings owned by the hospital and used in its normal day-to-day activities. Included in this account are the hospital buildings themselves, personnel residences, garages and storage houses, and utility structures such as an outlying heating and cooling plant. A building which has been donated to the hospital for endowment investment purposes, and is not used in regular hospital activities, should be reported among the assets of the endowment fund. All hospital buildings, of course, are depreciable.
- ***Fixed Equipment***. The fixed equipment account includes the cost of equipment that is affixed to, and constitutes a structural component of, the hospital building. Another characteristic of fixed equipment is that it is not subject to transfer or removal from its fixed location. Equipment in this classification includes such things as mechanical and electrical systems, elevators, generators, pumps,

boilers, and refrigeration machinery. All of this equipment is depreciable over a relatively long life.

• ***Major Movable Equipment***. The general characteristics of equipment included in this category are as follows:

1. A capability of being readily moved from one location to another in the hospital
2. A unit cost sufficiently large to justify the expense incident to control by means of a subsidiary equipment ledger
3. A minimum useful life of usually 3 years or more

Some examples of major movable equipment are desks, chairs, beds, automobiles and trucks, accounting machines, sterilizers, operating tables, and X-ray apparatus. Major movable equipment items are depreciable over lives generally much shorter than for fixed equipment.

• ***Minor Equipment***. Minor-equipment items include wastebaskets, bedpans, glassware, sheets, basins, buckets, silverware, and most surgical instruments. As a matter of expedience, many accounting systems provide that only the cost of the original supply of minor equipment should be charged to this asset account. This original cost generally is depreciated over a short period (perhaps 3 years), with all additional purchases being charged to expense at acquisition. Other hospitals record all minor equipment (both the original supply and replacement purchases) to the asset account, and depreciate it over a 3-year period. Since it is not feasible to attempt to inventory this equipment annually, and because the costs involved are relatively immaterial, no other accounting procedures are generally workable.

DETERMINATION OF COST

The "cost" of a purchased plant asset includes all expenditures related to acquiring the asset, bringing it to the desired location, and making it ready for use in hospital activities. Such costs include the following:

1. The billed price of the asset, net of any trade or cash discounts allowed
2. Freight charges
3. Sales taxes
4. Fees and commissions paid
5. Installation costs

The cost of a purchased asset, however, generally should not include interest. A hospital, for example, may acquire expensive equipment under a conditional sales or other deferred payment plan requiring a series of installment payments which include interest. Such interest charges should be excluded from asset cost, being recorded instead as interest expense.

When plant assets are acquired by gift or donation, the assets should be recorded at their fair market values at the date received. The offsetting credit is made directly to the unrestricted fund balance account, and not to a revenue account. All receipts of plant assets by donation are considered contributions to the permanent capital of the hospital. Depreciation should be recorded on donated plant assets as if the assets had been purchased.

ACCOUNTING PROCEDURE

To illustrate the accounting procedure for plant asset acquisitions, let us assume that on January 1, 1978, Hopewell Hospital purchased a new item of X-ray equipment for $75,000. This equipment has an estimated useful life of 5 years and an estimated salvage value of 20%, or $15,000. The necessary entries to record the acquisition are as follows:

Voucher Register

1/1/78	Major Movable Equipment	$75,000	
	Accounts Payable		$75,000
	To record voucher for purchase of new item of X-ray equipment.		

Cash Disbursements Journal

1/1/78	Accounts Payable	$75,000	
	Cash—General Checking Account		$75,000
	To record check issued for purchase of new item of X-ray equipment.		

The major movable equipment account, as you know, is a general ledger control account whose balance reflects the cost of all items of equipment in the major movable classification which are owned by the hospital. Detailed information concerning the individual items of equipment in this account must be provided by some form of subsidiary ledger record for plant assets.

Figure 100
Plant Asset Subsidiary Ledger Card

Description *Radiology Equipment (details)* I.D. No. *7040-8510-67*

Cost	*$75,000*	Life *5 years*		Method *SL*
Salvage value	*15,000*	Depreciation:		
		Per year	*$12,000*	
Depreciable cost	*$60,000*	Per month	*1,000*	

Date			Asset			Accumulated Depreciation			Book
			Dr.	Cr.	Balance	Dr.	Cr.	Balance	Value
1	*1*	*78*	*$75,000*		*$75,000*				*$75,000*

One form of subsidiary ledger record is illustrated in figure 100. When an item of equipment is acquired, it is entered on one of these cards as shown in the illustration. This provides a detailed record including a full description of the equipment, its cost, date of acquisition, salvage value, and estimated life, depreciation method and amounts, and whatever additional information may be desired. Such records support the periodic depreciation charges and the balance sheet asset valuations, provide the basis for insurance coverage and claims, permit the accurate recording of asset retirements and disposals, and assist in securing effective internal controls over the plant asset investment.

Notice that the plant ledger card indicates that the X-ray equipment was assigned identification number 7040-8510-67. (As you may recall, 7040 is the expense account number for the radiology department, and 8510 is the account number for depreciation expense. The *67* indicates that this equipment is the sixty-seventh item of equipment in the department. Numbering systems, of course, vary; this is simply an example.) A metal tag showing this number is attached to the equipment to facilitate its identification with the accounting records whenever an inventory is taken of the hospital's equipment.

Even where electromechanical accounting equipment is employed, however, it may not be feasible to attempt to maintain this type of separate subsidiary record for each individual item of equipment. Instead, similar items of equipment may be grouped on a single card. All beds in a particular nursing unit, for example, might be entered on one card. In other systems, a separate plant asset subsidiary record is maintained for the equipment in each department. When one of these variations is found, depreciation often can be computed on a group or composite basis such as is described later in this chapter.

Depreciation of Plant Assets

When Hopewell Hospital purchased the X-ray equipment, it acquired a "bundle of services" at a cost of $75,000. Each year, as this equipment is used in hospital activities, it gives off a portion of its total service capability. After 5 years of use, it is estimated that this bundle of services will have been exhausted. Clearly the cost of the services consumed each year should be recognized as an expense to be matched against the revenues produced by such services. This expiration of cost, or expense, is known as depreciation. It is as valid an expense as is the hospital payroll. But how is it measured?

The determination of periodic depreciation charges is dependent upon 3 important factors: (1) depreciable cost, (2) service life, and (3) choice of depreciation method. In past years, hospitals have employed a variety of depreciation methods, including the straight-line method and various accelerated methods such as the declining-balance method and the sum-of-years'-digits method. All these methods are in conformity with generally accepted accounting principles and are widely used by industrial and commercial firms for accounting and income tax purposes. Recently, however, the use of accelerated depreciation methods by hospitals for cost reimbursement purposes has been disallowed by governmental and certain other third-party payers. For this reason, the discussion in this book is limited to the straight-line depreciation method. A complete discussion of the accelerated depreciation methods can be found in the author's *Hospital Financial Accounting—Theory and Practice*.

DEPRECIABLE COST

The depreciable cost, sometimes called the depreciation base or basis, of a plant asset is its acquisition cost minus its estimated salvage value:

ACQUISITION COST − SALVAGE VALUE = DEPRECIABLE COST

The residual salvage value of a depreciable plant asset is the estimated amount for which the asset can be sold when it is retired from use in hospital activity. There is no simple formula by which salvage value determinations can be made. It is largely a matter of judgment applied by the individual hospital in view of its plant asset retirement policy and experience, expected future market conditions for used or scrapped equipment, and other factors. Some assistance, however, may be obtained from the hospital's auditors and from equipment manufacturers.

SERVICE LIFE

The useful service life of a plant asset ordinarily is expressed in terms of years. In selecting a service life, consideration should be given to both the functional and the physical factors that limit the service life. The functional factors include obsolescence resulting from technological change, growth in the scale of a hospital's activities, and major changes in methods of delivering health care services. The physical factors include wear and tear resulting from use and deterioration caused by the elements. As was true of salvage value determinations, however, the determination of service lives also is largely a matter of judgment, and is heavily dependent upon the individual hospital's plant asset retirement policy and experience. Although a plant asset remains in very sound condition, its economical service life may be at an end from the standpoint of a particular hospital. Various guides are published which offer assistance in establishing estimated useful lives.

BASIC STRAIGHT-LINE DEPRECIATION METHOD

The straight-line (often abbreviated as "SL") method of depreciation is a procedure under which an equal amount of depreciation is assigned to each year of useful life. The formula is the following:

$$\frac{\text{COST} - \text{SALVAGE VALUE}}{\text{ESTIMATED USEFUL LIFE}} = \text{ANNUAL DEPRECIATION EXPENSE}$$

Application of the formula to the data assumed above for the new item of X-ray equipment produces annual depreciation expense of $12,000, as follows:

$$\frac{\$75{,}000 - \$15{,}000}{5} = \underline{\underline{\$12{,}000}}$$

Thus, each year of the 1978–1982 period would be charged with $12,000 of depreciation expense for this item of equipment.

Since monthly financial statements should reflect all expenses, including depreciation, the following adjusting entry would be required at the end of each monthly reporting period:

General Journal

Depreciation Expense	$ 1,000	
Accumulated Depreciation—Major Movable Equipment		$ 1,000
To record monthly straight-line depreciation on item of X-ray equipment ($12,000 × 1/12).		

While the entry is posted to the general ledger accounts, no postings generally are made to the plant asset subsidiary ledger cards at this time. Postings to the ledger cards ordinarily are made only on an annual basis as illustrated in figure 101. The information on the subsidiary ledger cards is reconciled with that of the general ledger control accounts (for plant assets, depreciation expense, and accumulated depreciation) at the end of each fiscal year.

Mention should be made here of the fact that a special policy may be followed in recording depreciation on plant assets acquired during the course of a fiscal year. Because depreciation expense, after all, is merely an estimate, it is acceptable to adopt a policy of taking a half year's depreciation on all plant asset additions in the year acquired, regardless of the month of acquisition. Once this policy is adopted, however, it should be consistently followed.

Figure 101
Depreciation Posting to Plant Ledger Card

Description *Radiology Equipment (details)* I.D. No. *7040-8510-67*

Cost	*$75,000*	Life *5 years*		Method *SL*
Salvage value	*15,000*	Depreciation:		
		Per year	*$12,000*	
Depreciable cost	*$60,000*	Per month	*1,000*	

Date			Asset Dr.	Asset Cr.	Asset Balance	Accumulated Depreciation Dr.	Accumulated Depreciation Cr.	Accumulated Depreciation Balance	Book Value
1	1	78	$75,000		$75,000				$75,000
12	*31*	*78*					*$12,000*	*$12,000*	*63,000*

GROUP AND COMPOSITE STRAIGHT-LINE DEPRECIATION METHODS

The procedure described immediately above assumed *unit* depreciation; that is, the straight-line method was applied to a single unit or individual item. Since this procedure involves considerable clerical effort, hospitals often find it advantageous to associate depreciation computations with groups of plant assets rather than with each particular asset item. This procedure leads to so-called composite and group depreciation methods in which a single depreciation rate is applied to the total cost of a combined group of assets.

• ***Group Rates***. Under the group depreciation method, a number of *similar* plant assets are depreciated as a single unit. All the beds in a particular nursing unit, for example, might be grouped on a single subsidiary ledger record. Depreciation would then be computed as if these beds were a single asset. If these beds have a total depreciable cost of $45,000 and an average service life of 15 years, the annual depreciation expense would be $3,000 (i.e., $45,000/15).

• ***Composite Rates***. Under the composite depreciation method, a number of *dissimilar* assets may be depreciated as a single unit. To illustrate, assume that 6 different items of equipment are acquired on January 1, 1978, for a particular department of a hospital. Each equipment item has a different cost, salvage value, and useful life. When acquired, these items are entered on a single subsidiary ledger record, and a composite depreciation rate is determined as shown in figure 102. The composite rate of depreciation for this departmental group of assets is 11.2% (i.e., $8,000/$71,400); the composite life is 8.925 years (i.e., $71,400/$8,000). Thus, $8,000 of depreciation expense is taken each year so that, at the end of 8.925 years, accumulated depreciation will amount to $71,400.

Figure 102
Computation of Composite Depreciation Rate

Asset	Acquisition Cost	Salvage Value	Depreciable Cost	Useful Life (Years)	Annual Depreciation
A	$ 4,000	$ 400	$ 3,600	4	$ 900
B	22,000	2,000	20,000	20	1,000
C	9,000	-0-	9,000	5	1,800
D	20,000	4,000	16,000	8	2,000
E	6,000	1,200	4,800	6	800
F	19,000	1,000	18,000	12	1,500
	$80,000	$8,600	$71,400		$ 8,000

Composite depreciation rate = $8,000/$71,400 = 11.2%

FUNDING OF DEPRECIATION

The *funding* of depreciation refers to the process by which cash resources are set aside periodically and accumulated for the purpose of financing the renewal or replacement of plant assets. To illustrate the procedure, assume that Hopewell Hospital's depreciation expense for a particular year is $185,000:

	Debit	Credit
Depreciation Expense	$185,000	
Accumulated Depreciation		$185,000
To record depreciation expense for the year.		

Now assume that the funding of depreciation by the hospital is a voluntary action prescribed by the governing board. This is the appropriate entry, assuming 100% funding:

	Board-designated Assets—Cash	$185,000	
	Cash—General Checking Account		$185,000
	To record 100% funding of depreciation expense for the year.		

Thus, $185,000 is transferred from the hospital's general checking account and set aside in a special board-designated cash account *within* the unrestricted fund. Although earmarked for a specific purpose, the future use of this money remains entirely under the control of the board. It would be improper to transfer these monies to the plant replacement and expansion fund as if they were donor-restricted resources.

The hospital, of course, may fund more or less than the amount recorded as depreciation expense. The amount actually funded, however, has no bearing whatever on the amount of depreciation expense to be recorded. Naturally, the cash set aside in this way should be invested until such time as new plant assets are required. Income earned on such investments is accounted for as unrestricted resources and must be reported as nonoperating revenues in the hospital's income statement. This income, however, may be designated by the board for the purchase of new plant assets and added to the accumulated depreciation funds. It should be pointed out that the funding of depreciation is the only means through which the value of plant assets is maintained and converted into cash during the assets' useful lives. The alternative is to allow the asset value to become depleted over the useful life which, in reality, depletes and impairs the hospital's permanent capital.

DISPOSAL OF PLANT ASSETS

It is important that an accurate accounting be made of disposals of plant assets through normal retirement, sale, or exchange. Each of these possibilities is examined below. As a basis for the illustrations, we again assume that X-ray equipment was acquired on January 1, 1978, for $75,000. The equipment, which had an estimated useful life of 5 years and a $15,000 salvage value, has been depreciated under the straight-line method since the date of acquisition.

NORMAL RETIREMENT

If the equipment's useful service life ends on December 31, 1982, as was estimated, and its expected salvage value is realized, the entry to record the normal retirement of the equipment is

Cash Receipts Journal

12/31/82	Cash—General Checking Account	$15,000	
	Accumulated Depreciation—Major Movable Equipment	60,000	
	Major Movable Equipment		$75,000
	To record normal retirement of X-ray equipment, with proceeds of sale equal to salvage value.		

In addition to the general ledger postings arising from this entry, suitable notations are made on the plant ledger card as indicated in figure 103. The card is then removed to an inactive file and retained for the period of time which is required by the hospital's record retention policies.

Figure 103
Retirement Recorded on Plant Ledger Card

Description *Radiology Equipment (details)* I.D. No. *7040-8510-67*

Cost	*$75,000*	Life *5 years*		Method *SL*
Salvage value	*15,000*	Depreciation:		
		Per year	*$12,000*	
Depreciable cost	*$60,000*	Per month	*1,000*	

Date			Asset Dr.	Asset Cr.	Asset Balance	Accumulated Depreciation Dr.	Accumulated Depreciation Cr.	Accumulated Depreciation Balance	Book Value
1	1	78	$75,000		$75,000				$75,000
12	31	78					$12,000	$12,000	63,000
12	31	79					12,000	24,000	51,000
12	31	80					12,000	36,000	39,000
12	31	81					12,000	48,000	27,000
12	31	82					12,000	60,000	15,000
12	*31*	*82*		*$75,000*	*–0–*	*$60,000*			*–0–*

Retired 12/31/82; salvage value was $15,000.

Should the actual salvage value prove to be more or less than $15,000, the above entry would include an account for the recognition of a gain or loss on retirement of the asset. If the salvage proceeds proved to be $16,500, for example, the entry would include a credit to a "gain on retirement of plant assets" account for $1,500. This gain would be reported among the nonoperating revenues in the hospital's 1982 income statement.

In cases where fully depreciated assets remain in service, the usual practice is to take no further depreciation and to make no adjustment of previously recorded depreciation. The cost of such assets and the related accumulated depreciation remain on the books until the assets are eventually retired from service.

SALE OF PLANT ASSETS

A plant asset may be sold prior to the end of its scheduled useful service life for reasons not anticipated when it was acquired. Assume, for example, that the X-ray equipment is sold for $49,400 on May 1, 1980:

Cash Receipts Journal

5/1/80	Cash—General Checking Account	$49,400	
	Accumulated Depreciation—Major Movable Equipment	28,000	
	Major Movable Equipment		$75,000
	Gain on Sale of Plant Assets		2,400

To record sale of item of X-ray equipment as follows:	
Cost	$75,000
Accumulated depreciation	
1978 (12 months)	$12,000
1979 (12 months)	12,000
1980 (4 months)	4,000
Total	$28,000
Book value	$47,000
Sales proceeds	49,400
Gain	$ 2,400

If this equipment had been sold on this date for an amount less than its $47,000 book value, the transaction would have produced a "loss on sale of plant assets." Such losses usually are reported as negative figures in the nonoperating revenues section of the income statement.

EXCHANGES (TRADES) OF PLANT ASSETS

In certain instances, an old plant asset may be used as a trade-in, when a new plant asset is acquired. To illustrate, assume that the X-ray equipment along with $33,800 cash is given in exchange for a new item of X-ray equipment. The necessary accounting entry, assuming that the exchange occurs on May 1, 1980, is as follows:

Cash Receipts Journal

5/1/80	Major Movable Equipment		$80,800	
	Accumulated Depreciation—Major Movable Equipment		28,000	
	Major Movable Equipment			$75,000
	Cash—General Checking Account			33,800
	To record acquisition of new equipment in exchange for old equipment and cash as follows:			
	Book value of old equipment	$47,000		
	Cash paid	33,800		
	Cost of new equipment	$80,800		

The general accounting rule is that the "cost" of assets received in an exchange is the fair market value of the asset given up, plus cash paid—or the fair market value of the asset received—whichever is more clearly evident. An exception to that rule is made when, as above, the assets exchanged are similar in nature and use. In such cases, the "cost" of the asset received is the book value given up, plus cash paid, and no gain or loss is recognized.

PRICE-LEVEL ADJUSTMENTS

A new procedure recommended in the 1976 edition of the AHA's *Chart of Accounts for Hospitals* is that of formally adjusting the plant asset accounts to reflect the effects of inflation as measured by changes in the general purchasing power of the dollar. For this purpose, the AHA suggests the use of an index of the general level of prices known as the Gross National Product Implicit Price Deflator, published quarterly by an agency of the federal government.

To illustrate the procedure, again assume the purchase of an item of X-ray equipment for $75,000 (5-year estimated life; $15,000 salvage value) on January 1, 1978. Assume also that the GNP Deflator was reported to be 190 on January 1, 1978, and 200 on December 31, 1978. (At the time of this writing, this index uses the general level of prices in 1958 as the base year: 1958 = 100.) In addition to the 1978 entries based upon historical cost, the AHA recommendation would require entries such as the following:

General Journal

Major Movable Equipment—Price-Level Increment		$ 3,947	
Unrestricted Fund Balance—Price-Level Revaluations			$ 3,947
To record price-level adjustment of major movable equipment for 1978 increase in general price-level index			
($75,000 × 200/190)	$78,947		
Historical cost	75,000		
Price-level increment	$ 3,947		
Depreciation Expense—Price-Level Adjustment		$ 632	
Accumulated Depreciation—Major Movable Equipment—Price-Level Increment			$ 632
To record price-level adjustment of depreciation expense on major movable equipment for 1978 increase in general price-level index			
($12,000 × 200/190)	$12,632		
Depreciation expense based on historical cost	12,000		
Price-level increment	$ 632		

As a result, the December 31, 1978, balance sheet would report this equipment at $78,947 and the related depreciation accumulated at $12,632. The 1978 income statement would report depreciation expense in the amount of $12,632. In this way, the financial statements disclose the effects of inflation on the hospital's plant assets and operating results (to the extent of the depreciation charge). Similar adjustments would be made at the end of each subsequent year based upon the price-level index at those times. The procedure is intended to emphasize, and draw attention to, the fact that depreciation charges based upon historical costs are inadequate to provide for the replacement of hospital properties at the higher price levels which probably will prevail in the future.

You should recognize, however, that formal recognition of inflation in accounting is not as yet a generally accepted accounting principle. Historical cost still remains the only generally accepted method, though many approaches are currently being discussed by the Financial Accounting Standards Board and the AICPA. The AHA recommendation is only a partial approach to the problem of accounting for the effects of inflation. Other authorities are urging the adoption of more-comprehensive and -thorough solutions. Further discussion of this matter is beyond this book's scope.

QUESTIONS

1. Distinguish between *land* and *land improvements*.

2. Distinguish between fixed equipment and major movable equipment. Give examples of the types of equipment that are includable in each of these classifications.

3. Describe briefly the proper accounting procedure for minor equipment.

4. List 5 items which generally should be included in the cost of purchased equipment. Should interest be included in the cost of equipment purchased on an installment or deferred payment plan?

5. Reston Hospital obtained an item of equipment by donation. At the date received, the equipment had a fair market value of $25,000. This equipment has an estimated useful life of 8 years and a 20% salvage value.

   a. Make the entry to record the acquisition of the equipment.
   b. Compute the annual depreciation to be recorded on this equipment.

6. What are the advantages of maintaining a detailed subsidiary ledger for plant assets?

7. How are each of the following determined?

   a. Depreciable cost
   b. Useful life
   c. Salvage value

8. "Depreciation expense is a measure of the decline in the value of plant assets during an accounting period." Do you agree? Explain.

9. Distinguish briefly between the group depreciation method and the composite rate depreciation method.

10. What is meant by the "funding" of depreciation? What entry is made to record the funding of, say, $79,000 of depreciation?

11. Riggin Hospital purchased an item of equipment for $40,000 on January 1, 1975. This equipment has an estimated useful life of 8 years and a 10% salvage value. On June 30, 1978, the equipment is sold for $23,100 cash. Assuming straight-line depreciation, prepare the necessary entry to record the sale of the equipment.

12. Ruggle Hospital purchased an item of equipment for $60,000 on January 1, 1974. This equipment has an estimated useful life of 10 years and a 20% salvage value. On October 1, 1978, this equipment is traded, along with $26,000 cash, for similar equipment having a list price of $72,000. Assuming straight-line depreciation, prepare the necessary entry to record the trade.

13. Summarize briefly the accounting procedure to be followed when an existing item of equipment having a book value of $40,000 and a fair market value of $45,000 is traded, along with $13,000 cash, for a new item of equipment having a list price of $60,000.

14. Ragsdale Hospital purchased an item of equipment on April 1, 1974. This equipment has an estimated useful life of 12 years and a 10% salvage value. The accumulated depreciation on this equipment on March 31, 1977, was $18,000. Assuming straight-line depreciation has been recorded, what was the acquisition cost of the equipment?

PROBLEMS

A. On January 1, 1977, Rainbow Hospital acquired 5 items of equipment as follows:

Asset	Acquisition Cost	Salvage Value	Useful Life (Years)
#1	$10,000	$2,000	8
#2	45,000	5,000	10
#3	24,000	4,000	5
#4	30,000	6,000	12
#5	19,000	1,000	6

Required. Prepare a table, similar to the one illustrated in figure 102 of the text, showing a computation of the composite rate of depreciation and the composite life of these 5 items of equipment.

B. On January 1, 1977, Radiant Hospital acquired an item of equipment for $90,000. This equipment has an estimated useful life of 5 years and a 20% salvage value. On March 1, 1980, this equipment is sold for $44,000.

Required. Assume that Radiant Hospital's fiscal year ends on December 31 and that adjustments for depreciation are made only at the end of each year. (1) Prepare all necessary journal entries from January 1, 1977, through March 1, 1980. (2) Draw up and complete a plant ledger card for this equipment item.

C. Rayfield Hospital purchased a new item of equipment for $100,000 on January 1, 1978. This equipment has an estimated useful life of 8 years and a 10% salvage value. Assume that the index of the general price level was 200 on January 1, 1978, and 212 on December 31, 1978. Rayfield Hospital's fiscal year ends on December 31, and depreciation adjustments are made on an annual basis only.

Required. Prepare the necessary journal entries to (1) record the acquisition of the equipment on January 1, 1978, (2) record 1978 depreciation on historical cost, and (3) record price-level adjustments at December 31, 1978.

D. Rex Hospital purchased an X-ray machine on October 1, 1977, at a cost of $20,000. In addition, the hospital paid $200 for freight and $800 for the construction of a concrete base and for making the proper electrical connections. The estimated useful life of the machine is 6 years with no expected salvage value. The hospital's fiscal year ends September 30.

Required. Prepare journal entries to record (1) the purchase of the machine, (2) depreciation expense for the first year, (3) the write-off of the fully depreciated machine after 6 years, and (4) the funding of depreciation at the end of the first year.

E. Roeder Hospital's preadjusted trial balance at December 31, 1977 (the end of the hospital's fiscal year), includes the following accounts:

	Dr.	Cr.
Land	$ 13,000	
Land improvements	18,000	
Accumulated depreciation—land improvements		$ 2,000
Buildings	900,000	
Accumulated depreciation—buildings		28,800
Fixed equipment	300,000	
Accumulated depreciation—fixed equipment		20,000
Major movable equipment	445,000	
Accumulated depreciation—major movable equipment		60,000
Minor equipment	24,000	
Accumulated depreciation—minor equipment		16,000

The following additional information is available:

1. Roeder Hospital began operations on January 1, 1975, when (with the exception noted below) all its plant assets were acquired. The correct amounts of depreciation have been recorded for 1975 and 1976, but no depreciation entries have as yet been made for 1977.
2. The land improvements are being depreciated over an 18-year life with no expected salvage value.
3. The building has an estimated useful life of 50 years and an estimated salvage value of 20%.
4. The fixed equipment has an estimated useful life of 25 years and an estimated salvage value of $50,000.
5. An analysis of the major movable equipment account appears below.

1/1/75	Equipment purchased having an estimated useful life of 12 years and a 10% salvage value	$400,000
3/1/77	Equipment purchased having an estimated useful life of 8 years and a 20% salvage value	60,000
9/1/77	Proceeds from sale of equipment purchased on 1/1/75 for $20,000	(15,000)
		$445,000

6. Minor equipment is being depreciated over a 3-year period with no salvage value expected.

Required. (1) Prepare the necessary journal entries at December 31, 1977. (2) Prepare a presentation of the plant assets section of the hospital's December 31, 1977, balance sheet.

19 Long-Term Investments

Temporary, or short-term, investments in stocks and bonds are those which are readily marketable and which management intends to hold for only a brief period (generally not in excess of one year). The proceeds from their disposition ordinarily are used to meet current obligations. Security investments not meeting these tests are separately classified in the balance sheet under the caption *long-term investments*. Short-term investments were discussed in chapter 16; this chapter will be concerned with long-term investments.

Long-term investments may appear in any fund, but often they are found as assets of the endowment fund or of the plant replacement and expansion fund. The funding of depreciation by action of the hospital's governing board may result too in long-term investments which are properly carried as board-designated assets in the unrestricted fund. In any case, these investments typically consist of government bonds, corporate bonds, and corporate stocks.

When securities of a long-term investment nature are acquired by gift or by endowment, they are recorded in the appropriate fund at their fair market value when received. The cost of bonds and stocks purchased, on the other hand, will include the quoted purchase price, brokerage fees, and other expenditures that are necessary to the acquisition. Income from long-term investments, usually consisting of interest and dividends, should be recognized on the accrual basis and in the appropriate fund. All income on unrestricted fund investments and all unrestricted income on investments of the restricted funds must be reported as nonoperating revenues of the unrestricted fund. Donor-restricted investment income generally is recorded in either the specific purpose fund or the plant replacement and expansion fund. Gains and losses on the disposition of long-term investments usually are recorded within the fund where the investments were carried as assets.

Long-term security investments, regardless of the fund in which they are recorded, are normally carried in the accounts at cost. Departures from the cost basis are not currently acceptable unless there is clear evidence of a material and apparently permanent decline in the market value of such investments. Such "write-downs" to the lower market values are reported as losses of the period in which the decline in value occurs. In no event is it presently in accord with generally accepted accounting principles to adjust the carrying value of long-term investments upward to reflect higher market values. Certain authorities, however, are challenging this position. The AHA *Chart of Accounts for Hospitals* (in both the 1976 and the 1966 editions), for example, expresses a preference for the valuation of long-term security investments at market value, whether it be higher or lower than historical cost. Nevertheless, in spite of its merit, this procedure is not yet a generally accepted accounting principle. So, in this book we will assume that long-term investments are to be valued in accordance with the cost principle in the formal accounting records but that market values should be disclosed parenthetically in the balance sheet or as supplementary information in the hospital's financial statements.

INVESTMENTS IN BONDS

A major part of the hospital investment portfolio is likely to consist of investments in government and corporate bonds because of the emphasis usually put on safety of principal and stability of income. Both government and corporate bonds are available in varying types and different denominations, although bonds of $1,000 face, or "par," value are most common. Interest is quoted at annual percentage rates of face value but often is paid semiannually on specified dates 6 months apart.

ACQUISITION OF BONDS

To illustrate the accounting procedures for long-term investments in bonds, let us assume that Goodcare Hospital purchases 60 of the $1,000, 8%, 10-year bonds of National Company on September 1, 1978. The bonds have a May 1, 1985, maturity date (they were originally issued by National Company on May 1, 1975) and pay interest semiannually on May 1 and November 1. Although bonds may be purchased at face value at times, it is more likely that the acquisition price will be either more or less than face value; that is, the bonds will be purchased either at a premium or at a discount. This occurs largely because the current market rate of interest (which changes frequently) is higher or lower than the nominal or coupon rate of interest paid by the bonds (which is fixed).

• ***Discount Acquisition***. If the current market rate of interest is in excess of 8%, the National Company bonds may be quoted at a price that is less than face value. Assume, for example, that the bonds are quoted at 92 (i.e., at 92% of face value) or $55,200 (i.e., 92% of $60,000). Let us also assume that brokerage fees and other acquisition costs total $400. The entries for the acquisition of the bonds therefore are as follows:

Voucher Register

9/1/78	Investments—Bonds	$55,600	
	Accrued Interest Receivable	1,600	
	Accounts Payable		$57,200

To record voucher for purchase of
National Company bonds as follows:

Quoted price (92% of $60,000)	$55,200
Acquisition costs	400
Cost of bonds	$55,600
Accrued interest ($60,000 × .08 × 4/12)	1,600
Disbursement	$57,200

Cash Disbursements Journal

9/1/78	Accounts Payable	$57,200	
	Cash—General Checking Account		$57,200
	To record check issued for purchase of National Company bonds.		

Notice that the brokerage fees and other acquisition expenditures are treated as a part of the cost of the bonds. Note also that since these bonds were purchased between interest payment dates, the hospital must pay the seller the amount of interest accrued since the last interest payment date (May 1, 1978). This, however, will be recovered by the hospital on November 1, 1978, as National Company will always pay a full 6 months' interest on each interest payment date regardless of the number of months the bonds have been held by the investor. (This was explained earlier at page 296, chapter 16.) If these bonds had been purchased on an interest payment date (May 1 or November 1 in this example), no accrued interest would have been involved in the acquisition.

• ***Premium Acquisition***. In instances where the nominal or coupon rate of interest is higher than the current market rate of interest, bonds tend to sell at a "premium," a price greater than the face value. Assume, for example, that Goodcare Hospital purchased the above National Company bonds at 105 and that acquisition costs were $600. The necessary entries are as follows:

Voucher Register

9/1/78	Investments—Bonds	$63,600	
	Accrued Interest Receivable	1,600	
	Accounts Payable		$65,200
	To record voucher for purchase of National Company bonds at a premium as follows:		

Quoted price (105% of $60,000)	$63,000
Acquisition costs	600
Cost of bonds	$63,600
Accrued interest ($60,000 × .08 × 4/12)	1,600
Disbursement	$65,200

Cash Disbursements Journal

9/1/78	Accounts Payable	$65,200	
	Cash		$65,200
	To record check issued for purchase of National Company bonds.		

Observe that Goodcare Hospital will receive annual interest of $4,800 (i.e., 8% of $60,000). Since $63,600 was paid for the bonds, however, the effective (actual) rate of return on this investment to the hospital will be somewhat *less* than 8%. In the previous example, which assumed that the bonds were acquired at a cost of $55,600, the effective yield will be *greater* than 8%.

BOND INTEREST INCOME

The amount of bond interest to be recorded as investment income by Goodcare Hospital depends upon whether the bonds were purchased at a discount or premium. This is true because the amount of discount or premium must be *amortized* over the number of months between the date of acquisition and the maturity date of the bonds. Let us examine the amortization process through the following illustrations.

• ***Amortization of Discount***. Again assume the purchase of the National Company bonds (details provided at page 347) at a discount on September 1, 1978. At the end of September (and at the end of each ensuing month), Goodcare Hospital will make an adjusting entry to record bond interest income for the month. Assuming that the bond discount is amortized by the straight-line method, this is the necessary entry:

General Journal

9/30/78	Accrued Interest Receivable			$ 400	
	Investments—Bonds			55	
	Bond Interest Income				$ 455
	To record accrued interest and amortization of bond discount as follows:				
	Nominal interest ($60,000 × .08 × 1/12)		$400		
	Discount amortization				
	Maturity value of bonds	$60,000			
	Cost of bonds	55,600			
	Discount	$ 4,400			
	Divide by months to maturity	80	55		
	Monthly interest income		$455		

Note that the discount ($4,400) will be taken into the accounts as bond interest income over the 80 months from the acquisition date to the maturity date of the bonds at the rate of $55 per month. The resulting $455 credit to income is a rough approximation of the effective amount of interest earned each month on the investment.

Notice also that the above entry debits the monthly amortization to the investment account, thereby increasing its carrying value by $55 each month. By the maturity date (May 1, 1985), the investment account will have a balance of exactly $60,000—that is, $55,600 + ($55 × 80 months). So, when the face amount of the bonds is paid to the hospital on the maturity date by National Company, the following entry can be made:

Cash Receipts Journal

5/1/85	Cash—General Checking Account	$60,000	
	Investments—Bonds		$60,000
	To record receipt of face value of matured National Company bonds.		

If the discount were not amortized over the 80-month period, the entire $4,400 discount would have to be recorded as 1985 income in the above entry. It seems quite clear, however, that the discount is earned by the hospital ratably over the 80-month period rather than just in the year of maturity alone. Thus, long-term investments in bonds purchased at a discount are carried in the accounts at acquisition cost plus discount amortization to date.

On November 1, 1978, Goodcare Hospital will receive 6 months interest on its investment in National Company bonds:

Cash Receipts Journal

11/1/78	Cash—General Checking Account	$ 2,400	
	Accrued Interest Receivable		$ 2,400
	To record receipt of semiannual interest on investment in National Company bonds ($60,000 × .08 × 6/12).		

Remember that the accrued interest receivable account was debited for $1,600 on September 1, when the bonds were acquired; for $400 on September 30, in an adjusting entry; and for $400 again on October 31, in an adjusting entry. The resulting $2,400 debit balance is then cleared from the accounts by the credit in the above cash receipts journal entry on November 1. The adjusting entry required at the end of each month to record the nominal monthly interest income is also used to record the discount amortization for the month.

To assist you in understanding this process, figure 104 shows the postings of all 1978 entries relating to Goodcare Hospital's investment in the National Company bonds. The hospital's 1978 income statement will report bond interest income of $1,820. Its December 31, 1978, balance sheet will include $800 of accrued interest receivable and will report the long-term investment at $55,820 (acquisition cost plus discount amortization to date).

• ***Amortization of Premium.*** Refer to page 348 where the purchase of the National Company bonds on September 1, 1978, at a cost of $63,600 was described. At the end of each ensuing month, an adjusting entry will be required to record bond interest income and amortization of bond premium for the month. Assuming that the premium is amortized by the straight-line method, the entry at September 30, 1978, is

General Journal

9/30/78	Accrued Interest Receivable			$ 400	
	Investments—Bonds				$ 45
	Bond Interest Income				355
	To record accrued interest and amortization of bond premium as follows:				
	Nominal interest ($60,000 × .08 × 1/12)		$400		
	Premium amortization				
	Cost of bonds	$63,600			
	Maturity value of bonds	60,000			
	Premium	$ 3,600			
	Divide by months to maturity	80	45		
	Monthly interest income		$355		

Figure 104
Accounting for Bonds Purchased at a Discount

Cash— General Checking Account

Debit		Credit	
(5)	2,400	(2)	57,200

Accrued Interest Receivable

Debit		Credit	
(1)	1,600	(5)	2,400
(3)	400		
(4)	400		
(6)	400		
(7)	400		
Bal.	800		

Investments—Bonds

Debit		Credit	
(1)	55,600		
(3)	55		
(4)	55		
(6)	55		
(7)	55		
Bal.	55,820		

Accounts Payable

Debit		Credit	
(2)	57,200	(1)	57,200

Bond Interest Income

Debit		Credit	
		(3)	455
		(4)	455
		(6)	455
		(7)	455
		Bal.	1,820

Posting references:

(1) 9/1/78 acquisition of bonds—voucher register.
(2) 9/1/78 acquisition of bonds—cash disbursements journal.
(3) 9/30/78 adjusting entry—general journal.
(4) 10/31/78 adjusting entry—general journal.
(5) 11/1/78 receipt of interest—cash receipts journal.
(6) 11/30/78 adjusting entry—general journal.
(7) 12/31/78 adjusting entry—general journal.

Exactly the same entry will be made at the end of each month until May 1, 1985, the maturity date of the bonds. Note that the premium ($3,600) will be taken into the accounts as a reduction of bond interest income at the rate of $45 per month. The resulting $355 credit to income is roughly the effective amount of interest earned monthly on the investment.

Notice that the adjusting entry credits the monthly amortization of premium to the investment account, thereby decreasing its carrying value by $45 monthly. By the maturity date of the bonds, the investment account will have a balance of precisely $60,000—that is, $63,600 − ($45 × 80 months). Thus, long-term investments in bonds purchased at a premium are carried in the accounts at acquisition cost minus premium amortization to date.

Figure 105 presents the postings of all 1978 entries for Goodcare Hospital's investment (at a premium) in the National Company bonds. You should study this illustration in comparison with the entries provided in figure 104.

DISPOSAL OF BONDS

The entry to be made when bond investments are held to maturity has been illustrated earlier. Suppose, however, that bonds held as long-term investments are sold prior to their maturity. Refer to the facts at page 347 relating to the purchase of the National Company bonds for $55,600 on September 1, 1978, and now assume that the bonds are sold on April 1, 1980, at 102 and accrued interest. The required entry is as follows:

Cash Receipts Journal

4/1/80	Cash—General Checking Account	$62,725	
	Accrued Interest Receivable		$ 2,000
	Investments—Bonds		56,645
	Gain on Sale of Investments		4,080
	To record sale of National Company bonds at 102 and accrued interest, less brokerage fees, as follows:		

Sales price ($60,000 × 102)	$61,200
Less brokerage fees	475
Net sales proceeds	$60,725
Accrued interest ($60,000 × .08 × 5/12)	2,000
Cash received	$62,725
Net sales proceeds (above)	$60,725
Book value of bonds	
Acquisition cost	$55,600
Add amortized discount ($55 × 19 months)	1,045
Book value of bonds	$56,645
Gain on sale	$ 4,080

As can be seen, the cash account is debited for the quoted price at which the bonds were sold (net of brokerage fees) plus the 5 months of interest that had accrued since the last interest payment date (November 1, 1979). This accrued interest, of course, had previously been established in the accounts by the month-end adjusting entries. At the date of the sale, the bond investment account had a balance of $56,645, having been written up to that amount because of the amortization of discount at the rate of $55 per month for the 19 months since the date of acquisition. Then, the difference between this carrying value and the net sales proceeds was recorded as the gain on the sale. Make special note of the fact that the accrued interest at the date of sale has no bearing on the amount of gain or loss on the sale.

Instead of selling all the bonds, let us now assume that only 40% (face value of $24,000) of the bonds are sold on April 1, 1980, at 102 and accrued interest, with brokerage fees amounting to $200. The necessary entry is as follows:

Cash Receipts Journal

4/1/80	Cash—General Checking Account	$25,080	
	Accrued Interest Receivable		$ 800
	Investments—Bonds		22,658
	Gain on Sale of Investments		1,622
	To record sale of 40% of the National Company bonds at 102 and accrued interest, less brokerage fees, as follows:		

Sales price ($24,000 × 102)	$24,480
Less brokerage fees	200
Net sales proceeds	$24,280
Accrued interest ($24,000 × .08 × 5/12)	800
Cash received	$25,080
Net sales proceeds (above)	$24,280
Book value of bonds sold (40% × $56,645)	22,658
Gain on sale	$ 1,622

Interest and discount amortization, of course, will continue on the remaining $36,000 face value of the National Company bond investment until these bonds are either sold or reach maturity. The monthly interest and discount amortization, however, will be 60% of the amounts illustrated earlier; in other words, the monthly amortization will be $33 (i.e., 60% of $55) and the monthly credit to bond interest income $273 (i.e., 60% of $455), starting April 30, 1980.

Figure 105
Accounting for Bonds Purchased at a Premium

Cash—General Checking Account

(5) 2,400	(2) 65,200

Accrued Interest Receivable

(1) 1,600	(5) 2,400
(3) 400	
(4) 400	
(6) 400	
(7) 400	
Bal. 800	

Investments—Bonds

(1) 63,600	(3) 45
	(4) 45
	(6) 45
	(7) 45
Bal. 63,420	

Accounts Payable

(2) 65,200	(1) 65,200

Bond Interest Income

	(3) 355
	(4) 355
	(6) 355
	(7) 355
	Bal. 1,420

Posting references:

(1) 9/1/78 acquisition of bonds—voucher register.
(2) 9/1/78 acquisition of bonds—cash disbursements journal.
(3) 9/30/78 adjusting entry—general journal.
(4) 10/31/78 adjusting entry—general journal.
(5) 11/1/78 receipt of interest—cash receipts journal.
(6) 11/30/78 adjusting entry—general journal.
(7) 12/31/78 adjusting entry—general journal.

The procedures described here are also applicable to bonds acquired by the hospital as a gift or endowment. In these cases, the fair market value of such bonds at the date of donation is regarded to be their cost. If the fair market value is less than maturity value, accounting procedures are those described for bonds acquired at a discount. If the fair market value is greater than maturity value, the accounting procedure is that described for bonds acquired at a premium.

INVESTMENTS IN STOCKS

The investment of hospital resources in corporate stocks involves some degree of risk with regard to price declines, but such investments may offer large rewards in the form of dividends and appreciation in value if they are managed intelligently. Investments may be made in either preferred or common stocks. Preferred stock, has certain preferences over common stock, as the name implies, such as the fact that dividends must be paid to a company's preferred stockholders before any dividends may be paid to its common stockholders. Accounting procedures for investments in capital stocks, however, are not much affected by the particular type of stock involved.

ACQUISITION OF STOCKS

Assume that Goodcare Hospital purchases 400 shares of Bluchip Company's common stock for $22,000 (including brokerage fees and other acquisition costs) on January 2, 1978:

Voucher Register

1/2/78	Investments—Stocks	$22,000	
	Accounts Payable		$22,000
	To record purchase of 400 shares of Bluchip Company's common stock for $22,000 ($55 per share).		

Cash Disbursements Journal

1/2/78	Accounts Payable	$22,000	
	Cash—General Checking Account		$22,000
	To record check issued for purchase of Bluchip Company stock.		

For investments in both bonds and stocks, a subsidiary ledger record should be maintained to provide the details of each investment and to support the general ledger investment control accounts. These subsidiary records sometimes are kept in the form illustrated in figure 106.

RECEIPT OF DIVIDENDS

Hospitals having capital stocks in their investment portfolios may receive cash dividends and perhaps stock dividends. We will illustrate the receipt of both types of dividends below with respect to Goodcare Hospital's investment in Bluchip Company stock.

• ***Cash Dividends***. There are 3 important dates with respect to dividends. A typical cash dividend announcement would read somewhat as follows:

> On April 20, 1978, the board of directors of Bluchip Company declared a cash dividend of $1.50 per share payable on May 19, 1978, to common stockholders of record at May 5, 1978.

You can find dividend announcements of this sort in the financial pages of many newspapers, in business journals, and even in certain popular magazines. These announcements always provide 3 dates:

1. The *declaration date* (April 20 above), that is, the date on which the board of directors voted dividend payment approval
2. The *record date* (May 5 above), that is, the date on which a determination is made of the names of the stockholders entitled to the dividend on the basis of the company's records
3. The *payment date* (May 19 above), that is, the date on which the company will mail out the dividend checks

Figure 106
Subsidiary Ledger Record for Investments

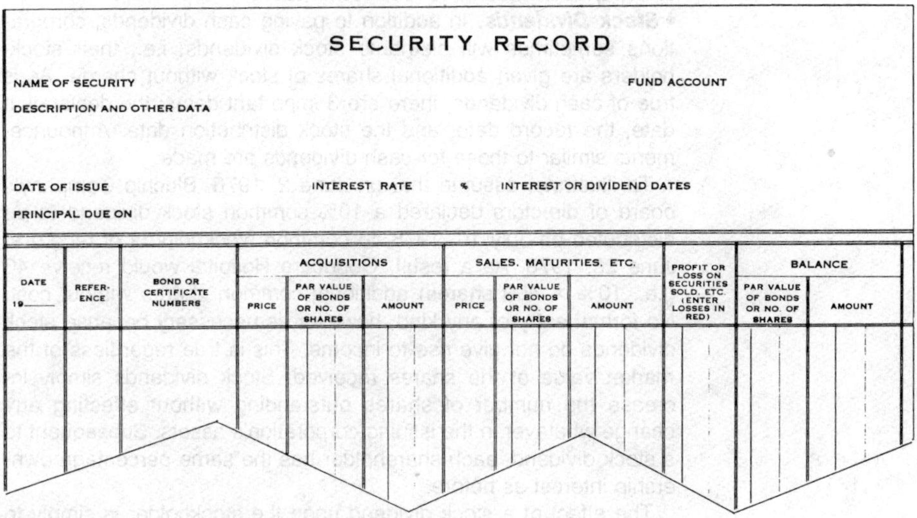
SECURITY RECORD

NAME OF SECURITY — FUND ACCOUNT
DESCRIPTION AND OTHER DATA
DATE OF ISSUE — INTEREST RATE % — INTEREST OR DIVIDEND DATES
PRINCIPAL DUE ON

DATE 19___	REFERENCE	BOND OR CERTIFICATE NUMBERS	ACQUISITIONS			SALES, MATURITIES, ETC.			PROFIT OR LOSS ON SECURITIES SOLD, ETC. (ENTER LOSSES IN RED)	BALANCE	
			PRICE	PAR VALUE OF BONDS OR NO. OF SHARES	AMOUNT	PRICE	PAR VALUE OF BONDS OR NO. OF SHARES	AMOUNT		PAR VALUE OF BONDS OR NO. OF SHARES	AMOUNT

Once a dividend has been declared, it must be paid. It also should be noted that all stockholders listed as such in the company's records on the record date will receive the dividend although they may sell their stock prior to the payment date. If the stock is purchased or sold between the declaration date and the record date, the quoted price per share will include the dividend. If the stock is purchased or sold after the record date, the quoted price per share does *not* include the dividend.

An entry for cash dividends should be made at the declaration date by the investor because the dividend has been earned at that time and because the payment of the declared dividend by the corporation is legally required. Goodcare Hospital's entry follows:

General Journal

4/20/78	Dividends Receivable	$ 600	
	Dividend Income		$ 600
	To record dividend income on Bluchip Company stock (400 shares × $1.50).		

Assuming that the hospital continues to hold the 400 shares of Bluchip stock, no entry will be necessary at the record date. But, when the dividend check is received on May 19, the following entry is made:

	Cash Receipts Journal		
5/19/78	Cash—General Checking Account	$ 600	
	Dividends Receivable		$ 600
	To record receipt of dividend on Bluchip Company stock.		

Carefully note that the dividend income was recorded in April (the month in which the dividend was earned) while the cash receipt was recorded in May. This, you see, is accrual basis accounting; income is recorded in the time period in which it is earned rather than in the time period in which it is received in cash.

• ***Stock Dividends***. In addition to paying cash dividends, corporations sometimes will distribute stock dividends; i.e., their stockholders are given additional shares of stock without charge. As is true of cash dividends, there are 3 important dates: the declaration date, the record date, and the stock distribution date. Announcements similar to those for cash dividends are made.

To illustrate, assume that on June 2, 1978, Bluchip Company's board of directors declared a 10% common stock dividend to be distributed on July 10, 1978, to common stockholders of record at June 26, 1978. As a result, Goodcare Hospital would receive 40 (i.e., 10% × 400 shares) additional common shares without cost. No formal entry of any kind, however, is necessary because stock dividends do not give rise to income. This is true regardless of the market value of the shares received. Stock dividends simply increase the number of shares outstanding without effecting any change whatever in the issuing corporation's assets. Subsequent to a stock dividend, each shareholder has the same percentage ownership interest as before.

The effect of a stock dividend upon the stockholder is simply to reduce the *cost per share* of stock. Goodcare Hospital, for example, had 400 shares of stock which had cost $22,000, or $55 per share. Upon receipt of the 40-share stock dividend, the hospital has 440 shares which cost $22,000, or $50 per share. Thus, the effect of the stock dividend in this example is simply an increase in the number of shares held and a decrease in the cost per share. Naturally, the subsidiary ledger investment records would be adjusted accordingly, but *no* journal entry is required.

DISPOSITION OF STOCKS

When stock is sold, the difference between the proceeds of sale (net of any brokerage fees and other expenses of sale) and the cost of the stock (as it may be adjusted for stock dividends, if any) is recorded as a gain or loss of the fund in which the stock was carried as an investment. Assume, for example, that Goodcare Hospital sells 100 shares of the Bluchip Company common stock for $6,425 on September 4, 1978. Assuming brokerage fees of $92, the entry to record the sale is as follows.

Cash Receipts Journal

9/4/78	Cash—General Checking Account	$6,333	
	Investments—Stocks		$5,000
	Gain on Sale of Investments		1,333
	To record sale of 100 shares of Bluchip Company common stock as follows:		
	Sales price $6,425		
	Less brokerage fees 92		
	Net sales proceeds $6,333		
	Less cost of stock (100 shares × $50) 5,000		
	Gain on sale $1,333		

The subsidiary ledger records should be properly adjusted for the shares sold. It should be clear that 340 (i.e., 440 − 100) shares of Bluchip stock remain in the investment account at a cost of $17,000 (i.e., $22,000 − $5,000, or 340 shares @ $50).

Suppose, however, that the Bluchip stock had been acquired at different times and at different costs per share. In such cases, to determine the cost of shares subsequently sold, it may be necessary to assume first-in–first-out (FIFO) or other costing methods (see chapter 17) in much the same manner as is done with respect to inventories of supplies. Of course, if the subsidiary record of investments provides a record of costs per share according to stock certificate numbers, a specific identification can be made to determine the cost of shares sold.

INTERNAL CONTROLS

Suitable internal controls should be maintained to safeguard the hospital's investments in stocks and bonds, as well as the related interest and dividend income, against loss through fraud, error, or mismanagement. It is important that all purchases and sales of investment securities be authorized by the hospital's governing board or by its investment committee. Once acquired, stock and bond certificates should be kept in a safe place, preferably in a bank safe-deposit box with entry requiring two hospital officials. Employees who have access to the accounting records or to cash should not, of course, have access to investment securities. Finally, regular reports of investments should be submitted to the hospital's governing board.

QUESTIONS

1. Distinguish between temporary and long-term investments.

2. When securities of a long-term investment nature are acquired by donation, at what amount are such assets initially recorded in the hospital's accounts?

3. When securities are purchased for long-term investment purposes by the hospital, what is their "cost"?

4. In what fund should the hospital record (a) income earned on long-term investments? (b) gains and losses on sales of long-term investments?

5. Explain what is meant by the declaration date, the rec-

ord date, and the payment date with respect to corporate dividend distributions on hospital investments in corporate stocks.

6. What are some of the major features of a satisfactory system of internal control over hospital investments in securities?

7. Towson Hospital holds an investment in the capital stock of an industrial corporation. The hospital receives 50 shares of the corporation's common stock as a dividend at a time when the stock is quoted on the market at $40 per share. Should Towson Hospital record $2,000 of dividend income? Explain.

8. Thomas Hospital owns investment securities which cost $100,000 but have a current market value of $140,000. At what amount should these securities be presented in the hospital's balance sheet? Explain.

9. A hospital owns 300 shares of stock which were acquired as follows:

1/1/76 100 shares purchased for $4,000
1/1/77 100 shares purchased for $5,000
1/1/78 100 shares purchased for $6,000

On 2/1/78, 150 of these shares are sold for $9,750. What is the amount of the gain on the sale?

10. When corporate bonds are purchased between interest payment dates, the hospital purchaser must pay accrued interest since the last interest payment date. Why?

11. When corporate bonds are purchased at a price higher or lower than face value, the premium or discount must be amortized by the purchaser. What is the purpose of amortizing bond premium or discount?

12. In what sections of the hospital balance sheet does one find the following accounts?

a. Temporary investments
b. Long-term investments—bonds
c. Accrued interest receivable
d. Long-term investments—stocks
e. Dividends receivable

PROBLEMS

A. Topmost Hospital purchased 90 of the $1,000, 8%, 10-year bonds of ABC Company on August 1, 1978, at 91 and accrued interest. Brokerage and other acquisition costs were $560. These bonds have an April 1, 1988, maturity date and pay interest semiannually on April 1 and October 1. The hospital's fiscal year ends on December 31.

Although the hospital intended to hold these bonds as long-term investments, the bonds were sold on January 1, 1979, at 98 and accrued interest. Brokerage and other expenses of sale amounted to $610.

Required. Prepare a chart, such as the one illustrated in figure 104 of the text, showing all necessary entries from August 1, 1978, through January 1, 1979.

B. Topville Hospital purchased 90 of the $1,000, 8%, 10-year bonds of ABC Company on August 1, 1978, at 108 and accrued interest. Brokerage and other acquisition costs were $572. These bonds have an April 1, 1988, maturity date and pay interest semiannually on April 1 and October 1. The hospital's fiscal year ends on December 31.

Although the hospital intended to hold these bonds as long-term investments, the bonds were sold on January 1, 1979, at 102 and accrued interest. Brokerage and other expenses of sale amounted to $520.

Required. Prepare a chart, such as the one illustrated in figure 105 of the text, showing all necessary entries from August, 1, 1978, through January 1, 1979.

C. Topsoil Hospital purchased $100,000 face value of XYZ Company bonds at 96 on May 1, 1978. These bonds pay 6% interest per year, payable semiannually on April 1 and October 1. The maturity date of these bonds is April 1, 1987. Brokerage fees and various other acquisition costs totaling $255 were paid. It was management's intention to hold these securities as long-term investments, but on January 1, 1979, 60% of the bonds were sold at 94 and accrued interest, less brokerage fees and other expenses of sale amounting to $210.

Required. Prepare all necessary entries relating to this investment from May 1, 1978, through January 1, 1979.

D. Topsail Hospital purchased $100,000 face value of XYZ Company bonds at 104 on May 1, 1978. Brokerage and other acquisition costs were $280. These bonds pay 7.5% interest per year, payable semiannually on April 1 and October 1. The maturity date of the bonds is April 1, 1987. It was management's intention to hold these securities as long-term investments, but on January 1, 1979, 40% of the bonds were sold at 106 and accrued interest, less brokerage fees of $310.

Required. Prepare all necessary entries relating to this investment from May 1, 1978, through January 1, 1979.

E. Topburgh Hospital purchased 200 shares of the $10 par value common stock of Mohawk Company on May 15, 1978, for $12,700. Brokerage fees amounted to $60. On June 1 the board of directors of Mohawk Company declared a cash dividend of $2.50 per share payable June 18 to stockholders of record at June 10. On August 4 the board of directors of Mohawk Company declared a 10% stock dividend payable August 30 to stockholders of record at August 15. At August 4 Mohawk stock was selling on the market at $80 per share. On September 19 Topburgh Hospital sold 120 shares of the Mohawk Company stock for $10,800, with brokerage fees amounting to $140.

Required. Prepare entries to record all matters relating to the investment in Mohawk Company stock for 1978.

F. Topvalue Hospital purchased Southcoast Company common stock as shown below:

Date	Shares	Price Per Share	Brokerage	Total Cost
1/1/77	20	$11.00	$20.00	$240.00
1/1/78	20	14.50	30.00	320.00

On April 1, 1978, Southcoast Company declared a cash dividend of $1.50 per share payable May 1, 1978, to stockholders of record at April 20, 1978. On July 2, 1978, Southcoast Company declared a 25% stock dividend payable August 15, 1978, to stockholders of record at July 21, 1978. On October 3, 1978, Topvalue Hospital sold 10 shares of the Southcoast Company stock for $160, less brokerage costs of $25.

Required. Prepare entries to record all matters relating to the investment in Southcoast Company stock for 1977 and 1978.

20
Long-Term Liabilities

In addition to the current liabilities described in chapter 17, a hospital will have economic obligations that will not be discharged with resources presently classified in the balance sheet as current assets. These obligations are variously referred to as *long-term*, *noncurrent*, or *fixed* liabilities. Whereas current liabilities generally arise from informal contractual arrangements, long-term liabilities are ordinarily based upon a written contract such as a mortgage document, bond indenture, or lease agreement. A proper distinction between current and noncurrent liabilities in the balance sheet is of considerable importance in evaluating the financial position of a hospital as well as in managing its financial affairs.

Long-term liabilities typically consist of mortgages and bonds payable, long-term contract and capital lease obligations, employee pension and retirement plan liabilities, and the noncurrent portion of deferred revenues. The discussion in this chapter will be limited, however, to accounting procedures relating to hospital bond issues. Since a majority of hospitals can no longer expect to obtain significant amounts of new long-term funds from philanthropy, public subscription, government grants, and other traditional sources, the only recourse is for the hospital to borrow through bond issues and then to repay with internally generated cash. The rapid increase in debt financing by hospitals in recent years provides sufficient documentation on this matter. This practice, encouraged by various state laws which enable hospitals to issue tax-free revenue bonds, naturally places a premium on superior financial management and its accounting prerequisites. It is largely for this reason that this chapter is devoted entirely to the subject of accounting for bonds payable. Accounting procedures relating to long-term leases, pension plans, and other noncurrent liabilities are described at length in the author's *Hospital Financial Accounting—Theory and Practice*.

Nature of Bonds

The power of a hospital corporation to issue bonds arises in the corporation laws of the state and is exercised by authorization of the governing board. In the case of state and municipal hospitals, bonded indebtedness also may require the approval of a majority of citizens. Many states have created statutory authority for issuing tax-exempt bonds to finance nonprofit hospitals' long-term capital needs.

Bonds ordinarily are issued in $1,000 denominations referred to as "face" (or "maturity") value. The terms of a bond issue are spelled out in a contract known as a *bond indenture*. It details the rights and obligations of the bondholders and the hospital, names the bank that is to act as trustee to protect the rights and enforce the covenants and obligations of both parties, and describes the bonds as to security, interest rate, maturity date, and other matters. While bonds may be sold directly to the general public, they more often are underwritten by investment bankers who either market the bonds on a commission basis or buy them at a discount and, in turn, sell them at face value.

Several different types of bonds may be issued by hospitals. *Registered* bonds are those on which interest is paid only to "bondholders of record" (that is, those whose holdings are recorded by the issuing hospital or its registrar agent). No record is kept of the owners of *coupon* bonds; rather, interest on coupon bonds is paid to all bondholders who present the periodic interest coupons which accompany the bond certificates. *Serial* bonds mature in installments over a period of years, while a *term* bond issue matures on a single fixed maturity date. Some bonds, at the option of the hospital, may be *callable* at specified times upon payment of a "call price" which usually is higher than the face value of the bonds.

In addition, bonds may be either secured or unsecured. *Secured* bonds, often known as "mortgage" bonds, involve the pledging of specific plant assets under liens as security to bondholders. Hospital bond issues may also be secured in the sense that payment of principal and/or interest may be guaranteed by a governmental authority or some parent organization. The security for a hospital bond issue may also arise from the accumulation of a bond "sinking fund" (a pool of resources earmarked for the payment of interest charges and for the retirement of the bonds). In many instances, hospitals have issued *revenue* bonds on which interest is paid from specified revenue sources. Finally, hospitals having extremely high credit ratings may sometimes issue general obligation bonds that are secured only by the hospital's reputation and general financial resources. Unsecured bonds of this type are called *debentures*.

The decision to issue bonds is a critical matter. All relevant factors must be carefully considered and evaluated. It should be apparent that the bond issue is the most desirable means of obtaining the necessary long-term funds at reasonable cost and on acceptable terms. There must be assurances that the debt burden, periodic interest charges and principal retirement, will not lead to financial embarrassment and endanger the hospital's ability to meet its social obligations to the community it serves. In all cases, the assistance of reputable professional firms specializing in hospital financing should be obtained.

ISSUANCE OF BONDS

When the hospital corporation issues bonds, it contracts to pay at periodic intervals usually each 6 months long (1) the face value of the bonds at a specified maturity date and (2) interest, expressed as a percentage of face value. This nominal, or coupon, interest rate is predetermined on the basis of expectations concerning the rate of interest investors will demand at the time the bonds are actually issued. The market rate of interest varies according to the degree of credit risk, the term of the bonds, the supply-and-demand situation for long-term money, and the taxability of the bond interest to investors, among other things.

If the nominal interest rate should equal the market rate, the hospital's bonds will sell at face value. There often will be a difference, however, between the nominal and market rates of interest. Bonds will sell at a *premium* (a price greater than face value) if the nominal interest rate is higher than the market rate; they will sell at a *discount* (a price lower than face value) if they pay interest at a rate less than the market rate. Thus, differences between the contractual and market rates of interest are reflected in the prices investors are willing to pay for the bonds, thereby eliminating the need to amend the bond contract. As issuing bonds at a discount or a premium is most common, we will discuss only those 2 possibilities.

ISSUANCE AT A DISCOUNT

To illustrate the accounting procedures for bonds issued at a discount, let us assume that Supercare Hospital issues $400,000 (face value) of 6%, 20-year bonds at 92.625 (92.625% of face value, or $370,500) on August 1, 1978. (Hospital bond issues generally are much larger amounts, but $400,000 is a convenient assumption for purposes of illustration.) These bonds pay interest semiannually on April 1 and October 1; semiannual interest payments are $12,000 (i.e., $400,000 × .06 × 6/12). The bonds are dated April 1, 1978, so the maturity date is April 1, 1998. Also assume that bond issue costs amount to $17,700, which consists of sales commissions paid to investment bankers, legal and accounting fees, registration and filing fees, appraisal costs, and printing expenses.

As noted above, the bond certificates are dated April 1, 1978, but the hospital postponed the actual sale of the bonds until August 1, 1978, in order to take advantage of an expected decline in the market rate of interest. Assuming that all the bonds are sold on August 1, 1978, then, the following entries will be made in the accounts of the hospital's unrestricted fund:

Cash Receipts Journal

8/1/78	Cash—General Checking Account	$378,500	
	Unamortized Bond Discount	29,500	
	Accrued Interest Payable		$ 8,000
	Bonds Payable		400,000
	To record issue of $400,000 of 6%, 20-year bonds at 92.625 and accrued interest, as follows:		

Face value	$400,000
Proceeds ($400,000 @ 92.625)	370,500
Discount	$ 29,500

Proceeds (above)	$370,500
Accrued interest ($400,000 × .06 × 4/12)	8,000
Total cash received	$378,500

Voucher Register

8/1/78	Unamortized Bond Issue Costs	$ 17,700	
	Accounts Payable		$ 17,700
	To record voucher issued for payment of bond issue costs.		

Cash Disbursements Journal

8/1/78	Accounts Payable	$ 17,700	
	Cash—General Checking Account		$ 17,700
	To record check issued in payment of bond issue costs.		

When bonds are issued or sold between interest payment dates, as these bonds were, the issuing hospital collects accrued interest from the purchasers as a part of the transaction. This procedure enables the hospital to pay a full 6 months' interest at each semiannual interest payment date regardless of the length of time individual bondholders may have held their bonds. It would be impractical for the hospital to try to compute the amount of interest actually due each bondholder at each interest payment date. Accrued-interest settlements are made between sellers and buyers of bonds at the trading date as an adjustment of the price to be paid by the buyers.

If a balance sheet were prepared immediately after the above bond issue, it would present the bonds as a long-term liability of Supercare Hospital's unrestricted fund in the following manner:

6% Bonds Payable, Due 1998	$400,000	
Less Unamortized Bond Discount	29,500	$370,500

Thus, the unamortized bond discount is deducted from the face amount of the outstanding bonds in the long-term liability section of the balance sheet. The unamortized bond issue costs of $17,700, on the other hand, should be included in the assets of the unrestricted fund in a "deferred charges" or "other assets" category. Only the unamortized bond discount should be shown in the contraliability position above. It is never correct to classify the bond discount as an asset. Finally, the balance sheet also would present the $8,000 of accrued interest payable among the current liabilities of the hospital.

ISSUANCE AT A PREMIUM

Where the nominal interest rate is higher than the market rate of interest, bonds will be issued at a premium. Assume, for example, that Supercare Hospital issues $400,000 (face value) of 9%, 20-year bonds at 108.85 (i.e., 108.85% of $400,000, or $435,400) on August 1, 1978. These bonds pay interest semiannually on April 1 and October 1, and mature April 1, 1998. Also assume that bond issue costs amounted to $23,600. Assuming that all the bonds are sold on August 1, 1978, the following entries will be made in the unrestricted fund accounts.

Cash Receipts Journal

8/1/78	Cash—General Checking Account	$447,400	
	Unamortized Bond Premium		$ 35,400
	Accrued Interest Payable		12,000
	Bonds Payable		400,000
	To record issue of $400,000 of 9%, 20-year bonds at 108.85 and accrued interest, as follows:		

Proceeds ($400,000 @ 108.85)	$435,400
Face value	400,000
Premium	$ 35,400
Proceeds (above)	$435,400
Accrued interest ($400,000 × .09 × 4/12)	12,000
Total cash received	$447,400

Voucher Register

8/1/78	Unamortized Bond Issue Costs	$ 23,600	
	Accounts Payable		$ 23,600
	To record voucher issued for payment of bond issue costs.		

Cash Disbursements Journal

8/1/78	Accounts Payable	$ 23,600	
	Cash—General Checking Account		$ 23,600
	To record check issued in payment of bond issue costs.		

If a balance sheet were prepared immediately after the above bond issue, it would present the bonds as a long-term liability of the unrestricted fund in the following manner:

9% Bonds Payable, Due 1998	$400,000	
Add Unamortized Bond Premium	35,400	$435,400

Note that unamortized bond premium is *added* to the face amount of bonds outstanding, whereas unamortized bond discount was *deducted* in the previous illustration. The balance sheet also will include the unamortized bond issue costs of $23,600 in a "deferred charges" or "other assets" classification and will report the $12,000 of accrued interest payable among the current liabilities.

BOND INTEREST AND AMORTIZATION

The amount of bond interest expense to be recorded each month is influenced by the premium or discount recorded at the time the bonds are issued. Amortization of bond discount is regarded as an addition to periodic interest expense, whereas the amortization of bond premium is treated as a reduction of interest expense. This system is followed in order to obtain at least a rough approximation of the effective (actual) interest cost of the bonds. In practice, bond discount and premium usually are amortized (allocated) evenly throughout the life of the bond issue by application of the straight-line, or average, method. (A theoretically superior procedure, called the compound-interest or effective-yield method, described in the author's *Hospital Financial Accounting—Theory and Practice*, is also used in actual practice.) The costs of the bond issue also are amortized to expense by application of the straight-line method.

INTEREST AND DISCOUNT

Refer to the example on page 363 where the proceeds of the $400,000, 6% bond issue amount to only $370,500. The resulting $29,500 of bond discount should be amortized by charges to interest expense over the 236-month life of the bond issue: the 236 months between August 1, 1978, and April 1, 1998. The idea is that since the hospital received only $370,500 but must repay $400,000 at maturity, the $29,500 represents a cost that is properly allocable to the period that is presumed to benefit from use of the resources provided by the bond issue. It is a matter of cost allocation and of matching costs and revenues on a periodic basis. A similar procedure applies to the $17,700 of bond issue costs.

At the end of each of the 236 months during which the bonds will be outstanding, adjusting entries will be made to amortize $125 (i.e., $29,500/236) of bond discount and $75 (i.e., $17,700/236) of bond issue costs. The necessary entries for August 31, 1978, will illustrate the procedure.

General Journal

8/31/78	Bond Interest Expense		$ 2,125	
	Unamortized Bond Discount			$ 125
	Accrued Interest Payable			2,000
	To record monthly amortization of bond discount, and to accrue monthly interest expense, as follows:			
	Nominal interest ($400,000 × .06 × 1/12)	$2,000		
	Discount amortization ($29,500/236)	125		
	Monthly interest expense	$2,125		
8/31/78	Amortization of Bond Issue Costs		$ 75	
	Unamortized Bond Issue Costs			$ 75
	To record monthly amortization of bond issue costs ($17,700/236).			

Notice that the amortization of bond discount is a part of the debit to the bond interest expense account which roughly approximates the real monthly interest cost. Amortization of bond issue costs, however, is charged to a separate expense account so titled. Such costs, being in the nature of prepaid expenses, should not be confused or combined with bond discount.

The same entries, of course, will be made on September 30, 1978. Then, on October 1, 1978, when Supercare Hospital pays 6 months' interest on the bonds, the interest payment entries are the following:

Voucher Register

10/1/78	Accrued Interest Payable	$ 12,000	
	Accounts Payable		$ 12,000
	To record voucher for payment of semiannual bond interest.		

Cash Disbursements Journal

10/1/78	Accounts Payable	$ 12,000	
	Cash—General Checking Account		$ 12,000
	To record checks issued to pay semiannual bond interest.		

Recall that the accrued interest payable account was credited for $8,000 in the bond issue entry on August 1, 1978, and was credited for $2,000 on August 31 and again on September 30, 1978, in the month-end adjusting entries. The resulting credit balance of $12,000 is eliminated by the debit in the above voucher register entry of October 1, 1978.

You also should recognize that the entire $29,500 of bond discount, and the $17,700 of bond issue costs, will have been charged to expense by April 1, 1998, the maturity date of the bonds. So, when the maturity date arrives, the entries to record the retirement of the bonds are simply these:

Voucher Register

4/1/98	Bonds Payable	$400,000	
	Accounts Payable		$400,000
	To record voucher issued for payment of maturity value of bonds.		

Cash Disbursements Journal

4/1/98	Accounts Payable	$400,000	
	Cash—General Checking Account		$400,000
	To record checks issued to retire bonds at maturity date.		

In certain circumstances, all or part of a bond issue may be retired prior to its normal maturity date. This matter will be pursued in a subsequent section of this chapter.

Let us return for a moment to 1978 and summarize all the entries which will be made during the year for the $400,000 bond issue. These 1978 entries are provided in the general ledger accounts presented in figure 107. Take note of the year-end account balances. The 1978 income statement of Supercare Hospital will report $10,625 of bond interest expense and $375 of bond issue cost amortization (an expense). The December 31, 1978, balance sheet will present the bonds as a long-term liability as follows:

6% Bonds Payable	$400,000	
Less Unamortized Bond Discount	28,875	$371,125

This balance sheet also will report $17,325 of unamortized bond issue costs as an asset and $6,000 of accrued interest payable as a current liability.

INTEREST AND PREMIUM

Refer to the example on page 365 where the proceeds of the $400,000, 9% bond issue amount to $435,400. At the end of each of the 236 months during which the bonds will be outstanding, adjusting entries such as the following will be made to amortize $150 (i.e., $35,400/236) of bond premium and $100 (i.e., $23,600/236) of bond issue costs.

General Journal

8/31/78	Bond Interest Expense	$ 2,850	
	Unamortized Bond Premium	150	
	Accrued Interest Payable		$ 3,000
	To record monthly amortization of bond premium, and to accrue monthly interest expense, as follows:		

Figure 107
Accounting for Bonds Issued At A Discount

Cash—General Checking Account

(1)	378,500	(3)	17,700
		(9)	12,000

Unamortized Bond Issue Costs

(2)	17,700	(5)	75
		(7)	75
		(11)	75
		(13)	75
		(15)	75
Bal.	17,325		

Accounts Payable

(3)	17,700	(2)	17,700
(9)	12,000	(8)	12,000

Accrued Interest Payable

(8)	12,000	(1)	8,000
		(4)	2,000
		(6)	2,000
		(10)	2,000
		(12)	2,000
		(14)	2,000
		Bal.	6,000

Bonds Payable

		(1)	400,000

Unamortized Bond Discount

(1)	29,500	(4)	125
		(6)	125
		(10)	125
		(12)	125
		(14)	125
Bal.	28,875		

Bond Interest Expense

(4)	2,125		
(6)	2,125		
(10)	2,125		
(12)	2,125		
(14)	2,125		
Bal.	10,625		

Amortization of Bond Issue Costs

(5)	75		
(7)	75		
(11)	75		
(13)	75		
(15)	75		
Bal.	375		

Posting references:

(1) 8/1/78 bond issue—cash receipts journal.
(2) 8/1/78 payment of bond issue costs—voucher register.
(3) 8/1/78 payment of bond issue costs—cash disbursements journal.
(4) 8/31/78 interest accrual and discount amortization—general journal.
(5) 8/31/78 amortization of issue costs—general journal.
(6) 9/30/78 interest accrual and discount amortization—general journal.
(7) 9/30/78 amortization of issue costs—general journal.
(8) 10/1/78 payment of semiannual interest—voucher register.
(9) 10/1/78 payment of semiannual interest—cash disbursements journal.
(10) 10/31/78 interest accrual and discount amortization—general journal.
(11) 10/31/78 amortization of issue costs—general journal.
(12) 11/30/78 interest accrual and discount amortization—general journal.
(13) 11/30/78 amortization of issue costs—general journal.
(14) 12/31/78 interest accrual and discount amortization—general journal.
(15) 12/31/78 amortization of issue costs—general journal.

Nominal interest ($400,000 × .09 × 1/12)	$3,000		
Premium amortization ($35,400/236)	150		
Monthly interest expense	$2,850		

8/31/78	Amortization of Bond Issue Costs	$ 100	
	Unamortized Bond Issue Costs		$ 100
	To record monthly amortization of bond issue costs ($23,600/236).		

Notice that the amortization of bond premium reduces the amount to be debited to bond interest expense so as to obtain an approximation of the true monthly interest cost.

The same entries, of course, will be made on September 30, 1978. Then, on October 1, 1978, when Supercare Hospital pays 6 months' interest on the bonds, the interest payment entries are as follows:

Voucher Register

10/1/78	Accrued Interest Payable	$ 18,000	
	Accounts Payable		$ 18,000
	To record voucher for payment of semiannual bond interest ($400,000 × .09 × 6/12).		

Cash Disbursements Journal

10/1/78	Accounts Payable	$ 18,000	
	Cash—General Checking Account		$ 18,000
	To record checks issued to pay semiannual bond interest.		

Following this, the previously described monthly adjusting entries will be made on October 31, November 30, and December 31, 1978. All the 1978 entries for the $400,000 of 9% bonds issued at a premium are summarized in figure 108.

Notice the year-end balances in figure 108. The December 31, 1978, balance sheet will present the bonds as a long-term liability as follows:

9% Bonds Payable	$400,000	
Add Unamortized Bond Premium	34,650	$434,650

This balance sheet also will report $23,100 of unamortized bond issue costs as an asset and $9,000 of accrued interest payable as a current liability. The 1978 income statement of Supercare Hospital will report $14,250 of bond interest expense and $500 of bond issue cost amortization (an expense).

RETIREMENT OF BONDS

The normal retirement of term bonds at the scheduled maturity date has previously been illustrated. Let us examine here the procedure to be followed when term bonds are reacquired and retired prior to the normal retirement date. Also, we want to consider the issue and retirement of serial bonds. Accounting for the *refunding* of bond issues (the replacement of an outstanding bond issue with a new bond issue) and for the operation of bond sinking funds, however, will not be covered in this book. These matters are dealt

Figure 108
Accounting for Bonds Issued At A Premium

General Checking Account

(1)	447,400	(3)	23,600
		(9)	18,000

Unamortized Bond Issue Costs

(2)	23,600	(5)	100
		(7)	100
		(11)	100
		(13)	100
		(15)	100
Bal.	23,100		

Accounts Payable

(3)	23,600	(2)	23,600
(9)	18,000	(8)	18,000

Accrued Interest Payable

(8)	18,000	(1)	12,000
		(4)	3,000
		(6)	3,000
		(10)	3,000
		(12)	3,000
		(14)	3,000
		Bal.	9,000

Bonds Payable

		(1)	400,000

Unamortized Bond Premium

(4)	150	(1)	35,400
(6)	150		
(10)	150		
(12)	150		
(14)	150		
		Bal.	34,650

Bond Interest Expense

(4)	2,850		
(6)	2,850		
(10)	2,850		
(12)	2,850		
(14)	2,850		
Bal.	14,250		

Amortization of Bond Issue Costs

(5)	100		
(7)	100		
(11)	100		
(13)	100		
(15)	100		
Bal.	500		

Posting references:

(1) 8/1/78 bond issue—cash receipts journal.
(2) 8/1/78 payment of bond issue costs—voucher register.
(3) 8/1/78 payment of bond issue costs—cash disbursements journal.
(4) 8/31/78 interest accrual and premium amortization—general journal.
(5) 8/31/78 amortization of issue costs—general journal.
(6) 9/30/78 interest accrual and premium amortization—general journal.
(7) 9/30/78 amortization of issue costs—general journal.
(8) 10/1/78 payment of semiannual interest—voucher register.
(9) 10/1/78 payment of semiannual interest—cash disbursements journal.
(10) 10/31/78 interest accrual and premium amortization—general journal.
(11) 10/31/78 amortization of issue costs—general journal.
(12) 11/30/78 interest accrual and premium amortization—general journal.
(13) 11/30/78 amortization of issue costs—general journal.
(14) 12/31/78 interest accrual and premium amortization—general journal.
(15) 12/31/78 amortization of issue costs—general journal.

with at length in the author's *Hospital Financial Accounting—Theory and Practice*.

TERM BONDS REACQUIRED PRIOR TO MATURITY

A hospital may sometimes reacquire its own bonds in the market prior to normal maturity when bond prices and other factors make such action desirable. To illustrate, refer to the facts of the example on page 365 where a $400,000 bond issue is sold at a premium on August 1, 1978. Assume that Supercare Hospital reacquires $80,000 (face value) of these bonds at 98 and accrued interest on June 1, 1984, with brokerage and other reacquisition costs of $115 being paid. At the reacquisition date, the relevant accounts on the hospital's books will have the following balances:

Accrued Interest Payable ($3,000 × 2 months)	$ 6,000 Cr.
Bonds Payable	400,000 Cr.
Unamortized Bond Premium	
($35,400) – ($150 × 70 months)	24,900 Cr.
Unamortized Bond Issue Costs	
($23,600) – ($100 × 70 months)	16,600 Dr.

The 70 months used in the above computations of account balances is the number of months between the bond issue date (August 1, 1978) and the bond reacquisition date (June 1, 1984).

The entry to record the reacquisition requires the recognition of a gain (or loss) of the difference between the amount paid for such bonds (exclusive of accrued interest) and their book value at the date of reacquisition. The book value of the bonds reacquired and retired is computed as follows:

Book value of all bonds outstanding		
Face value	$400,000	
Unamortized premium	24,900	
Unamortized issue costs	(16,600)	
Total		$408,300
Percentage of bonds reacquired		
($80,000/$400,000)		20%
Book value of bonds reacquired		$ 81,660

The amount paid (exclusive of interest) to reacquire these bonds will be $78,515 (i.e., 98% of $80,000 plus $115 of brokerage fees and other reacquisition costs). So, the gain on the reacquisition will be $3,145 (i.e., $81,660 – $78,515).

The necessary entries to record the reacquisition and retirement of the bonds on June 1, 1984, therefore are these.

Voucher Register

6/1/84	Bonds Payable		$80,000	
	Accrued Interest Payable		1,200	
	Unamortized Bond Premium		4,980	
	Unamortized Bond Issue Costs			$ 3,320
	Gain on Reacquisition of Bonds			3,145
	Accounts Payable			79,715
	To record voucher for reacquisition and retirement of 20% of bond issue as follows:			
	Face value (20% × $400,000)	$80,000		
	Unamortized premium (20% × $24,900)	4,980		

Unamortized issue costs (20% × $16,600)	(3,320)	
Book value of bonds reacquired	$81,660	
Reacquisition cost ($80,000 @ 98)	$78,400	
Brokerage fees	115	
Total	78,515	
Accrued interest (20% × $6,000)	1,200	
Cash disbursement	$79,715	

Cash Disbursements Journal

6/1/84	Accounts Payable	$79,715	
	Cash—General Checking Account		$79,715
	To record check issued for reacquisition and retirement of 20% of bond issue.		

After this reacquisition, accounting continues as before until maturity with respect to the remaining $320,000 of bonds. The monthly amount of amortization and interest, however, will be reduced by 20%: the monthly interest expense will be $2,280, monthly premium amortization will be $120, and monthly amortization of bond issue costs will be $80 (rather than $2,850, $150, and $100, respectively). Similarly, the monthly addition to accrued interest payable will be $2,400 (i.e., $320,000 × .09 × 1/12).

RETIREMENT OF SERIAL BONDS

The illustrations to this point have assumed that the bonds in question have been term bonds; that is, that all bonds in the issue have had a fixed single maturity date. Some hospital bond issues, however, are serial bonds which mature in periodic installments. To illustrate, assume a simplified case in which Supercare Hospital issues $400,000 of 5% serial bonds on January 1, 1978, at 94. These bonds pay interest annually on January 1, and mature at the rate of $80,000 annually, starting January 1, 1979. Issue costs totaled $14,400.

Figure 109
Summary of Discount Amortization and Interest
Bonds Outstanding Method

Year	Bonds Outstanding	(1) Fraction	(2) Bond Discount	(3) Discount Amortization	(4) 5% Nominal Interest	(5) Interest Expense
1978	$ 400,000	40/120	$24,000	$ 8,000	$20,000	$28,000
1979	320,000	32/120	24,000	6,400	16,000	22,400
1980	240,000	24/120	24,000	4,800	12,000	16,800
1981	160,000	16/120	24,000	3,200	8,000	11,200
1982	80,000	8/120	24,000	1,600	4,000	5,600
	$1,200,000			$24,000	$60,000	$84,000

(1) × (2) = (3) and (3) + (4) = (5)

Figure 109 provides a summary of annual discount amortization and bond interest expense as computed by the "bonds outstanding" method. This method, rather than the straight-line method described earlier in this chapter, is used because the face amount of bonds outstanding each year varies. It provides for an amortization pattern which corresponds to the amount of bonds outstanding. Bond issue costs are amortized in the same pattern.

To illustrate the entries to be made for serial bonds, let us assume that Supercare Hospital makes entries for amortization and interest accruals only once each year, on December 31. All the necessary entries for 1978 and 1979 are summarized in figure 110.

Figure 110
Entries for Serial Bonds

	Cash Receipts Journal		
1/1/78	Cash—General Checking Account	$376,000	
	Unamortized Bond Discount	24,000	
	Bonds Payable		$400,000
	To record issuance of 5% serial bonds at 94.		
	Voucher Register		
1/1/78	Unamortized Bond Issue Costs	$ 14,400	
	Accounts Payable		$ 14,400
	To record voucher issued for payment of bond issue costs.		
	Cash Disbursements Journal		
1/1/78	Accounts Payable	$ 14,400	
	Cash—General Checking Account		$ 14,400
	To record check issued for payment of bond issue costs.		
	General Journal		
12/31/78	Bond Interest Expense	$ 28,000	
	Unamortized Bond Discount		$ 8,000
	Accrued Interest Payable		20,000
	To record bond discount amortization and accrual of interest as follows:		
	Nominal interest ($400,000 × 5%) — $20,000		
	Discount amortization ($24,000 × 40/120) — 8,000		
	1978 interest expense — $28,000		
12/31/78	Amortization of Bond Issue Costs	$ 4,800	
	Unamortized Bond Issue Costs		$ 4,800
	To record amortization of bond issue costs for 1978 ($14,400 × 40/120).		

(Figure 110 continued)

	Voucher Register			
1/1/79	Accrued Interest Payable		$ 20,000	
	Bonds Payable		80,000	
	Accounts Payable			$100,000
	To record vouchers issued for payment of 1978 accrued interest and for retirement of bonds due January 1, 1979.			
	Cash Disbursements Journal			
1/1/79	Accounts Payable		$100,000	
	Cash—General Checking Account			$100,000
	To record checks issued for payment of 1978 accrued interest and for retirement of bonds due January 1, 1979.			
	General Journal			
12/31/79	Bond Interest Expense		$ 22,400	
	Unamortized Bond Discount			$ 6,400
	Accrued Interest Payable			16,000
	To record bond discount amortization and accrual of interest as follows:			
	Nominal interest ($320,000 × 5%)	$16,000		
	Discount amortization ($24,000 × 32/120)	6,400		
	1979 interest expense	$22,400		
12/31/79	Amortization of Bond Issue Costs		$ 3,840	
	Unamortized Bond Issue Costs			$ 3,840
	To record amortization of bond issue costs for 1979 ($14,400 × 32/120).			

QUESTIONS

1. Distinguish between current and long-term liabilities.
2. Briefly identify each of the following:
   a. Bond indenture
   b. Registered bond
   c. Coupon bond
   d. Serial bond
   e. Term bond
   f. Callable bond
   g. Secured bond
   h. Revenue bond
   i. Debentures
3. How should (a) unamortized bond discount, (b) unamortized

bond premium, and (c) unamortized bond issue costs be presented in the hospital's balance sheet?

4. On January 1, 1978, a hospital issued serial bonds with a total face value of $1,000,000. These bonds mature annually in $200,000 amounts, beginning January 1, 1979. Indicate how these bonds should be presented in the hospital balance sheet at December 31, 1978.

5. A hospital bond issue, dated April 1, 1978, is actually issued for cash on June 1, 1978. The purchasers of these bonds will pay the hospital for 2 months of accrued interest. Why?

6. Distinguish between the nominal (or coupon) rate of interest and the effective rate of interest with respect to a hospital bond issue.

7. For what reasons might a hospital bond issue sell at a price that is higher or lower than face value?

8. If a hospital bond issue is sold at a discount, will the monthly charge to bond interest expense be greater or less than the nominal amount of interest per month? Explain.

9. A hospital bond issue is sold at a premium on January 1, 1978. Interest on the bonds is payable annually on December 31. Will the annual interest expense recorded on the hospital's books be greater or less than the amount of annual interest actually paid to the bondholders? Explain.

10. If the market rate of interest is higher than the nominal (or coupon) rate of interest specified in a hospital bond issue, will the hospital's bonds sell at a price that is higher or lower than face value? Explain.

PROBLEMS

A. Saltville Hospital issued $1,000,000 of 5-year, 6% bonds at 100 and accrued interest on August 1, 1978. Issue costs were $56,000. Interest is payable semiannually, April 1 and October 1. The maturity date of the bonds is April 1, 1983. On February 1, 1979, $200,000 of these bonds are reacquired at 98 and accrued interest.

Required. Prepare entries to record all matters relating to the bond issue from August 1, 1978, through February 1, 1979.

B. Saltlick Hospital issued $500,000 (face value) of 6%, 10-year bonds at 97.7 and accrued interest on October 1, 1978. Bond issue costs amounted to $20,700. The bonds pay interest semiannually on May 1 and November 1, and mature May 1, 1988. The hospital's fiscal year ends on December 31.

On January 1, 1979, Saltlick Hospital reacquires 20% of these bonds by purchase in the open market at 92 and accrued interest, with brokerage and other reacquisition costs of $280 being paid.

Required. (1) Prepare a chart, such as the one illustrated in figure 107, showing entries for all matters relating to this bond issue through December 31, 1978. (2) Indicate how all matters relating to this bond issue should be presented in the hospital's 1978 financial statements. (3) Prepare the necessary entry to record the reacquisition of 20% of the bonds on January 1, 1979. (4) Compute the amount of bond interest expense for January, 1979.

C. Salty Hospital issued $500,000 (face value) of 6%, 10-year bonds at 102.3 and accrued interest on October 1, 1978. Bond issue costs amounted to $16,100. The bonds pay interest semiannually on May 1 and November 1, and mature May 1, 1988. The hospital's fiscal year ends on December 31.

On January 1, 1979, Salty Hospital reacquires 20% of these bonds by purchase in the open market at 101 and accrued interest, with brokerage and other reacquisition costs of $260 being paid.

Required. (1) Prepare a chart, such as the one illustrated in figure 108, showing entries for all matters relating to this bond issue through December 31, 1978. (2) Indicate how all matters relating to this bond issue should be presented in the hospital's 1978 financial statements. (3) Prepare the necessary entry to record the reacquisition of 20% of the bonds on January 1, 1979. (4) Compute the amount of bond interest expense for January, 1979.

D. Saltrock Hospital issued $500,000 (face value) of 6% serial bonds on January 1, 1978, at 94. These bonds pay interest annually on January 1 and mature at the rate of $100,000 annually, starting January 1, 1979. Issue costs amounted to $15,000. The hospital's fiscal year ends on December 31, at which time annual entries are made for amortization and accruals.

Required. (1) Prepare a table, such as the one illustrated in figure 109, to summarize discount amortization and interest expense for the 1978–1982 period. (2) Prepare the necessary journal entries for 1978 and 1979 only. (3) Indicate how all matters relating to these bonds should be presented in the hospital's 1979 financial statements.

E. Saltmine Hospital issued $600,000 (face value) of 8% serial bonds on January 1, 1978, at 106. These bonds pay interest annually on January 1 and mature at the rate of $120,000 annually, starting January 1, 1979. Issue costs amounted to $18,000. The hospital's fiscal year ends on December 31, at which time annual entries are made for amortization and accruals.

Required. (1) Prepare a table, such as the one illustrated in figure 109, to summarize premium amortization and interest expense for the 1978–1982 period. (2) Prepare the necessary journal entries for 1978 and 1979 only. (3) Indicate how all matters relating to these bonds should be presented in the hospital's 1979 financial statements.

F. Saltless Hospital issued $600,000 (face value) of 6%, 10-year bonds at 94 and accrued interest on June 1, 1978. Bond issue costs were $18,000. The bonds pay interest annually on June 1 and mature June 1, 1988. The hospital's fiscal year ends on December 31.

On January 1, 1980, Saltless Hospital reacquires $150,000 (face value) of these bonds by purchase in the open market at 90 and accrued interest, with brokerage and other reacquisition costs of $300 being paid.

Required. Prepare the necessary journal entries at (1) June 1, 1978, (2) June 30, 1978, (3) June 1, 1979, (4) January 1, 1980.

21
Statement of Changes in Financial Position

An *income statement* presents the results of a hospital's operations in terms of revenues earned and expenses incurred during a given time period. The *balance sheet* presents the hospital's financial position in terms of the assets, liabilities, and fund balances existing at a given point in time. The *statement of changes in fund balances* provides a summary analysis of the factors causing increases and decreases in the individual fund balances over a given period of time. For many years, these 3 financial statements were considered sufficient for the purposes of external financial reporting.

In 1971, however, the American Institute of Certified Public Accountants recognized the *statement of changes in financial position* as a fourth statement to be required when reporting the financial activities and affairs of an economic enterprise.[1] This position subsequently was affirmed and specifically made applicable to hospital financial reporting by the Institute's Committee on Health Care Institutions.[2] In this chapter, we will examine the nature of this required statement and illustrate the procedure for its preparation.

This statement has variously been referred to as the "statement of sources and applications of funds," the "statement of source and disposition of working capital," the "statement of resources provided and applied," or simply the "funds statement." In the following discussion, we will use the technically correct name specified by the AICPA—the *statement of changes in financial position*—and that title should be employed in hospital financial reports. Properly understood and used, this statement can be one of the most valuable of all 4 required statements, since it provides so much information about the reasons for financial changes—both of an operating and a capital nature—in the total hospital entity during the year.

---

[1]APB Opinion No. 19, "Reporting Changes in Financial Position" (New York: American Institute of Certified Public Accountants, 1971).

[2]*Hospital Audit Guide* (New York: American Institute of Certified Public Accountants, 1972), p. 38.

NATURE OF THE STATEMENT

Comparative income statements and balance sheets for Hopeful Hospital are presented in figures 111 and 112. (The changes in the unrestricted fund balance are assumed to consist only of the net income figures as shown within the fund balance section of the balance sheets. Consequently, a separate statement of changes in fund balances is not presented here.) Clearly, these statements provide a considerable amount of essential information concerning the operating results and financial position of Hopeful Hospital. Intelligent decision making, either by the hospital's management or by interested external parties, requires such information. Is the information provided in these statements alone sufficient to the needs of management and external users? Is the information complete: does it clearly reflect all significant investing and financing activities of the hospital during 1977 and 1978? Do income statements and balance sheets alone adequately depict the flow of resources into and out from the hospital enterprise? In each instance, the answer is no.

Figure 111
Hopeful Hospital
Comparative Income Statements
Years Ended December 31, 1978 and 1977

	1978	1977
Gross patient service revenues	$9,490	$8,870
Less deductions from revenues	890	780
Net patient service revenues	8,600	8,090
Other operating revenues	633	519
Total operating revenues	9,233	8,609
Less operating expenses:		
Nursing services	3,188	2,995
Other professional services	2,030	1,920
General services	1,610	1,540
Fiscal and administrative services	1,460	1,370
Depreciation	540	465
Other	315	292
Total operating expenses	9,143	8,582
Operating income	90	27
Nonoperating income	195	154
Net income for the year	$ 285	$ 181

Certain important changes in financial position and certain vital aspects of the financing and investing (capital) activities of Hopeful Hospital are not disclosed by or made clearly apparent from an examination of its income statements and balance sheets. Consider, for example, the following items drawn from the balance sheets in figure 112:

	1978	1977
Long-term investments	$1,010	$ 600

You might conclude from this presentation that new long-term investments costing $410 were purchased during 1978. As you will shortly see, however, Hopeful Hospital purchased new long-term investments costing $450 and sold long-term investments (which had cost $40) for $49! Thus, the apparent $410 increase in long-term investments actually is the net difference between the costs of investments purchased and sold during 1978.

Figure 112
Hopeful Hospital
Comparative Balance Sheets—Unrestricted Fund
December 31, 1978 and 1977

Assets	1978	1977
Cash	$ 124	$ 280
Accrued interest receivable	45	30
Accounts receivable, net of allowance for uncollectible accounts of $210 at 12/31/78 and $160 at 12/31/77	1,536	1,340
Inventories	175	140
Prepaid expenses	32	40
Total current assets	1,912	1,830
Long-term investments	1,010	600
Plant assets, net of accumulated depreciation of $1,850 at 12/31/78 and $1,340 at 12/31/77	5,250	4,920
Total assets	$8,172	$7,350
Liabilities and Fund Balance		
Accounts payable	$ 302	$ 370
Accrued expenses payable	208	220
Deferred revenues	77	60
Total current liabilities	587	650
Bonds payable	3,000	2,400
Total liabilities	3,587	3,050
Fund balance, January 1	4,300	4,119
Add net income for the year	285	181
Fund balance, December 31	4,585	4,300
Total liabilities and fund balance	$8,172	$7,350

Similar offsetting transactions typically are found in many of the other financial position accounts. These offsetting transactions, however, ordinarily are not determinable from the information provided in the balance sheet and income statement alone. If these financial statements are not to be misleading, such "hidden" information must be fully disclosed in some manner.

The necessary disclosure is accomplished through the preparation of a statement of changes in financial position. It provides a summary of all operations and all financing and investing activities of the hospital by accounting for all changes in financial position as reported in successive balance sheets. As noted above, certain of these changes may not be readily determined simply by studying balance sheet and income statement information alone. In disclosing these changes in financial position, the statement depicts the inflows and outflows of resources. It presents the sources and amounts of resources which became available to the hospital as well as the uses made of these during a given period of time.

The information in the statement of changes in financial position has important implications for the hospital's creditors, reimbursement and planning agencies, and other external groups as well as for internal management decisions. It can be used in estimating the resources that will be generated in the future and the growth potential of the hospital in terms of its ability to finance expansion and meet added indebtedness. The statement is most useful, of course, when presented in comparative form for 2 or more years.

It should be noted that the term *funds* has been defined in several ways for purposes of the statement of changes in financial position. In its narrowest sense, the term *funds* might be used simply to denote cash. The statement, in that case, would become a statement of the sources and uses of cash. Correctly viewed, the term *funds* means working capital (current assets minus current liabilities), and when this definition is used, the statement of changes in financial position presents the sources and uses of the hospital's working capital. The "working capital" concept of *funds* will be the main thrust of this chapter; further on in the chapter, however, a "cash flow" statement will be illustrated.

Illustration Data

Figure 113 presents a summary of the financial activity of Hopeful Hospital for the year ended December 31, 1978. This summary worksheet begins with the December 31, 1977, postclosing balances which you saw earlier in the hospital's December 31, 1977, balance sheet (figure 112). The following 2 columns of the worksheet provide a summary of the 1978 transactions; the next 2 columns show the adjustments required at December 31, 1978; and the final 2 columns contain the preclosing account balances at the end of the year. These preclosing balances appeared in the hospital's 1978 financial statements illustrated in figures 111 and 112.

To assist you in your study of this worksheet, the 1978 transactions and adjustments are presented below in general journal form:

(1) Accounts Receivable	$ 9,490	
Patient Service Revenues		$ 9,490
To record gross revenues from services to patients.		
(2) Cash	$ 8,404	
Deductions from Revenues	840	
Accounts Receivable		$ 9,244
To record revenue deductions and cash collections on patients' accounts.		

(3)	Cash	$ 49	
	Gain on Sale of Investments		$ 9
	Long-Term Investments		40
	To record sale of long-term investments (cost $40) for $49.		
(4)	Cash	$ 54	
	Loss on Sale of Plant Assets	16	
	Accumulated Depreciation	30	
	Plant Assets		$ 100
	To record sale of plant assets (cost $100; accumulated depreciation $30) for $54.		
(5)	Cash	$ 3,830	
	Other Operating Revenues		$ 650
	Nonoperating Revenues		180
	Bonds Payable		3,000
	To record other cash receipts, including proceeds of new 6% bond issue.		
(6)	Nursing Services Expenses	$ 3,000	
	Other Professional Services Expenses	1,900	
	General Services Expenses	1,100	
	Fiscal and Administrative Services Expenses	1,400	
	Other Operating Expenses	300	
	Accounts Payable		$ 7,700
	To record vouchering of operating expenses other than supplies.		
(7)	Inventories	$ 935	
	Long-Term Investments	450	
	Plant Assets	940	
	Bonds Payable	2,400	
	Accounts Payable		$ 4,725
	To record other vouchers issued for purchase of inventory, purchase of long-term investments, purchase of plant assets, and retirement of old 7% bond issue.		
(8)	Accounts Payable	$12,493	
	Cash		$12,493
	To record checks issued in payment of vouchers.		
(9)	Nursing Services Expenses	$ 200	
	Other Professional Services Expenses	130	
	General Services Expenses	510	
	Fiscal and Administrative Services Expenses	60	
	Inventories		$ 900
	To record cost of supplies used.		
(10)	Depreciation Expense	$ 540	
	Accumulated Depreciation		$ 540
	To record depreciation expense for 1978.		
(11)	Accrued Interest Receivable	$ 15	
	Nonoperating Revenues		$ 15
	Adjustment for increase in accrued interest receivable.		
(12)	Deductions from Revenues	$ 50	
	Allowance for Uncollectible Accounts		$ 50

Adjustment for required increase in allowance for uncollectible accounts.

(13) Other Operating Expenses	$ 8	
Prepaid Expenses		$ 8
Adjustment for decrease in prepaid expenses.		
(14) Accrued Expenses Payable	$ 12	
Nursing Services Expenses		$ 12
Adjustment for decrease in accrued expenses (*assuming* that expense items relate solely to nursing services).		
(15) Other Operating Revenues	$ 17	
Deferred Revenues		$ 17
Adjustment for increase in balance of deferred revenues.		

You recognize, of course, that certain liberties have been taken in these entries in an effort to simplify and reduce the size of the illustration. As you trace these entries through the worksheet (figure 113), however, you should concern yourself only with acquiring a knowledge of Hopeful Hospital's 1978 financial activities.

FORMULA FOR THE STATEMENT

Since the term *funds* is defined as working capital (current assets minus current liabilities), an analysis of the changes in the noncurrent asset, noncurrent liability, and fund balance accounts will provide the information necessary for preparation of the statement of changes in financial position. First, however, you must be able to identify which of these changes are sources of funds and which are applications of funds. The formula for identification of the elements entering into the statement is derived as follows:

1. A = L + FB. This is the basic accounting equation upon which the balance sheet rests: assets = liabilities + fund balance.
2. CA + NCA = CL + NCL + FB. This is simply an expansion of the above equation by substitution of CA (current assets) and NCA (noncurrent assets) for A (assets) and, similarly, CL (current liabilities) and NCL (noncurrent liabilities) for L (liabilities).
3. CA + NCA − CL = NCL + FB. Here current liabilities (CL) have been subtracted from each side of equation 2 above.
4. CA − CL = NCL + FB − NCA. Now noncurrent assets (NCA) have been subtracted from each side of equation 3 above.

Since CA − CL is working capital, equation 4 is the formula for the statement of changes in financial position: working capital = NCL + FB − NCA. Given this formula, it follows that an increase in working capital occurs when the value of the right-hand side of the equation increases. It also is clear that a decrease in working capital occurs when the value of the right-hand side of the equation decreases.

SOURCES OF WORKING CAPITAL

In terms of the equation (working capital = NCL + FB − NCA), there are but 3 possible sources of working capital:

1. *Increases in NCL*. Increases in noncurrent liability accounts are sources of working capital. Hopeful Hospital, for example, issued $3,000 of 6% bonds in 1978 (see worksheet entry number 5). This

Figure 113
Hopeful Hospital
Worksheet for Year Ended December 31, 1978

	12/31/77 Balances	
	Dr.	Cr.
Cash	280	
Accrued interest receivable	30	
Accounts receivable	1,500	
Allowance for uncollectible accounts		160
Inventories	140	
Prepaid expenses	40	
Long-term investments	600	
Plant assets	6,260	
Accumulated depreciation		1,340
Accounts payable		370
Accrued expenses payable		220
Deferred revenues		60
Bonds payable		2,400
Fund balance		4,300
Patient service revenues		
Deductions from revenues		
Other operating revenues		
Nursing services expenses		
Other professional services expenses		
General services expenses		
Fiscal and administrative services expenses		
Depreciation expense		
Other operating expenses		
Gain on sale of investments		
Loss on sale of plant assets		
Nonoperating revenues		
Totals	8,850	8,850

increase in a noncurrent liability account (bonds payable) provided the hospital with $3,000 of additional working capital. In the 1978 statement of changes in financial position, this bond issue will be reported as a source of working capital in the amount of $3,000.

2. *Increases in FB.* Increases in the fund balance are sources of working capital; for example, net income or transfers of resources from

1978 Transactions		12/31/78 Adjustments		12/31/78 Balances	
Dr.	Cr.	Dr.	Cr.	Dr.	Cr.
(2) 8,404	(8) 12,493			124	
(3) 49					
(4) 54					
(5) 3,830					
		(11) 15		45	
(1) 9,490	(2) 9,244			1,746	
			(12) 50		210
(7) 935	(9) 900			175	
			(13) 8	32	
(7) 450	(3) 40			1,010	
(7) 940	(4) 100			7,100	
(4) 30			(10) 540		1,850
(8) 12,493	(6) 7,700				302
	(7) 4,725				
		(14) 12			208
			(15) 17		77
(7) 2,400	(5) 3,000				3,000
					4,300
	(1) 9,490				9,490
(2) 840		(12) 50		890	
	(5) 650	(15) 17			633
(6) 3,000			(14) 12	3,188	
(9) 200					
(6) 1,900				2,030	
(9) 130					
(6) 1,100				1,610	
(9) 510					
(6) 1,400				1,460	
(9) 60					
		(10) 540		540	
(6) 300		(13) 8		308	
	(3) 9				9
(4) 16				16	
	(5) 180		(11) 15		195
48,531	48,531	642	642	20,274	20,274

the plant replacement and expansion fund are reported as sources of working capital in the statement of changes in financial position.

Working capital, of course, is generated by hospital operations, but the net income figure does *not* indicate the amount of working capital generated from that source. This is true because certain items that did not require (provide) working capital were deducted (added) in the income statement determination of net income. The reported net income therefore must be adjusted for these items to arrive at the amount of working capital provided by operations.

Hopeful Hospital, for example, reported a 1978 net income of $285 (see figure 111). This net income figure is adjusted for various items as follows:

Net income for the year		$285
Add items deducted in income statement but not requiring the use of working capital		
Depreciation expense	$540	
Loss on sale of plant assets	16	556
Total		841
Less items included in income statement but not providing working capital		
Gain on sale of long-term investments		9
Working capital provided by operations		$832

In other words, since depreciation ($540) and the loss ($16) were deducted, and since the gain ($9) was added, in the determination of the 1978 net income, the net income figure *understates* the amount of working capital generated from the hospital's operating activities. This is not to say, however, that either depreciation or losses on the sale of plant assets are sources of working capital; they are not sources of funds. They are added back to net income only because they previously have been deducted in computing net income.

3. *Decreases in NCA*. Decreases in noncurrent asset accounts are sources of working capital. Hopeful Hospital, for example, sold long-term investments for $49 and sold plant assets for $54 in 1978. These 2 items will be reported as sources of working capital in the hospital's 1978 statement of changes in financial position.

   Notice that the amounts to be shown as sources of working capital arising from decreases in noncurrent asset accounts are not the costs of the assets sold but the sales proceeds figures. The sales proceeds figures are the amounts by which such sales increased the hospital's working capital. Gains and losses from such sales, as noted above, are treated as adjustments of the net income figure.

Thus, sources of working capital arise only from increases in noncurrent liability accounts, increases in the fund balance account, or decreases in noncurrent asset accounts. Hospitals, of course, sometimes have noncurrent accounts other than those included in this illustration. The principles outlined here, however, generally apply to changes in all types of noncurrent accounts with few exceptions. Such exceptions are beyond the scope of this discussion.

APPLICATIONS OF WORKING CAPITAL

In terms of the equation (working capital = NCL + FB − NCA), there are but 3 possible applications or uses of working capital:

1. *Decreases in NCL*. Decreases in noncurrent liability accounts are applications (uses) of working capital. Hopeful Hospital, for example, retired $2,400 of 7% bonds in 1978 (see worksheet entry number 7). This decrease in a noncurrent liability account (bonds payable) required the use of $2,400 of working capital and will be reported in the 1978 statement of changes in financial position as an application of working capital.

2. *Decrease in FB*. Decreases in the fund balance account are applications of working capital; a net loss from operations is an application of working capital, therefore. As Hopeful Hospital had a net income in 1978 (and not a net loss), and because no other negative changes in the fund balance were included in the illustration, there are no applications of working capital in this category for the hospital.

   Let us assume, however, that Hopeful Hospital reported a net loss of $285. The net loss would be adjusted for various items as follows:

Net loss for the year		$(285)
Less items deducted in income statement but not requiring the use of working capital:		
Depreciation expense	$540	
Loss on sale of plant assets	16	556
Balance		$271
Less items included in income statement but not providing working capital:		
Gain on sale of long-term investments		9
Working capital provided by operations		$262

   Although there was a $285 net loss, the adjustments are large enough to produce a positive figure of $262 which would be reported in a statement of changes in financial position as the amount of working capital provided by operations. If the adjusted figure had been negative, however, such a negative amount would be reported as an application of working capital.

3. *Increases in NCA*. Increases in noncurrent asset accounts are applications of working capital. During 1978, for example, Hopeful Hospital purchased $450 of new long-term investments and $940 of new plant assets (see worksheet entry number 7). These increases in noncurrent asset accounts will be reported as applications of working capital in the hospital's 1978 statement of changes in financial position. Acquisition of these assets required the use of working capital.

Thus, the "working capital equation" may be used as an analytical tool for the identification of changes in noncurrent accounts, including the fund balance account, as sources or as applications of working capital. The results of this analysis may be seen in figure 114 in the statement of changes in financial position illustrated.

Notice that sources exceeded applications of working capital by $145. This means that there was a $145 net increase in Hopeful Hospital's working capital during 1978. The amount of this increase is verified by the schedule of changes in working capital accompanying the statement. A schedule of this kind should always be presented as an integral part of the statement of changes in financial position. The computation of the amount of working capital generated by operations also should be included in the statement presentation.

Statement Worksheet

In addition to the equation approach to the preparation of the statement of changes in financial position, a worksheet approach also is available. This approach is illustrated in figure 115, using the Hopeful Hospital data previously provided. Notice that the worksheet begins with a listing of the postclosing account balances at

Figure 114
Hopeful Hospital
Statement of Changes in Financial Position
Year Ended December 31, 1978

Sources of Working Capital:		
Funds generated by operations (schedule 1)	$ 832	
Issue of 6% bonds	3,000	
Sale of long-term investments	49	
Sale of plant assets	54	
Total sources		$3,935
Applications of Working Capital:		
Retirement of 7% bonds	2,400	
Purchase of long-term investments	450	
Purchase of plant assets	940	
Total applications		3,790
Increase in working capital (schedule 2)		$ 145

Schedule 1:

Net income for the year		$285
Add items deducted in income statement but not requiring the use of working capital		
Depreciation expense	$540	
Loss on sale of plant assets	16	556
Total		841
Less items included in income statement but not providing working capital		
Gain on sale of long-term investments		9
Working capital provided by operations		$832

Schedule 2:

	December 31		Increase
	1978	1977	(Decrease)
Cash	$ 124	$ 280	$ (156)
Accrued interest receivable	45	30	15
Accounts receivable (net)	1,536	1,340	196
Inventories	175	140	35
Prepaid expenses	32	40	(8)
Total current assets	1,912	1,830	82
Accounts payable	302	370	(68)
Accrued expenses payable	208	220	(12)
Deferred revenues	77	60	17
Total current liabilities	587	650	(63)
Working capital	$1,325	$1,180	$ 145

the end of 1978 and 1977, but not including the current asset and current liability accounts. The current accounts for each year are netted to the working capital figure which is entered on the first line of the worksheet. (These working capital figures were seen in schedule 2 of figure 114.) This procedure eliminates unnecessary detail from the worksheet and concentrates attention on an analysis of the noncurrent accounts—where, of course, the sources and applications of working capital are to be found.

The next 2 columns of the worksheet show the net changes in each of the accounts listed. The long-term investments account, for example, increased by $410 (net) during 1978. Note that the net changes are classified as net debit changes or net credit changes. Increases in accounts having debit balances are net debit changes, and increases in accounts having credit balances are listed as net credit changes. And, as you can see, the net changes columns balance at totals of $1,395.

In the adjustments columns, entries are made to eliminate each of the net changes. Entry number 1 credits the working capital line for $145 to eliminate the $145 net debit change in working capital; the offsetting debit is made under the working capital applied column to the line designated "increase in working capital." Adjustments 2 through 8 *reverse* the transaction entries which gave rise to the net changes in the noncurrent accounts. This procedure eliminates the net changes in the noncurrent accounts and identifies the amounts to be entered in the applied and provided columns under "working capital."

In 1978, for example, Hopeful Hospital purchased new long-term investments for $450, making the following entry:

Long-Term Investments	$450	
Cash		$450

Adjustment 2 reverses this entry by *crediting* long-term investments for $450. Since the worksheet does not include a cash account, however, a reversing debit cannot be made to cash. Instead, the debit is made under the applied column on the line designated "purchase of long-term investments."

Hopeful Hospital also sold certain long-term investments during 1978, making the following entry:

Cash	$ 49	
Long-Term Investments		$ 40
Gain on Sale of Investments		9

Adjustment 3 reverses this entry by *debiting* long-term investments for $40. Since the worksheet does not include a cash account, however, a reversing credit cannot be made to cash. Instead, the credit for $49 is made under the working capital provided column on the line designated "sale of long-term investments." The $9 gain, as no gain account appears on the worksheet, is debited to the fund balance T account at the upper right-hand side of the worksheet.

Now, notice that the $410 net *debit* change on the long-term investments line has been eliminated by adjustments 2 and 3 which

Figure 115
Statement of Changes in Financial Position Worksheet
Year Ended December 31, 1978

	Balances 12/31/78	Balances 12/31/77	Net Changes Dr.	Net Changes Cr.
Debits				
Working capital	1,325	1,180	145	
Long-term investments	1,010	600	410	
Plant assets	7,100	6,260	840	
Totals	9,435	8,040		
Credits				
Accumulated depreciation	1,850	1,340		510
Bonds payable	3,000	2,400		600
Fund balance	4,585	4,300		285
Totals	9,435	8,040	1,395	1,395
Increase in working capital				
Purchase of long-term investments				
Sale of long-term investments				
Purchase of plant assets				
Sale of plant assets				
Retirement of 7% bonds payable				
Issue of 6% bonds payable				
Working capital generated from operations				
Totals				

net to a *credit* of $410 ($450 − $40). In addition, the adjustments have established the $450 purchase of investments as an application of working capital and the $49 sale of investments as a source of working capital. A similar procedure (adjustments 4–8) is followed for each of the other noncurrent accounts.

After the 8 adjustments are entered on the worksheet, the fund balance T account is totaled. The debit total ($9) is then offset against the credit total ($556) to determine the net adjustment of $547 (credit). This $547 net adjustment is then transferred as a credit to the fund balance line under the adjustments columns of the

Adjustments Dr.		Adjustments Cr.	
		(1)	145
(3)	40	(2)	450
(5)	100	(4)	940
(6)	540	(5)	30
(8)	3,000	(7)	2,400
(9)	832	(T)	547

Fund Balance

Dr.		Cr.	
(3)	9	(5)	16
		(6)	540
	9		556
			9
		(T)	547

Working Capital

Applied		Provided	
(1)	145		
(2)	450		
		(3)	49
(4)	940		
		(5)	54
(7)	2,400		
		(8)	3,000
		(9)	832
	3,935		3,935

Key to adjustments:

(1) Increase in working capital.
(2) Reversal of entry for purchase of investments.
(3) Reversal of entry for sale of investments.
(4) Reversal of entry for purchase of plant assets.
(5) Reversal of entry for sale of plant assets.
(6) Reversal of entry for depreciation.
(7) Reversal of entry for retirement of bonds.
(8) Reversal of entry for issue of bonds.
(9) Working capital generated from operations.

worksheet. To eliminate the net credit change of $285 in the fund balance account, a debit adjustment of $832 is now required ($285 + $547). So, adjustment 9 debits the fund balance line and credits working capital provided for $832. This $832, of course, is the amount of working capital provided by operations (see schedule 1 of figure 114).

Finally, observe that the working capital applied and provided columns balance at totals of $3,935. The information contained in these columns can now be used in the preparation of a formal statement of changes in financial position.

"Cash" Concept of Funds

The preceding discussion has assumed that, in the context of the statement of changes in financial position, the term *funds* was defined as working capital. In other words, sources of funds were identified as increases in working capital and applications of funds seen as decreases in working capital. This "working capital" concept of funds is the correct concept for financial reporting purposes.

Another useful concept of funds, however, is the "cash" concept. In other words, the term *funds* is defined as cash. Sources of funds, then, are receipts of cash; applications of funds are cash disbursements. A funds statement, assuming the cash concept of funds, is illustrated for Hopeful Hospital in figure 116. This statement is referred to as a "cash-flow" statement because it accounts for the net change in the cash balance during a given period.

Figure 116
Hopeful Hospital
Cash-Flow Statement
Year Ended December 31, 1978

Sources of Cash:		
Funds generated by operations (schedule 1)	$ 531	
Issue of 5% bonds	3,000	
Sale of long-term investments	49	
Sale of plant assets	54	
Total sources		$3,634
Applications of Cash:		
Retirement of 7% bonds	2,400	
Purchase of long-term investments	450	
Purchase of plant assets	940	
Total applications		3,790
Decrease in cash balance		$ 156

Schedule 1:		
Net income for the year		$285
Add:		
Depreciation expense	$540	
Loss on sale of plant assets	16	
Decrease in prepaid expenses	8	
Increase in deferred revenues	17	581
Total		866
Less:		
Gain on sale of long-term investments	9	
Increase in accrued interest receivable	15	
Increase in accounts receivable (net)	196	
Increase in inventories	35	
Decrease in accounts payable	68	
Decrease in accrued expenses payable	12	335
Funds generated by operations		$531

Under the cash concept of funds, the increases and decreases in the current asset and liability accounts are treated (see schedule 1 of figure 116) as adjustments of net income in order to arrive at the amount of cash generated by the operations of the period. Under the working capital concept of funds, this schedule (see figure 114) computed the amount of *working capital* generated by operations. Other than this very significant difference, figures 114 and 116 are quite similar. The net result of the statement in figure 114, however, was the $145 increase in working capital; the net result of the statement in figure 116 is the $156 decrease in the cash balance during 1978.

QUESTIONS

1. If a hospital's annual financial report includes an income statement, balance sheet, and statement of changes in fund balances, why should a statement of changes in financial position also be included?

2. State the formula (equation) for the statement of changes in financial position.

3. In the context of the statement of changes in financial position, list the 3 possible sources of working capital. Give an example of each.

4. In the context of the statement of changes in financial position, list the 3 possible applications of working capital. Give an example of each.

5. Is depreciation a source of working capital? Explain.

6. Uptown Hospital reported a net income of $87,400 for 1977. The income statement included the following items, among others:

Loss on sale of long-term investments	$ 13,900
Depreciation expense	141,600
Gain on sale of plant assets	8,300

In the hospital's 1977 statement of changes in financial position, what amount should be reported as "working capital provided by operations"?

7. Refer to question 6 but assume that Uptown Hospital reported a *net loss* of $87,400 for 1977. In the hospital's 1977 statement of changes in financial position, what amount should be reported as "working capital provided by operations"?

8. Distinguish between a cash-flow statement and a statement of changes in financial position.

9. Downtown Hospital's balance sheets provide the following information:

	12/31/78	12/31/77
Long-term investments	$288,300	$262,700

During 1978, the hospital sold certain long-term investments at a gain of $14,600 and purchased new long-term investments at a cost of $87,500. In the hospital's 1977 statement of changes in financial position, what amount should be reported as a source of working capital from the sale of long-term investments?

10. Explain why the annual provision for bad debts (a noncash item included in the income statement) is not added again to reported net income (as depreciation expense is) to arrive at the amount of working capital provided by operations in a hospital's statement of changes in financial position.

PROBLEMS

A. Swelltown Hospital provides you with the following comparative balance sheets at December 31, 1978, and 1977:

	12/31/78	12/31/77
Current assets	$ 600	$ 500
Long-term investments	440	450
Plant and equipment	7,900	7,600
Accumulated depreciation	(1,740)	(1,550)
Total	$7,200	$7,000
Current liabilities	$ 534	$ 250
7% bonds payable	2,800	3,000
Fund balance	3,866	3,750
Total	$7,200	$7,000

The following additional information is available:

1. The 1978 income statement reports a net income of $116.
2. Long-term investments which had cost $60 were sold for $75 in 1978.
3. In 1978 plant and equipment was purchased for $500.
4. Depreciation expense for 1978 was $280.
5. During 1978 plant and equipment items were sold for $100.

Required. Prepare, in good form, a statement of changes in financial position for Swelltown Hospital for the year ended December 31, 1978.

B. Goodtown Hospital provides you with the following comparative balance sheets at December 31, 1978 and 1977:

	12/31/78	12/31/77
Current assets	$ 200	$ 100
Long-term investments	400	350
Plant and equipment	2,000	1,860
Accumulated depreciation	(900)	(780)
Total	$1,700	$1,530
Current liabilities	$ 90	$ 40
8% long-term notes payable	---	500
7% long-term notes payable	600	---
Fund balance	1,010	990
Total	$1,700	$1,530

The 1978 income statement shows a net income of $80. Long-term investments were purchased at a cost of $90; certain other investments were sold for $54. Plant and equipment which had cost $100 (and was 60% depreciated) was sold for $32. In 1976, $60 of reimbursed depreciation restricted by third-party payers was transferred to the hospital's plant replacement and expansion fund.

Required. Prepare, in good form, a statement of changes in financial position for Goodtown Hospital for the year ended December 31, 1978.

C. Finetown Hospital's preclosing trial balance at December 31, 1977, is presented below:

	Dr.	Cr.
Cash	$ 310	
Accrued interest receivable	40	
Accounts receivable	1,460	
Allowance for uncollectible accounts		$ 170
Inventories	180	
Prepaid expenses	35	
Long-term investments	990	
Plant assets	6,100	
Accumulated depreciation		1,300
Accounts payable		390
Accrued expenses payable		210
Deferred revenues		50
Bonds payable		2,500
Fund balance		3,225
Patient service revenues		8,900
Deductions from revenues		800
Other operating revenues		670
Nursing services expense	3,200	
Other professional services expense	2,100	
General services expense	1,600	
Fiscal and administrative services expense	1,500	
Depreciation expense	570	
Other expenses	320	
Nonoperating income		190
	$18,405	$18,405

The following information relates to 1978 activities:

1. Patient service revenues totaled $9,600.
2. Collections were as follows on accounts receivable.

Cash	$8,600
Deductions from revenues	750
Credited to accounts receivable	$9,350

3. The hospital sold long-term investments (cost $50) for $58.
4. The hospital sold plant assets (cost $250, accumulated depreciation $170) for $65.
5. Other cash receipts were as follows.

Other operating revenues	$ 680
Nonoperating revenues	170
Proceeds of new bond issue	3,500

6. Operating expenses vouchered were as follows.

Nursing services	$3,100
Other professional services	2,000
General services	900
Fiscal and administrative services	1,500
Other operating expenses	260

7. Depreciation expense for the year was $550.
8. Vouchers issued for other items were as follows.

Purchase of inventory	$ 900
Purchase of long-term investments	500
Purchase of plant assets	1,500
Retirement of long-term debt (bonds payable)	2,500

9. Checks issued in payment of vouchers totaled $12,300.
10. Cost of supplies used during the year was as follows.

Nursing services	$ 210
Other professional services	140
General services	490
Fiscal and administrative services	70

11. Accrued interest receivable at December 31, 1978, is $55.
12. The allowance for uncollectible accounts at December 31, 1978, should be adjusted to a balance of $195.
13. Prepaid expenses at December 31, 1978, total $49.
14. Accrued expenses payable at December 31, 1978, total $234 (make the necessary adjustment through nursing services expense).
15. Deferred revenues at December 31, 1978, total $75 (make the necessary adjustment through other operating revenues).

Required. (1) Prepare a summary worksheet, such as the one in figure 113, for the year ended December 31, 1978. (2) Prepare a statement of changes in financial position worksheet, such as the one in figure 115, for the year ended December 31, 1978. (3) Prepare a formal statement of changes in financial position for the year ended December 31, 1978.

D. Righttown Hospital provides you with the following comparative balance sheets:

	12/31/78	12/31/77
Cash	$ 140	$ 290
Accrued interest receivable	50	40
Accounts receivable	1,800	1,600
Allowance for uncollectible accounts	(200)	(180)
Inventories	170	130
Prepaid expenses	60	70
Long-term investments	1,000	750
Plant assets	7,000	6,800
Accumulated depreciation	(1,900)	(1,300)
Total	$8,120	$8,200
Accounts payable	$ 300	$ 290
Accrued expenses payable	210	240
Deferred revenues	80	90
Bonds payable	3,000	3,000
Fund balance	4,530	4,580
Total	$8,120	$8,200

The following additional information is available:

1. During 1978 certain long-term investments were sold at a loss of $40, and new long-term investments were purchased for $400.
2. During 1978 certain plant assets (cost $250, accumulated depreciation $240) were sold for $22.

3. During 1978 an old $3,000, 7% bond issue was retired at face value, and a new $3,000, 6% bond issue was sold at face value.
4. The 1978 income reported a net loss of $50.

Required. (1) Prepare a statement of changes in financial position worksheet for 1978. (2) Prepare a formal statement of changes in financial position for 1978.

V
Selected Managerial Accounting Topics

22
Principles of Budgeting

The preparation and use of a budget is essential to the successful management of today's hospital. It is an absolutely necessary requirement in the administration of all hospitals, regardless of size, type, or other characteristics. Securing adequate financing and keeping expenses below revenues are universal and increasingly complex problems that cannot be solved merely by reacting on a day-to-day basis to changing conditions and events. Objectives must be established, long-range plans must be developed, and controls must be instituted, to assure the realization of those objectives and plans. A well-conceived program of budgetary planning and control, properly integrated with the accounting system, is one of the most important tools available to hospital management.

Budgeting is a major topic; entire books have been written on the subject. It deserves more space than can be given to it in this volume. In this one chapter, however, we can introduce you to some of the general principles and basic procedures of budgeting as practiced by hospitals. The purpose of this chapter is therefore limited to the presentation of a broad view of hospital budgeting, with selected illustrations of budgetary procedures.

Comprehensive Budgeting

A *budget* is, simply stated, a formal plan of future operations expressed in quantitative terms and serving as a basis of measurement for subsequent control of such operations. It is a written document in which the objectives and plans of the hospital are translated into dollars and various nonmonetary statistical terms. The dietary department budget for a given future period of time, for example, may be expressed as $360,000 and as 225,000 served meals. Budgeting is the process by which these forecasts are developed and used not only as a device for planning but also as a measurement tool for managerial review and control.

The term *comprehensive budget* refers to the total management plan for the hospital as a whole and for each of its departmental subdivisions. It is an overall master budget comprised of individual budgets for revenues, expenses, assets, and liabilities. This includes all sources of revenues, all types of expenses, cash flow, levels of receivables and inventories, requirements for purchasing and personnel, plant asset additions, and debt retirement schedules. The comprehensive budget brings together all these individual budgets, consolidating them into a coordinated and complete plan for the conduct of operations so as to achieve desired objectives. Comprehensive budgeting permits the development of projected financial statements as goals to be attained at various points in the future.

Prerequisites for Effective Budgeting

A number of conditions are essential to the development and operation of an effective budgetary program. Some of the fundamental prerequisites are briefly discussed below.

Sound Organizational Structure

Effective budgeting requires a sound organizational structure in which authority and lines of responsibility are clearly identified and understood at all levels of management. Every employee must know for what and to whom he or she is responsible. Each must be granted sufficient authority to perform assigned tasks. A departmentalization of activities must exist in which department managers and supervisors know the scope of their responsibility and authority within the overall organizational framework of the hospital. Such relationships are best presented by formal organization charts such as those illustrated earlier in this book.

Budgets are developed in a manner to conform with the existing pattern of authority and responsibility as reflected by the organization chart. Individual plans are established for the achievement of specified objectives for each area of responsibility. Each department manager or supervisor is responsible for the development of the departmental plan and for controlling departmental operations so as to conform to that plan. These individual plans are combined and coordinated into the comprehensive budget for the hospital as a whole.

Appropriate Chart of Accounts

Effective budgeting requires an appropriate chart of accounts—that is, one designed to conform to the plan of organization. It should provide for the accumulation of revenues and expenses according to the organizational units responsible for producing the revenues and incurring the expenses. The revenues associated with each unit are subclassified by activity source; the expenses of each unit are subclassified by object of expenditure. This facilitates the budgeting process because historical revenue and expense data are accumulated in the same classifications in which future revenues and expenses are budgeted. The classification of historical data and budgeted data thus conforms to the same chart of accounts which, in turn, conforms to the plan of organization.

Adequate Statistical Data

The availability of reliable nonmonetary statistical data relating to the volume and scope of services in prior periods is as essential for effective hospital budgeting as historical financial information. In budgeting, analyses are made of previously accumulated general statistics such as number of admissions, patient days of service, percentage of occupancy, and average length of stay as a basis for projecting the future level of activity in overall terms. Once a forecast is made of the expected general level of activity, studies are made of historical departmental occasions (units) of service statistics such as meals served, laboratory examinations, nursing hours, and pounds of laundry. This permits a projection of the probable volume of service, in statistical terms, in each department or organizational unit of the hospital. To be useful in projecting future volumes, of course, the statistics must have been accurately compiled and classified in a manner parallel to and consistent with the chart of accounts and organizational structure.

SUPPORT OF MANAGEMENT

To be successful, a budget program must have the full support of management at all levels, starting with the hospital administrator. Token support by top management personnel is not sufficient to obtain the cooperation and interest that is necessary at lower levels. Although impetus must come from the very top of the hospital organization, budgets must not be developed at that level alone. All department managers and supervisors should participate actively in the formulation of the budgets by which their future performances will be evaluated.

FORMAL BUDGETING PROCEDURES

Effective results will not be achieved if budgeting is approached in a haphazard, disorganized manner. While the budget is a cooperative endeavor, a specific individual must be assigned responsibility for the development of the various departmental inputs and for their integration into a coordinated and comprehensive master plan. This individual, sometimes called the budget officer, generally is the chairman of the hospital's budget committee. Among other things, this committee prepares a budget manual for the guidance of department managers and supervisors, establishes a budget calendar as a time schedule for completion of each step in the budgeting procedure, and reviews, amends, and presents departmental budgets for approval. And, as an end result, the committee produces a comprehensive budget for the administrator's presentation to the hospital's governing board.

BUDGETING OPERATING RESULTS

To know whether or not operating results are satisfactory, hospital revenues and expenses must be budgeted. Management control of operating results can be effective only if the hospital's managers are aware of what revenues and expenses *ought to be*, as well as what they actually are. Let us turn our attention, then, to the procedure by which the operating budget is developed.

REVENUE BUDGETING

Revenue is the very lifeblood of any organization, and it is particularly vital to the hospital enterprise which generally has a narrow profit margin or is conducted on a break-even basis. Since relatively small miscalculations of anticipated revenues may result in operating losses, careful attention must be given to the preparation of an accurate revenue budget. The revenue budget is the foundation too of the entire budgetary program; all other budgets are formulated on the basis of the revenue budget.

• ***Patient Service Revenues***. The budgeting of revenues from services to patients begins with the gathering of historical revenue dollars and nonmonetary statistics of volume of service. These data should be scheduled by months and should embrace a sufficient number of years to disclose significant trends. The data should be classified by individual revenue centers, with subclassification into inpatient and outpatient totals where appropriate. After a thorough study and analysis of this information, an evaluation should be made of the factors likely to have a material influence upon the volume and types of revenue-producing services to be provided during the coming budget period. This procedure permits a realistic projection of statistical data which, when multiplied by the charges to be made for the various services, results in a budget of gross revenues from services to patients.

The revenue to be derived from room, board, and routine nursing services obviously is dependent upon the daily rates for such services and the occupancy of the hospital's inpatient accommodations. Given the rates to be charged, the budgeting problem is one of forecasting occupancy in terms of patient days of service for the budget period. This forecast is developed for each nursing unit for each month of the period to facilitate subsequent budget versus actual comparisons on a monthly basis and to permit the preparation of a monthly cash budget.

The forecast of patient days is based upon an analysis of historical data, adjusted for trends and the probable impact of variations in the factors which affect occupancy. Factors include changes in certain characteristics of the population served, in hospital capacity, in types of services offered, in medical practices, in characteristics of the medical staff, in capabilities of other hospitals in the area, and in insurance coverages.

An illustration of the budgeting of daily inpatient service revenues for a medical and surgical nursing unit appears in figure 117. The format provides for a tabulation of historical data—patient days, revenue dollars, and average revenue per patient day—for a 5-year period, 1973–1977. Since the 1978 budget is developed before the end of the 1977 year, the 1977 data include estimates for the remaining month or so of the year. An analysis of these data leads to the budgeting of 15,400 patient days of service for 1978. Since it is assumed that statistics for patient days are not accumulated according to accommodation type, budgeted patient days are multiplied by the 1977 average revenue per patient day to obtain an unadjusted budget of revenue dollars, or $693,000. This assumes no change in room rates and no change in accommodation mix (the relative proportions of private and semiprivate occupancies, for example). If changes in these factors were anticipated, the impact of such changes would be shown as adjustments (either plus or minus) to the $693,000 budget.

The budgeting of revenues from other professional services is a

Figure 117
Wellrun Hospital
Comparative Historical Data and 1978 Revenue Budget
Daily Inpatient Service—Medical and Surgical Acute Nursing Unit #1

	Total	January	December
Historical Data			
Patient Days:			
1973	14,262	1,284	1,192
1974	15,140	1,363	1,238
1975	14,980	1,348	1,216
1976	15,474	1,393	1,257
1977 (current year)*	15,250	1,310	1,240
Revenue Dollars:			
1973	$577,896	$52,567	$48,729
1974	638,302	58,241	52,850
1975	642,642	57,977	52,252
1976	684,724	61,835	55,660
1977 (current year)*	686,250	59,553	56,234
Average Revenue per Patient Day:			
1973	$40.52	$40.94	$40.88
1974	42.16	42.73	42.69
1975	42.90	43.01	42.97
1976	44.25	44.39	44.28
1977 (current year)*	45.00	45.56	45.35
1978 Revenue Budget			
Patient Days	15,400	1,320	1,250
X 1977 Average Revenue per Patient Day	$45.00	$45.56	$45.35
Unadjusted Revenue Dollars**	$693,000	$60,100	$56,700
Adjustments:			
(none)			
1978 Revenue Budget	$693,000	$60,100	$56,700

*Actual to date plus estimate for remainder of year.

**Rounded to nearest $100.

similar procedure. Many of these services, however, are provided to both inpatients and outpatients. In such cases, historical dollar and statistical occasions of service data must be available in inpatient and outpatient classifications so that a separate revenue budget may be developed for each patient group. After a careful study of these historical data and an evaluation of the effects of anticipated changes in underlying factors, forecasts of activity are made for each of the patient service departments or revenue centers. These departmental activity forecasts are made in terms of statistical occasions or units of service such as hours in operating rooms, procedures or films in radiology, and examinations in the laboratory. In some cases, however, such general statistics can be refined into more specific or weighted units of measurement. Where this can be done, the resulting revenue budgets tend to be more accurate and more useful to department heads in planning personnel requirements, determining equipment needs, and evaluating productivity.

Figures 118 and 119 illustrate the development of inpatient and outpatient revenue budgets for the laboratory department of Wellrun Hospital for 1978. The inpatient revenue budget anticipates 106,000 occasions of service. This, when multiplied by the 1977 average revenue per occasion of service, produces an unadjusted revenue dollar budget of $689,000. A rate increase, however, is scheduled to go into effect on January 1, 1978, and it is estimated that this will provide $55,100 of additional revenues. Also, a new procedure (examination) is to be added to the services of the laboratory, and this adjustment increases the revenue budget to $748,000. Similar adjustments may be noted in figure 119 for the outpatient revenue budget.

• ***Deductions from Patient Service Revenues***. After budgeting gross revenues from services to patients, budgets are developed for the amounts of such revenues that will not be collected due to bad debts, contractual adjustments, and the provision of charity care. These budgets of revenue deductions are based upon an analysis of historical data with suitable modifications being made for trends and changes in factors such as hospital operating policies, reimbursement contract provisions, availability of specific-purpose grants for charity work, and economic conditions in the community. Each category of deductions should be separately budgeted and classified into inpatient and outpatient totals.

Figure 120 illustrates the budgeting of 1978 contractual adjustments related to inpatient services for Wellrun Hospital. Note that the contractual adjustments are budgeted as a percentage of budgeted gross inpatient service revenues. (Other types of revenue deductions also may be budgeted on a percentage basis.) Since no significant changes are expected in either the provisions of third-party contracts or in patient mix, the percentages experienced in 1977 are used in developing the 1978 budget. If material changes were anticipated, the impact of such changes would be shown as adjustments (plus or minus) in figure 120.

• ***Other Revenues***. The budgeting of other operating and nonoperating revenues should not be regarded lightly. These revenues often are substantial and must be accurately estimated to establish appropriate rates for various hospital services. Since historical data may not be available or indicative of the amounts to be

Figure 118
Wellrun Hospital
Comparative Historical Data and 1978 Revenue Budget
Other Professional Services—Laboratory Department
Inpatients

	Total	January		December
Historical Data				
Occasions of Service:				
1973	105,642	10,035		8,980
1974	102,075	9,697		8,676
1975	106,908	10,156		9,087
1976	105,259	9,905		8,947
1977 (current year)*	106,400	10,100		9,050
Revenue Dollars:				
1973	$642,303	$61,414		$53,611
1974	603,263	57,988		51,015
1975	659,622	63,069		55,340
1976	686,024	65,571		57,887
1977 (current year)*	691,600	66,155		57,920
Average Revenue per Occasion of Service:				
1973	$6.08	$6.12		$5.97
1974	5.91	5.98		5.88
1975	6.17	6.21		6.09
1976	6.58	6.62		6.47
1977 (current year)*	6.50	6.55		6.40
1978 Revenue Budget				
Occasions of Service	106,000	10,000		9,000
X 1977 Average Revenue per Occasion of Service	$6.50	$6.55		$6.40
Unadjusted Revenue Dollars**	$689,000	$65,500		$57,600
Adjustments:				
Rate Increase	55,100	5,200		4,600
New Laboratory Procedure	3,900	400		200
1978 Revenue Budget	$748,000	$71,100		$62,400

*Actual to date plus estimate for remainder of year.

**Rounded to nearest $100.

received in the future, the budgeting of some of these revenue items may be relatively difficult. Where reasonable certainty cannot be obtained, it is prudent to make conservative estimates.

Figure 119
Wellrun Hospital
Comparative Historical Data and 1978 Revenue Budget
Other Professional Services—Laboratory Department
Outpatients

	Total	January	December
Historical Data			
Occasions of Service:			
1973	14,677	1,321	1,027
1974	13,908	1,252	974
1975	14,482	1,303	1,014
1976	14,156	1,274	991
1977 (current year)*	14,620	1,316	1,020
Revenue Dollars:			
1973	$101,858	$9,300	$7,076
1974	95,409	8,689	6,623
1975	102,967	9,356	7,149
1976	106,028	9,631	7,393
1977 (current year)*	108,919	9,870	7,550
Average Revenue per Occasion of Service:			
1973	$6.94	$7.04	$6.89
1974	6.86	6.94	6.80
1975	7.11	7.18	7.05
1976	7.49	7.56	7.46
1977 (current year)*	7.45	7.50	7.40
1978 Revenue Budget			
Occasions of Service	14,800	1,330	1,030
X 1977 Average Revenue per Occasion of Service	$7.45	$7.50	$7.40
Unadjusted Revenue Dollars**	$110,300	$10,000	$7,600
Adjustments:			
Rate Increase	11,900	1,100	600
New Laboratory Procedure	1,200	100	100
1978 Revenue Budget	$123,400	$11,200	$8,300

*Actual to date plus estimate for remainder of year.

**Rounded to nearest $100.

Each of these revenue items is budgeted on the best basis available. The revenue from educational programs, for example, is budgeted on the basis of expected enrollments and tuition fees to be charged. Budgets of revenues to become available from unre-

Figure 120
Wellrun Hospital
Comparative Historical Data and 1978 Revenue Deductions Budget
Contractual Adjustments—Inpatients

	Total	January	December
Historical Data			
Gross Inpatient Service Revenues:			
1973	$7,462,893	$671,660	$622,403
1974	7,855,107	714,815	698,246
1975	8,172,783	727,378	701,494
1976	7,906,449	711,580	696,338
1977 (current year)*	8,256,000	751,300	738,100
Contractual Adjustments — Inpatients:			
1973	$276,127	$25,523	$21,784
1974	274,929	25,019	23,740
1975	277,875	24,003	22,448
1976	245,099	22,771	20,890
1977 (current year)*	247,700	23,300	21,400
Percentage of Contractual Adjustments to Gross Inpatient Service Revenues:			
1973	3.7%	3.8%	3.5%
1974	3.5	3.5	3.4
1975	3.4	3.3	3.2
1976	3.1	3.2	3.0
1977 (current year)*	3.0	3.1	2.9
1978 Budget			
Budgeted Gross Inpatient Service Revenues for 1978	$8,589,200	$773,000	$687,100
X 1977 Contractual Adjustments Percentage	3.0%	3.1%	2.9%
Unadjusted Contractual Adjustments Budget**	$ 257,700	$ 24,000	$ 19,900
Adjustments:			
(none)			
1978 Contractual Adjustments Budget — Inpatients	$ 257,700	$ 24,000	$ 19,900

*Actual to date plus estimate for remainder of year.

**Rounded to nearest $100.

stricted gifts and specific-purpose funds may be determined from an analysis of past experience, existing contracts, fund-raising programs, and requests made to granting organizations. Rentals of hospital space to doctors and employees may be estimated from a study of lease agreements. The budget of cafeteria sales and the sales of gift shops often are related to projected patient days and outpatient visits. A similar relationship also may be found with respect to telephone and television service, nonpatient sales of supplies, and medical record transcript fees. Budgeting investment income requires making an analysis of the hospital's current investments and an estimate of the changes likely to occur in the amounts of such investments during the budget period.

EXPENSE BUDGETING

A primary management objective is to keep expenses at a level consistent with anticipated revenues in order to maintain necessary financial integrity in operating results. This requires expense budgeting, and, since labor represents about two-thirds of hospital operating expenses, particular attention must be given to the development of accurate budgets for salaries and wages. Supplies, purchased services, and other nonlabor costs are significant, however, and they also should be budgeted with appropriate care.

• ***Salaries and Wages***. Salary and wage budgets should be developed in the classifications provided in the hospital's chart of accounts, assuming that the chart conforms to the organization plan that is required for responsibility accounting. Each departmental cost center supervisor should be given responsibility for the preparation of the salary and wage budget relating to personnel over whose employment and performance he or she has primary control. These department heads or supervisors should be supplied with adequate information concerning forecasted levels of activity, authorized numbers of employees in each job classification, and the approved rates of pay for each position. Staffing levels should be carefully monitored and controlled in relation to service volume.

Given a firm projection of the amount of work to be done, these supervisors are asked to determine the number of personnel in each classification that will be needed to meet expected workloads in an efficient manner. In this way, major emphasis is placed on the control of labor costs at the lowest levels of organization where decision authority and responsibility for the performance of personnel exists. While much of the salaries and wages paid by hospitals is relatively fixed within wide ranges of activity, the number of employees and the manner in which their services are utilized can vary considerably in areas with changes in volume of activity.

In addition to a cost center classification, the labor budget also must be broken down by months of the year. This permits determining the amounts and times of cash disbursements for salaries and wages that are needed for cash budgeting purposes. It also permits the necessary month-by-month comparison of budgeted and actual costs during the budget period. The labor hours budgeted for each cost center also should be classified by months for comparison with actual hours in subsequent budget versus actual reports. Comparisons on a dollar basis alone are not nearly so indicative of employee utilization and efficiency as are comparisons also made on the basis of hours.

Figure 121 illustrates a worksheet for development of the 1978 salaries and wages budget for the radiology department of Wellrun Hospital. A similar worksheet is prepared for each department or cost center of the hospital. The worksheet lists each authorized position by job classification code and employee name. Note that Wellrun Hospital has an "03" position vacant but expects to fill this position before the budget period begins. The current compensation rate for each position is indicated along with the budgeted increase and the date the increase becomes effective.

The scheduled work hours at straight-time pay are entered for each position. Assuming a 40-hour work week, the number of scheduled hours normally is 2,080, (i.e., 40 hours × 52 weeks). Employee Buzby, however, is scheduled for an additional 200 hours (4 overtime hours per week for 50 weeks). This employee will be paid time and a half for these excess hours, so the premium pay of $360 (i.e., 200 hours × ½ × $3.60) is listed as one of the adjustments on the worksheet. Since the hours involved in this type of premium pay are nonproductive hours, they are not shown as scheduled work hours. Note, however, that vacation hours are included in the scheduled work hours column.

In addition to the adjustment for the dollar amount of premium pay, adjustments also are listed for estimated work hours and dollar amounts relating to vacation relief, holiday relief, and on-call requirements. In each case, the costs are determined by multiplying the budgeted hourly rate by the number of hours required for each month. These hours and computed dollar amounts are distributed to the months during which vacations are scheduled, holidays occur, and on-call duty may be necessary.

Budgets also must be prepared for payroll-related costs such as FICA taxes, unemployment taxes, and workmen's compensation insurance. The budgeting of these expense items involves application of the tax or insurance rates to the budgeted amounts of salaries and wages subject to those rates. Other employee benefits such as the hospital's share of employee insurance and pension programs are budgeted on the basis of the payroll budget and the provisions of such programs.

• ***Supplies and Other Nonlabor Expense***. In budgeting nonlabor expenses, each cost center supervisor should be supplied by the accounting department with an analysis of the major categories of supplies and other expenses that have been charged to the center in the last few years. This analysis should show dollars and, where feasible, units such as dozens, pounds, and gallons. In addition, the historical dollars should be compared to historical statistical data such as patient days of service or departmental occasions of service, as appropriate.

Nonlabor expenses generally are more responsive than salaries and wages to changes in service volume, particularly in departments that render services directly to patients. As volume increases, nonlabor expenses tend to increase proportionately; as volume declines, these expenses tend to decrease at about the

Figure 121
Wellrun Hospital
Salaries and Wages Budget Worksheet
Radiology Department
1978

Authorized Positions		Compensation			Scheduled Work Hours	Vacation Hours
		Current	Budgeted Increase			
Code	Name	Rate*	Amount*	Eff. Date		
01	Hartmann, J.	$ 1,800PM	$ 150 PM	11/1	2,080	120
02	Noble, B.	1,500PM	90 PM	4/1	2,080	80
02	Biagioni, L.	1,500PM	90 PM	2/1	2,080	80
03	Thomas, P.	1,000PM	60 PM	12/1	2,080	80
03	Heitger, E.	1,000PM	60 PM	3/1	2,080	80
03	Hansen, J.	800PM	40 PM	2/1	2,080	80
03	(position vacant)	800PM	--	--	2,080	80
04	Baker, R.	700PM	30 PM	4/1	2,080	80
04	Buzby, T.	3.60PH	--	--	2,280	80
	Totals				18,920	760
	Adjustments:					
	Premium Pay					
	Vacation Relief				600	
	Holiday Relief				90	
	On Call				2,400	
	Total Adjustments				3,090	
	1978 Salaries and Wages Budget - Dollars					
	1978 Salaries and Wages Budget - Hours				22,010	760

*PM = Per Month
PH = Per Hour

same rate. Assuming that a close relationship of this kind exists for Wellrun Hospital's laboratory department, the budgeting of that department's supplies and other nonlabor expenses for 1978 may proceed as illustrated in figure 122. Note, however, that the tenta-

Total	January	February	March	April	November	December
$ 21,900	$ 1,800	$ 1,800	$ 1,800	$ 1,800	$ 1,950	$ 1,950
18,810	1,500	1,500	1,500	1,590	1,590	1,590
18,990	1,500	1,590	1,590	1,590	1,590	1,590
12,060	1,000	1,000	1,000	1,000	1,000	1,060
12,600	1,000	1,000	1,060	1,060	1,060	1,060
10,040	800	840	840	840	840	840
9,600	800	800	800	800	800	800
8,670	700	700	700	730	730	730
8,208	684	684	684	684	684	684
120,878	9,784	9,914	9,974	10,094	10,244	10,304
360	30	30	30	30	30	30
3,000	1,400					
540	45			90		270
4,800	400	400	400	400	400	400
8,700	1,875	430	430	520	430	700
$129,578	$11,659	$10,344	$10,404	$10,614	$10,674	$11,004
	2,100	1,650	1,810	1,780	1,760	1,850

tive dollar budget must be adjusted for the effects of expected cost price changes and for the effects of changes in the types of patient services provided or supply usage patterns.

A close correlation between nonlabor expenses and activity level,

Figure 122
Wellrun Hospital
Supplies and Expense Budget
Laboratory Department
1978

	Total	January	December
Inpatients			
1977 Supplies and Expense	$128,744	$11,587	$ 9,656
÷ 1977 Occasions of Service	106,400	10,100	9,050
1977 Expense Per Occasion of Service	$1.21	$1.15	$1.07
X 1978 Budgeted Occasions of Service	106,000	10,000	9,000
Unadjusted 1978 Dollar Budget*	$128,300	$11,500	$ 9,600
Adjustments:			
Estimated 8% Price Increase	10,300	900	800
New Laboratory Procedure	2,400	200	200
1978 Supplies and Expense Budget— Inpatients	$141,000	$12,600	$10,600
Outpatients			
1977 Supplies and Expense	$ 13,597	$ 1,198	$ 908
÷ 1977 Occasions of Service	14,620	1,316	1,020
1977 Expense Per Occasion of Service	$.93	$.91	$.89
X 1978 Budgeted Occasions of Service	14,800	1,330	1,030
Unadjusted 1978 Dollar Budget*	$ 13,800	$ 1,200	$ 900
Adjustments:			
Estimated 8% Price Increase	1,100	100	100
New Laboratory Procedure	600	100	100
1978 Supplies and Expense Budget— Outpatients	$ 15,500	$ 1,400	$ 1,100
Total 1978 Supplies and Expense Budget	$156,500	$14,000	$11,700

*Rounded to nearest $100.

such as that assumed in figure 122, will not be found in all departments of the hospital. This is likely to be the case in many of the hospital's indirect service departments. The amount of supplies used by the housekeeping department in servicing a given area, for example, probably would not vary greatly with changes in the number of patient days. Given no change in cleaning methods and assuming no changes in supply prices, the cost of housekeeping supplies should vary mainly with the square footage serviced.

Where nonlabor expenses are not closely related to volume, these expenses must be budgeted on an item-by-item basis in each department or cost center. A careful study is made of historical dollars by major category of expense. And, taking into account expected price changes, changes in the types of services provided, and changes in the methods of providing those services, each department manager determines for each expense item the amount the department *should* incur to accomplish the department's objective, usually with written justification for each amount budgeted.

Repairs and routine maintenance work to be performed may be estimated by the hospital engineer on the basis of his experience, knowledge of current costs, and condition of the facilities. Heat, light, power, and other utilities are budgeted in terms of past and projected usage and anticipated prices or service rates. Budgets for rent and insurance expense may be developed from an analysis of lease agreements and insurance policies. Items such as depreciation and interest are budgeted on the basis of plant asset records, plans for asset acquisitions and retirements, current debt service schedules, and plans for new borrowings.

SUMMARIZING THE OPERATING BUDGET

It should be understood that the expense and revenue budgets prepared by department heads and supervisors are preliminary in nature. The initial drafts of these budgets are consolidated by the hospital's budget officer into a projected income statement for the budget year. This tentative operating plan, after careful evaluation by the budget committee, is likely to undergo several revisions (1) to secure the desired relationship between revenues and expense for the hospital as a whole, (2) to achieve the necessary degree of coordination among the many departmental segments of the plan, and (3) to obtain compatibility between the operating plan and the hospital's financial-position objectives, requirements, and limitations. Department heads who disagree with budget committee amendments should be given an opportunity to present their views for further consideration by the committee. All such differences should be resolved to the fullest extent possible so that the resulting final budget is generally accepted and supported by those responsible for its implementation.

The final 1978 operating budget for Wellrun Hospital is illustrated in projected income statement form in figure 123. As indicated by this illustration, detailed information relating to the condensed totals in the statement should be provided in supporting schedules (schedules A through 0). All revenue and expense items should be budgeted in as much detail as is practicable and useful. Here, however, we present illustrations only of schedules B (figure 124) and J (figure 125). Note that the departmental budgets include statistical units as well as dollars.

Figure 123
Wellrun Hospital
1978 Operating Budget

Gross revenues from services to patients:
Nursing services
Other professional services
Total
Less deductions from revenues:
Bad debts
Contractual adjustments
Charity service
Total deductions from revenues
Net revenues from services to patients
Other operating revenues:
Cafeteria sales
Other
Total other operating revenues
Total operating revenues
Less operating expenses:
Nursing services
Other professional services
General services
Fiscal services
Administrative services
Unassigned expenses
Total operating expenses
Operating income
Add nonoperating revenues:
General contributions
Other
Total nonoperating revenues
Net income
*Only Schedules B and J are illustrated; see figures

BUDGETING FINANCIAL POSITION

As stated earlier, the operating budget is not established in final form until its impact on the hospital's financial position is determined. The tentative operating budget, in other words, must be translated into balance sheet terms. This requires the development of a projected balance sheet and a statement of changes in financial position for the end of each month of the budget year. The

Detail Schedule*	1978 Total	January	December
A	$6,082,300	$552,400	$487,600
B	2,506,900	220,600	199,500
	8,589,200	773,000	687,100
C	94,200	8,200	9,300
D	257,700	24,000	19,900
E	421,300	38,200	32,700
	773,200	70,400	61,900
	7,816,000	702,600	625,200
F	307,400	30,800	24,900
G	606,600	53,300	52,800
	914,000	84,100	77,700
	8,730,000	786,700	702,900
H	3,038,400	255,200	241,500
I	1,580,500	142,300	139,400
J	1,176,000	115,800	100,700
K	604,800	54,400	48,000
L	740,000	66,600	59,400
M	1,260,300	100,200	104,300
	8,400,000	734,500	693,300
	330,000	52,200	9,600
N	105,000	6,300	5,200
O	42,000	3,100	2,500
	147,000	9,400	7,700
	$ 477,000	$ 61,600	$ 17,300

124 and 125.

revenue budget, which was prepared on an accrual basis, is converted to a cash basis to allow a forecast of monthly cash receipts and accounts receivable figures. The expense budget, which also was prepared on an accrual basis, is similarly converted to a cash basis to permit estimates of monthly cash disbursements, inventory, and accounts payable figures. When this information is combined

Figure 124
Wellrun Hospital
Other Professional Services Revenues
1978 Budget
Schedule B

			Statistical Units
Inpatient revenues:			
Laboratory			Examinations
Radiology			Procedures
Pharmacy			Requisitions
Anesthesia			Hours
Total inpatient revenues			
Outpatient revenues:			
Laboratory			Examinations
Radiology			Procedures
Pharmacy			Requisitions
Anesthesia			Hours
Total outpatient revenues			
Total revenues			

with the hospital's plans for plant asset additions and disposals, investments and sales of securities, retirement of debt, and new borrowings, monthly balance sheets can be projected for the budget year. This will indicate whether the budgets for operating,

1978		January		December	
Units	Dollars	Units	Dollars	Units	Dollars
106,000	$ 748,000	9,600	$ 67,300	8,400	$ 59,800
54,000	815,300	4,900	73,400	4,300	65,200
43,000	346,200	3,800	31,200	3,400	27,700
9,300	239,100	900	23,100	700	17,900
	2,148,600		195,000		170,600
14,800	123,400	1,300	7,400	1,100	11,400
9,100	136,500	800	9,300	700	8,600
8,600	72,300	800	6,500	800	6,500
1,000	26,100	100	2,400	100	2,400
	358,300		25,600		28,900
	$2,506,900		$220,600		$199,500

plant and equipment, debt retirement, and other plans are compatible with the hospital's current and projected financial resources. If not, appropriate adjustments must be made in one or more of the preliminary budgets. Possible adjustments include an increase in

Figure 125
Wellrun Hospital
General Services Expenses
1978 Budget
Schedule J

		Statistical Units
Administrative office:		
Salaries and wages		Hours
Supplies and expenses		Hours
Total		
Dietary:		
Salaries and wages		Hours
Supplies and expenses		Number of meals
Total		
Plant operation and maintenance:		
Salaries and wages		Hours
Supplies and expenses		Square feet
Total		
Housekeeping:		
Salaries and wages		Hours
Supplies and expenses		Square feet
Total		
Laundry:		
Salaries and wages		Hours
Supplies and expenses		Pounds
Total		
Total salaries and wages		
Total supplies and expenses		
Total general services expenses		

hospital service rates, a reduction of tentative expense budgets, an increase in the amounts of planned borrowings, and the postponement of budgeted additions to plant assets.

Assuming that all necessary coordinating adjustments have been

1978		January		December	
Units	Dollars	Units	Dollars	Units	Dollars
6,300	$ 28,500	600	$ 2,600	500	$ 2,400
6,300	8,100	600	700	500	600
	36,600		3,300		3,000
40,000	97,100	3,600	8,800	3,400	8,200
325,000	511,800	31,400	47,100	29,800	44,300
	608,900		55,900		52,500
14,600	53,700	1,300	4,300	1,200	4,800
315,000	288,100	315,000	25,900	315,000	22,300
	341,800		30,200		27,100
28,000	71,900	2,500	7,500	2,400	6,800
260,000	44,600	260,000	12,300	260,000	4,300
	116,500		19,800		11,100
15,200	49,400	1,400	4,500	1,300	4,700
148,000	22,800	13,300	2,100	13,600	2,300
	72,200		6,600		7,000
	300,600		27,700		26,900
	875,400		88,100		73,800
	$1,176,000		$115,800		$100,700

made, figure 126 provides a somewhat simplified illustration of Wellrun Hospital's projected balance sheets in condensed form for the 1978 budget year. This chapter, however, is intended only as an introduction to budgeting, with emphasis on the operating

Figure 126
Wellrun Hospital
Projected Balance Sheets
1978 Budget Year

	1/31/78	2/28/78	3/31/78	12/31/78
Current assets:				
Cash	$ 95,100	$ 37,400	$ 49,800	$ 74,500
Short-term investments	105,000	105,000	180,000	45,000
Receivables from patients (net)	694,600	682,400	699,000	715,000
Inventories	100,600	110,000	112,800	118,000
Total current assets	995,300	934,800	1,041,600	952,500
Plant and equipment (net)	7,442,500	7,416,900	7,383,500	7,366,500
Total assets	$8,437,800	$8,351,700	$8,425,100	$8,319,000
Current liabilities:				
Notes payable	$ 120,000	$ -0-	$ -0-	$ 35,000
Accounts payable	83,000	93,200	94,500	98,600
Payroll taxes withheld and accrued	143,300	136,200	148,900	134,700
Accrued interest payable	16,500	25,000	37,500	60,300
Current portion of long-term debt	500,000	500,000	500,000	500,000
Total current liabilities	862,800	754,400	780,900	828,600
Long-term debt (bonds payable)	2,000,000	2,000,000	2,000,000	1,500,000
Total liabilities	2,862,800	2,754,400	2,780,900	2,238,600
Fund balance, 12/31/77	5,513,400	5,513,400	5,513,400	5,513,400
Add net income to date	61,600	83,900	130,800	477,000
Fund balance, end of month	5,575,000	5,597,300	5,644,200	5,990,400
Total liabilities and fund balance	$8,437,800	$8,351,700	$8,425,100	$8,319,000

budget. Consequently, the budgeting of each balance sheet item will not be described here; our attention is limited largely to the development of the cash budget.

A cash budget is a detailed estimate of future cash receipts from all sources and cash disbursements for all purposes. By budgeting these cash flows, the cash balance at various future places in time can be predicted in a reasonably accurate manner. In this way, the need for additional funds can be foreseen, and plans can be made for the investment of excess funds, if any. Cash budgeting also tends to provide assurance that money will be available in the amounts and at the times needed but, at the same time, avoids the holding of cash balances in excessive amounts.

To illustrate cash budgeting procedure, let us assume the 1978 operating budget previously presented in figure 123 and the December 31, 1977, balance sheet in figure 127. The completed 1978 cash budget for Wellrun Hospital is presented in figure 128.

Figure 127
Wellrun Hospital
Balance Sheet
December 31, 1977

Current assets:		
Cash	$ 94,700	
Short-term investments	55,000	
Receivables from patients (net)	680,000	
Inventories	105,700	
Total current assets		$ 935,400
Plant and equipment (net)		7,502,500
Total assets		$8,437,900
Current liabilities:		
Notes payable	$ 120,000	
Accounts payable	88,800	
Payroll taxes withheld and accrued	137,500	
Accrued interest payable	78,200	
Current portion of long-term debt	500,000	
Total current liabilities		$ 924,500
Long-term debt (bonds payable)		2,000,000
Total liabilities		2,924,500
Fund balance		5,513,400
Total liabilities and fund balance		$8,437,900

BUDGETING CASH RECEIPTS

It is assumed that the December 31, 1977, accounts receivable (net of allowances for uncollectible accounts) originated from charges made for services rendered during the previous 3 months:

1977	Charges to Patients*		12/31/77 Receivables
October	$680,000	× 10% =	$ 68,000
November	660,000	× 30% =	198,000
December	690,000	× 60% =	414,000
			$680,000

*Net of revenue deductions.

Figure 128
Wellrun Hospital
1978 Cash Budget

	1978 Total
Beginning cash balance	$ 94,700
Budgeted cash receipts:	
Collections on patients accounts receivable	7,781,000
Other operating revenues	914,000
Nonoperating revenues	147,000
Other receipts	
Proceeds from sales of investment securities	275,000
Proceeds from sales of plant assets	32,000
Short-term borrowings	95,000
Total budgeted cash receipts	9,244,000
Estimated cash available	9,338,700
Budgeted cash disbursements:	
Salaries and wages (net)	4,258,800
Payroll taxes withheld and accrued	1,640,300
Supplies	1,008,500
Interest	157,200
Other expenses	824,400
Other disbursements	
Purchases of new investment securities	265,000
Purchases of new plant and equipment	430,000
Repayment of short-term borrowings	180,000
Retirement of long-term debt	500,000
Total budgeted cash disbursements	9,264,200
Ending cash balance	$ 74,500

A study must be made of the hospital's collection experience in order to determine the pattern in which its receivables generally are collected in cash. Let us assume that Wellrun Hospital's analysis shows that about 40% of a given month's net charges (to inpatients and outpatients) is collected in the same month, an additional 30% is collected in the first following month, another 20% is collected in

January	February	March	Second Quarter	Third Quarter	Fourth Quarter
$ 94,200	$ 95,100	$ 37,400	$ 49,800	$ 106,800	$ 71,400
688,000	683,200	695,800	1,999,900	1,771,300	1,942,800
84,100	76,300	81,200	242,100	201,700	228,600
9,900	7,900	8,800	44,700	35,100	41,100
				275,000	
20,000					12,000
			95,000		
802,000	767,400	785,800	2,381,700	2,283,100	2,224,500
896,200	862,500	823,200	2,431,500	2,389,900	2,295,900
372,300	354,300	387,300	1,132,200	974,900	1,037,800
137,500	143,300	136,200	440,400	367,000	415,900
88,800	83,000	93,200	267,700	223,000	252,800
75,000	4,800			75,000	2,400
77,500	69,700	81,700	214,400	178,600	202,500
50,000		75,000	100,000		40,000
	50,000		170,000		210,000
	120,000				60,000
				500,000	
801,100	825,100	773,400	2,324,700	2,318,500	2,221,400
$ 95,100	$ 37,400	$ 49,800	$ 106,800	$ 71,400	$ 74,500

the second following month, and the remaining 10% is collected in the month after that. Thus, at December 31, 1977, 10% of October charges, 30% of November charges, and 60% of December charges remain uncollected and in receivables as shown in the preceding illustration.

Assuming that this collection pattern is valid for 1978, month-end

Figure 129
Budgeting Cash Collections and
Month-End Receivables Balances

Receivables originating in:			
October, 1977 — $680,000 X 10%			
November, 1977 — $660,000 X 20%			
$660,000 X 10%			
December, 1977 — $690,000 X 30%			
$690,000 X 20%			
$690,000 X 10%			
January, 1978 — $702,600 X 40%			
$702,600 X 30%			
$702,600 X 20%			
$702,600 X 10%			
February, 1978 — $671,000 X 40%			
$671,000 X 30%			
$671,000 X 20%			
$671,000 X 10%			
March, 1978 — $712,400 X 40%			
$712,400 X 30%			
$712,400 X 20%			
$712,400 X 10%			
Budgeted cash collections on patients' accounts			
Budgeted end-of-month accounts receivable			

balances of receivables and cash collections on patients' accounts may be budgeted for the first 3 months of the year as illustrated in figure 129. These are the budgeted cash collections and receivables balances which appear in figures 126 and 128 for January, February, and March of 1978. Budgeted amounts for other months of the year would be developed in the same way.

Collected During			Uncollected At		
January	February	March	January 31	February 28	March 31
$ 68,000					
132,000					
	$ 66,000		$ 66,000		
207,000					
	138,000		138,000		
		$ 69,000	69,000	$ 69,000	
281,000					
	210,800		210,800		
		140,500	140,500	140,500	
			70,300	70,300	$ 70,300
	268,400				
		201,300		201,300	
				134,200	134,200
				67,100	67,100
		285,000			
					213,700
					142,500
					71,200
$688,000	$683,200	$695,800			
			$694,600	$682,400	$699,000

Cash receipts relating to other operating and nonoperating revenues also should be accurately budgeted on the best basis available. This often requires an account-by-account analysis of each revenue source of major significance, giving consideration to projected accrued and deferred revenues. In figure 128, however, it is assumed that these revenue items are collected largely in the month that they are earned and recorded as revenues. Note, for example, that the operating budget statement in figure 123 includes $84,100 of other operating revenues and $9,400 of nonoperating revenues for January of 1978. These amounts also appear in figure 128 as the cash budget statement for the month. This procedure likely will be satisfactory when there are no material variations from month to month in the amounts of accrued and deferred revenues.

The other cash receipts in figure 128 are budgeted on the basis of management plans for the sale of investment securities, for the occasional sales of plant assets, and for new short-term borrowings. Certain of these plans, of course, are based upon the results of the cash budgeting process. So, the budgeting of cash receipts from these sources generally is postponed until all other segments of the cash budget have been formulated.

BUDGETING CASH DISBURSEMENTS

The estimates for cash disbursements are derived from previously established budgets for departmental salaries and wages, supplies and other expenses, and plant asset acquisitions. With a knowledge of payroll periods, the monthly cash requirements for salaries and wages are easily determined. The budgeted amount of a month's payroll *plus* the estimated accrued payroll at the beginning of the month *minus* the accrued payroll at the end of the month produces the necessary figures. Taxes and other payroll withholdings are excluded from the budgeted monthly payroll disbursement and are instead included in budgeted cash disbursements of the month in which such taxes and withholdings are to be remitted to governmental and other agencies.

Cash requirements also must be estimated by months with regard to the purchase of supplies and payments for insurance, interest, and purchased services such as utilities and telephone. (Of course, depreciation expense is omitted from the budget of cash expenditures unless it is being "funded," as described in chapter 18.) These determinations may be based on budgets for purchasing, insurance expiration and debt retirement schedules, and other relevant data provided by the operating budget. Cash requirements for planned investments in securities and new plant assets must also be estimated.

A number of simplifying assumptions were made in developing Wellrun Hospital's budget for 1978 cash disbursements. The general procedure followed appears in figure 130 for the first 3 months of 1978. Similar computations would be made for other months.

Figure 130 begins with total monthly operating expenses which are drawn from the operating budget (figure 128). Monthly gross salaries and wages are assumed, for the purposes of this illustration, to be 65% of total operating expenses. In actual practice, of course, the operating budget would provide the monthly salaries and wages figures. The same is true of supplies expense, but here we simply assume that this expense item is a flat 12% of total operating expenses budgeted for each month. The monthly depreciation expense amounts appearing in figure 130 are assumed, although in an actual case the information would be available in the detailed operating budget. The hospital's share of payroll taxes is assumed to be 8% of gross salaries and wages. Finally, monthly interest expense figures are deducted. In this illustration, the amounts of interest expense include $12,500 interest on the bonds ($2,500,000 × 6% × 1/12) and $800 interest on the short-term notes payable (which were paid off at the end of February).

Figure 130
Budgeting Cash Disbursements*

	1978 January	1978 February	1978 March
Total operating expenses	$734,500	$698,300	$763,900
Less salaries and wages (assumed 65% of operating expenses)	477,400	454,200	496,500
Balance	257,100	244,100	267,400
Less supplies expense (assumed 12% of operating expenses)	88,100	83,800	91,700
Balance	169,000	160,300	175,700
Less depreciation expense	40,000	41,000	41,800
Balance	129,000	119,300	133,900
Less payroll taxes (assumed 8% of salaries and wages)	38,200	36,300	39,700
Balance	90,800	83,000	94,200
Less interest expense	13,300	13,300	12,500
Other expenses (assumed paid in same month)	$ 77,500	$ 69,700	$ 81,700
Payroll taxes withheld (assumed 22% of salaries and wages)	$105,100	$ 99,900	$109,200
Accrued payroll taxes (above)	38,200	36,300	39,700
Total payroll taxes withheld and accrued (assumed paid in following month)	$143,300	$136,200	$148,900
Salaries and wages (above)	$477,400	$454,200	$496,500
Less payroll taxes withheld (above)	105,100	99,900	109,200
Net salaries and wages (assumed paid in same month)	$372,300	$354,300	$387,300
Supplies expense (above)	$ 88,100	$ 83,800	$ 91,700
Desired ending inventory (assumed 120% of following month's budgeted supplies expense)	100,600	110,000	112,800
Total	$188,700	$193,800	$204,500
Less opening inventory	105,700	100,600	110,000
Purchases of supplies (assumed paid in following month)	$ 83,000	$ 93,200	$ 94,500

* Rounded to nearest $100

After deducting the expense items mentioned above, an amount labeled "other expenses" remains in each column of figure 130. It is assumed for purposes of this example that these amounts are paid in the same month that they are budgeted as expenses. It would be useful to trace these figures back to the cash disbursements section of figure 128.

The next section of figure 130 shows the computation of total payroll taxes withheld and accrued during each month. It is assumed that withholdings are 22% of gross salaries and wages and that the hospital's share of payroll taxes are 8% of gross salaries and wages. It also is assumed that these amounts are paid (remitted to governmental agencies) in the following month, as may be seen in the cash budget (figure 128).

Figure 130 also includes a computation of the net salaries and wages of each month. It is assumed that the full amount of the net payroll is paid each month, that there is no accrued payroll either at the beginning or end of any month. You will want to locate these net payroll figures in the cash disbursements section of figure 128.

Finally, figure 130 shows the computation of required monthly purchases of supplies, assuming that Wellrun Hospital's policy is to maintain month-end inventories in a dollar amount equal to 120% of the following month's budgeted supplies expense. It is assumed that all purchases of supplies during a given month are paid for in the following month. This computation provides cash disbursement amounts for the cash budget (figure 128) and accounts payable figures for the budgeted balance sheets (figure 126).

The budgeted interest payments in figure 128 were developed with the assumption that the bonds pay interest semiannually on January 1 and July 1. It also is assumed that $500,000 (face amount) of the bonds are retired annually on July 1. The remaining interest payments in the cash budget are assumed interest payments on the hospital's short-term notes payable. The other disbursements listed in the budget reflect management plans for the purchase of investment securities, the purchase of new plant assets, and the repayment of short-term borrowings.

Finally, notice that Wellrun Hospital's cash budget is detailed by months for the first quarter of the year and by quarters only for the remainder of the year. This is often the practice because it may be impractical to try to prepare a detailed monthly cash budget which projects beyond 3 months into the future. As the year progresses, however, these quarterly budgets are adjusted to more-current expectations and are converted into detailed monthly budgets. On the other hand, some hospitals have found it possible and useful to budget cash on a daily basis for a month into the future; that is, as a new month approaches, the cash budget for that month is converted to a detailed daily budget.

This chapter has been concerned almost entirely with the *planning* aspect of budgeting. The uses of the budget as a means of *controlling* a hospital's operating results and financial position are described in chapter 24.

QUESTIONS

1. What are the 5 major prerequisites for effective budgeting?

2. Define the term *budget*. Why is budgeting essential to the successful management of a hospital?

3. What is meant by "comprehensive budgeting"?

4. Describe, in general terms, how you would go about developing a budget for daily patient service revenues for a particular nursing unit.

5. Upon what factors is the budget for deductions from patient service revenues based?

6. Indicate briefly the bases upon which the following "other revenues" might be budgeted:

   a. Tuition from educational programs
   b. Rental income
   c. Cafeteria sales
   d. Income from unrestricted fund investments
   e. Unrestricted contributions

7. Describe, in general terms, how you would go about developing a budget for the salaries and wages of a laboratory department of the hospital.

8. Describe, in general terms, how you would go about developing a budget for supplies and other nonlabor expenses for the dietary department of the hospital.

9. Why are the tentative departmental budgets consolidated into a projected income statement and converted into projected balance sheet terms?

10. Describe, in general terms, how you would go about developing a budget of cash receipts and disbursements for a hospital's unrestricted fund.

PROBLEMS

A. The July 1 accounts receivable of Vinson Hospital originate from charges made to patients during the previous 3 months as follows:

Month	Charges	Accounts Receivable
June	$300,000	$300,000
May	320,000	96,000
April	270,000	27,000

The hospital's past experience shows that about 70% of charges in any month are collected in the following month. An additional 20% are collected in the next following month, 8% are collected in the third month, and the remaining 2% prove to be uncollectible.

Required. Calculate the probable collections on accounts receivable during July for purposes of cash budgeting.

B. Verywell Hospital provides you with the following information:

	May	June	July	August	Sept.
Revenues	$100,000	$120,000	$ 90,000	$ 80,000	$110,000
Purchases of supplies	10,000	15,000	12,000	8,000	20,000
Other expenses	80,000	93,000	69,000	64,000	79,000

Eighty percent of revenues are collected in the month following the month in which services are rendered. The remaining 20% are collected in the second following month. Fifty percent of purchases are made for cash. The remainder is paid, net of a 1% discount, in the month following the month of purchase. Other expenses are paid in cash in the month incurred. Depreciation of $5,000 per month is included in the expenses given above; depreciation, however, is not funded by the hospital. A short-term bank loan of $40,000 falls due on September 1, and the hospital plans to purchase new equipment for $75,000 cash on August 1. The cash balance at June 30 is $25,000.

Required. Prepare a cash budget for July, August, and September, showing the projected cash balance at the end of each month.

C. Various information relating to the laboratory department of Virginia Hospital is presented below:

1. The hospital establishes charges for services at an amount that will approximate costs as nearly as possible. Total budgeted income for a department should be within a range of $1,000 of total budgeted expenses. A relative unit system is used in the laboratory department. During the fiscal year ended June 30, 1977, the average charge per unit was $1.02.
2. Deductions from revenues should be assumed to be 10% of gross revenues.
3. In budget preparation it is assumed that the laboratory department will continue to grow at the same rate, as far as the number of relative units of service is concerned, as it has in the past 2 years.
4. The 2 pathologists are guaranteed a base salary of $20,000 each, plus a pool of 10% of net revenue (gross revenue less deductions) which is divided equally.
5. The budget committee of the hospital has instructed you to allow for a 5% salary increase to all eligible personnel except the pathologists. These increases are to become effective for each employee on the first of the month following the anniversary of each employee's employment date.
6. Because of the increased workload, the budget committee has approved the addition of one new technologist to begin at the approved starting rate.
7. Overtime, vacation and holiday relief, and on-call pay should be computed at 15% of the technologists' and aides' salaries. The indirect cost ratio, laboratory department, is 25% of direct expenses.
8. The nonsalary direct expenses for the laboratory department in the year ended June 30, 1977, amounted to $50,000. It is expected that the 1977–78 nonsalary direct expenses will continue at approximately 25¢ per unit of service.

	Year Ended June 30		
	1975	1976	1977
Units of service	165,300	181,820	200,000
Gross charges	$175,218	$189,093	$204,000
Deductions	17,500	18,900	20,300
Net charges	157,718	170,193	183,700

Selected wage range for year ending June 30, 1978:

Job Code		Range in Dollars per Month
23	Secretary	$325–$450
44	Laboratory technologists	375– 525
67	Aides	300– 400

Analysis of personnel, July 1, 1977:

Authorized Positions		Current	Monthly	Employment
Job Code	Name	Annual Rate	Rate	Date
01	M. Apple, Pathologist	$20,000		7/1/69
01	W. Orange, Pathologist	20,000		9/1/68
23	P. Pine	4,800	$400	1/15/73
44	G. Gerber	6,120	510	8/5/66
44	D. Dudley	6,000	500	7/9/65
44	R. Ratterman	5,520	460	9/14/70
44	S. Smith	4,680	390	12/13/73
67	O. Otteson	4,560	380	6/12/69
67	T. Thompson	4,080	340	7/13/73

Required. Prepare an annual income-and-expense budget for the laboratory department of Virginia Hospital for the year ending June 30, 1978.

D. The following is information relating to the radiology department of Variety Hospital concerning the preparation of a budget of revenue and expense for the year ending December 31, 1978:

1. A relative unit value system has been adopted to account for the activities of the radiology department. Below is a schedule of these relative unit values:

	1976 Actual	1977 Actual	1978 Budget
January	10,500	11,000	11,500
February	10,000	10,500	11,000
March	12,500	12,500	13,500
April	11,500	12,000	13,000
May	13,500	14,500	15,000
June	14,500	14,500	15,500
July	10,500	11,000	12,000
August	13,000	13,500	14,000
September	15,500	16,000	16,500
October	14,500	15,500	16,500
November	12,500	14,000	14,500
December	10,000	11,000	11,500
	148,500	156,000	164,500

2. A review of management's overall plans does not indicate any changes which will affect the radiology department in the coming year.
3. The average revenue per relative unit value for the budget year is estimated to be 85¢.
4. Past experience indicates that a 2% rate of gross revenue combined with bad debt and contractual adjustment will prevail during 1978.
5. Salary increases in accordance with approved personnel policies are indicated on the following page:

Position	Name	Present Salary	Date of Increase	Monthly Increase
Supervisor	Alton	$7,680	2/1/78	$40
Sr. technician	Baker	7,020	7/1/78	30
Sr. technician	Carson	5,820	7/1/78	30
Jr. technician	Dowd	4,320	3/1/78	20
Jr. technician	Early	4,440	10/1/78	20
Jr. technician	French	4,080	1/1/78	10
Student technician	Gordon	3,840	7/1/78	10
Student technician	Hadley	3,780	1/1/78	10

6. An allowance of 5% of each monthly budgeted salary should be provided for on-call and overtime pay.
7. Supplies and expenses for the budget year have been determined to be 15¢ per relative unit value.
8. Radiologists' fees are determined at 40% of net income. Indirect expenses have been determined to be 8% of direct expenses excluding radiologists' fees.

Required. Prepare a revenue and expense budget for the radiology department in dollar detail for the first 3 months of 1978. Show all computations, rounding out all figures to the nearest dollar.

23
Cost Finding

In the typical accounting system, controllable expenses are classified and accumulated according to the organizational units or departments with which they are directly associated and by which they are incurred. The expenses recorded in the accounts of a given medical and surgical nursing unit, for example, consist largely of the salaries and wages paid to personnel working in the unit and the costs of certain supplies consumed in the unit. These expenses clearly are related to the operation of the nursing unit, and the unit supervisor can exercise a high degree of control over the amounts in which such expenses are incurred. This is accomplished mainly by controlling the labor hours and quantities of supplies used.

The operation of the nursing unit, however, requires services from other departments of the hospital. Meals for patients, for example, must be prepared and served by the dietary department. Cleaning and linen services are obtained from the housekeeping and laundry departments. Utilities and repair services are provided the nursing unit by the plant operation and maintenance departments. The expenses related to the provision of these and other departmental services, however, are not recorded in the nursing unit expense accounts but in the expense accounts of the departments providing the services.

In addition, certain other hospital expenses such as depreciation, insurance, and employee benefits often may be recorded as *unassigned expenses*, since they are not routinely recorded as direct expenses of any organizational unit. Yet, the incurrence of these expenses is necessary to the operation of all organizational units of the hospital.

The emphasis of the general accounting process, then, is upon expense control through the classification and accumulation of expenses according to the organizational units primarily responsible for their incurrence. No attempt is made within the formal accounting records to measure the full cost of operating any particular organizational unit or department. Expense accounts in the general ledger include only those direct, controllable expenses incurred by a particular department; the accounts exclude the costs of services provided that department by other departments of the hospital. The departmental expense accounts also exclude an appropriate share of the costs which are recorded in the unassigned expense classification.

Full cost information, however, is needed by hospital management for many important purposes. To develop the necessary full cost information, a procedure known as *cost finding* is performed at least annually, preferably monthly. This chapter will provide an introductory discussion of the nature of cost finding and a somewhat-simplified illustration of the techniques involved in a cost-finding procedure for a hospital of modest size. Should your interest in this subject extend beyond the materials of this chapter, a reading of the AHA's *Cost Finding and Rate Setting for Hospitals* manual is recommended.[1]

Nature of Cost Finding

General cost finding may be defined as a procedure in which unassigned expenses and the expenses of nonrevenue-producing departments are allocated to the revenue-producing departments of the hospital for the purpose of determining the full costs of providing various hospital services to patients. It is a procedure that is performed apart from, but supplemental to, the formal accounting system. Cost-finding results are not recorded in the hospital's accounts nor do they appear in its income statement. The results of the cost-finding procedure are presented, however, in a cost report as illustrated later in this chapter.

The prerequisites for a satisfactory cost-finding procedure include a sound organizational structure, an appropriate classification of accounts, and statistical data which adequately measure the amounts of service provided by each nonrevenue-producing department to all other departments of the hospital. These statistics, however, need not always be complete, actual counts; estimates derived from a sampling process frequently are used. And, in certain cases, the use of weighted statistics may be necessary to produce more equitable allocations to the various departments.

A major objective of general cost finding is to provide full cost information for use in determining rates. Also, cost finding is generally employed to determine the amount of reimbursable costs and to aid in negotiating reimbursement contracts with third-party agencies. This should not be regarded, however, as the sole purpose of the cost-finding procedure. Cost finding, like responsibility accounting and budgeting, is a basic tool of management and is valuable for managerial decision making in other areas to which full cost information is relevant.

Methods of Cost Finding

Several different methods of cost finding have been developed over the years. Those most widely used at the present time are (1)

[1]*Cost Finding and Rate Setting for Hospitals* (Chicago: American Hospital Association, 1968).

the step-down method and (2) the double-distribution method. To illustrate these 2 methods in a greatly simplified manner, let us assume a Handy Hospital having the following: one item of unassigned expense only; 3 nonrevenue-producing departments to be called departments 1, 2, and 3; and 3 revenue-producing departments to be referred to as departments A, B, and C. A trial balance of the hospital's expenses is presented in figure 131 shown in the illustration which follows:

Figure 131
Handy Hospital
Trial Balance of Expenses
Year Ended December 31, 1977

Unassigned expense	$ 80,000
Department 1	100,000
Department 2	60,000
Department 3	40,000
Department A	200,000
Department B	250,000
Department C	150,000
Total	$880,000

Let us also assume that the nonrevenue-producing departments (departments 1, 2, and 3) rendered services during 1977 to each other and to the revenue-producing departments (departments A, B, and C) as shown in figure 132. Department 1, for example, rendered 25% of its services to department 2, 15% to department 3, 30% to department A, 20% to department B, and 10% to department C. The indicated percentages are based upon an analysis of statistical data such as number of employees, labor hours, pounds of laundry, and square footage.

STEP-DOWN METHOD

A cost-finding worksheet, using the step-down method, is illustrated in figure 133. Column 1 consists of the trial balance of expenses shown in figure 131. The objective of the cost finding is to allocate the unassigned expense to all departments and to allocate the expenses of the nonrevenue-producing departments to each other and to the revenue-producing departments so that, at the end of the allocation process, all expenses will be located in departments A, B, and C. As a result, the total cost of the patient services provided by Handy Hospital's revenue-producing departments will be determined.

Column 2 of the worksheet shows the allocation of unassigned expense to the nonrevenue-producing and revenue-producing departments. It is assumed here that the appropriate allocation basis is departmental direct expenses as shown in the illustration which follows:

Department	Direct Expenses	Percentage of Total Direct Expenses	×	Unassigned Expenses	=	Allocated Expense
1	$100,000	12.50%		$80,000		$10,000
2	60,000	7.50		80,000		6,000
3	40,000	5.00		80,000		4,000
A	200,000	25.00		80,000		20,000
B	250,000	31.25		80,000		25,000
C	150,000	18.75		80,000		15,000
	$800,000	100.00%				$80,000

Depending upon the nature of the unassigned expense item, it may be more appropriate to use other allocation bases such as number of employees, gross salaries and wages, or square footage in the various departments. It also is assumed that the unassigned expense in this illustration is properly allocable to all departments.

Figure 132
Handy Hospital
Services Rendered by Nonrevenue-Producing Departments
Year Ended December 31, 1977

	Departments Rendering Services		
Departments Receiving Services:	Dept. 1	Dept. 2	Dept. 3
Department 1	---	10%	---
Department 2	25%	---	20%
Department 3	15	20	---
Department A	20	40	35
Department B	20	---	45
Department C	10	30	---
Totals	100%	100%	100%

The next step is to allocate the expenses of the nonrevenue-producing departments to each other and to the revenue-producing departments. In what sequence, however, should departments 1, 2, and 3 be allocated? Generally, the department which renders the greatest amount of service to the greatest number of other departments, and receives the least in services from other departments, is the first department whose expenses are allocated. The department which provides the next greatest amount of service to the next greatest number of other departments, and receives the next least in services from other departments, is the second department whose expenses are allocated, and so on. The nonrevenue-producing department whose expenses are allocated last is the one which renders the least service to the smallest number of other departments and receives the greatest amount of service from other departments. Where the sequence of allocation cannot be determined on this basis, the sequence may be established on the basis of accumulated expenses; that is, the department having the largest amount of expense is allocated first, the department having the next largest amount of expense is allocated second, and so on.

This means that the allocation sequence will not be identical in all hospitals—nor will it necessarily be consistent from year to year in the same hospital. Similarly, the allocation bases employed will differ among hospitals and may not necessarily be consistent from year to year in a given hospital. When an allocation sequence that is more logical and defensible can be determined, or when improved allocation bases become available, appropriate changes should be made in the cost-finding procedure. But these should be made only after careful consideration.

In figure 133 it is assumed that the nonrevenue-producing departments are properly allocable in this sequence: first department 1, second department 2, and third department 3. Notice, in column 4, the allocation of the expenses of department 1. The allocation, based on the percentages in figure 133, is 25% to department 2, 15% to department 3, 30% to department A, 20% to department B, and 10% to department C. The allocation to department 2, for example, is 25% of $110,000, or $27,500. Note also that the expenses of department 1 are allocated to all departments to which department 1 renders services. This includes other nonrevenue-producing departments and the revenue-producing departments.

Once the expenses of a nonrevenue-producing department have been allocated under the step-down method of cost finding, that department is considered to be *closed*. That department will not receive any portion of the expenses of the other nonrevenue-producing departments, therefore, whose expenses are yet to be allocated. Department 1 is now closed; it will receive no allocation of the expenses of departments 2 and 3. This is the procedure even though departments 2 and 3 may have rendered services to department 1 during 1977.

The allocation of the accumulated expenses ($60,000 + $6,000 + $27,500 = $93,500) of department 2 is shown in column 6 of figure 133. As noted above, although department 2 rendered 10% of its services to department 1, no allocation of department 2 expenses is made to department 1. So, the allocation of department 2 expenses is made as follows:

Department	Percent of Dept. 2's Services Received*	Fraction	×	Accum. Expenses of Dept. 2	=	Expense Allocation
3	20%	2/9		$93,500		$20,778
A	40	4/9		93,500		41,556
C	30	3/9		93,500		31,166
	90%	9/9				$93,500

*See figure 132.

Similarly, in column 8, the $81,278 of accumulated expenses in department 3 are allocated only to the revenue-producing departments since both the other nonrevenue-producing departments (departments 1 and 2) have previously been closed. The allocation of department 3 expenses is 35/80ths to department A and 45/80ths to department B. As indicated by figure 132, department 3 rendered no services to department C during 1977.

Figure 133
Handy Hospital
Cost-Finding Worksheet—Step-Down Method
Year Ended December 31, 1977

	(1) Trial Balance	(2) Unassigned Expense	(3) Subtotal
Unassigned expense	$ 80,000	$ 80,000	
Nonrevenue-producing departments:			
Department 1	100,000	$ 10,000	$110,000
Department 2	60,000	6,000	66,000
Department 3	40,000	4,000	44,000
Revenue-producing departments:			
Department A	200,000	20,000	220,000
Department B	250,000	25,000	275,000
Department C	150,000	15,000	165,000
Totals	$880,000	$ 80,000	$880,000

*For revenue-producing departments only.

The results of the cost finding are shown in column 9. Here, you see that Handy Hospital's total expenses of $880,000 are located in the revenue-producing departments only. The full costs of operating these departments are found to be $330,115 for department A, $342,719 for department B, and $207,166 for department C. The

(4)	(5)	(6)	(7)	(8)	(9)
Dept. 1	Subtotal	Dept. 2	Subtotal	Dept. 3	Full Cost Totals*
$110,000					
$ 27,500	$ 93,500	$ 93,500			
16,500	60,500	$ 20,778	$ 81,278	$ 81,278	
33,000	253,000	41,556	294,556	$ 35,559	$330,115
22,000	297,000		297,000	45,719	342,719
11,000	176,000	31,166	207,166		207,166
$110,000	$880,000	$ 93,500	$880,000	$ 81,278	$880,000

step-down method of cost finding, however, does *not* produce full cost information about the nonrevenue-producing departments.

DOUBLE-DISTRIBUTION METHOD

A cost-finding worksheet using the double-distribution method is presented for Handy Hospital in figure 134. Under this method,

Figure 134
Handy Hospital
Cost-Finding Worksheet—Double-Distribution Method
Year Ended December 31, 1977

	(1) Unassigned Expenses	(2) Nonrevenue Dept. 1
Trial balance, December 31, 1977	$ 80,000	$100,000
Allocation of unassigned expenses	-80,000	+10,000
Subtotals	$ -0-	110,000
Initial allocation of Department 1		-110,000
Subtotals		-0-
Initial allocation of Department 2		+ 9,350
Subtotals		9,350
Initial allocation of Department 3		-0-
Subtotals		9,350
Final allocation of Department 1		- 9,350
Subtotals		$ -0-
Final allocation of Department 2		
Subtotals		
Final allocation of Department 3		
Full cost totals		

greater recognition is given the fact that nonrevenue-producing departments render services to each other as well as to revenue-producing departments. The nonrevenue-producing departments are not closed after their expenses have been allocated. Instead, they remain open to receive expense allocations from other

(3)	(4)	(5)	(6)	(7)	(8)
Producing Departments		Revenue Producing Departments			
Dept. 2	Dept. 3	Dept. A	Dept. B	Dept. C	Total
$ 60,000	$ 40,000	$200,000	$250,000	$150,000	$880,000
+ 6,000	+ 4,000	+20,000	+25,000	+15,000	-0-
66,000	44,000	220,000	275,000	165,000	880,000
+27,500	+16,500	+33,000	+22,000	+11,000	-0-
93,500	60,500	253,000	297,000	176,000	880,000
-93,500	+18,700	+37,400	-0-	+28,050	-0-
-0-	79,200	290,400	297,000	204,050	880,000
+15,840	-79,200	+27,720	+35,640	-0-	-0-
15,840	-0-	318,120	332,640	204,050	880,000
+ 2,337	+ 1,403	+ 2,805	+ 1,870	+ 935	-0-
18,177	1,403	320,925	334,510	204,985	880,000
-18,177	+ 4,309	+ 8,079	-0-	+ 6,059	-0-
$ -0-	5,442	329,004	334,510	211,044	880,000
	- 5,442	+ 2,381	+ 3,061	-0-	-0-
	$ -0-				
		$331,385	$337,571	$211,044	$880,000

nonrevenue-producing departments. As a result, after an initial allocation of the accumulated expenses of the nonrevenue-producing departments, a second round of expense allocations must be made. The second-round allocations usually are made in accordance with the step-down method. When a department is closed in the second round, in other words, it remains closed. There are other variations of the double-distribution method of cost finding, but these variations will not be described in this book.

The worksheet illustrated in figure 134 is arranged in a vertical format (the figure 133 worksheet is arranged in a horizontal format). In figure 134, the unassigned expenses are allocated in exactly the same manner as they were in the step-down method. The initial allocation of department 1 expenses also is the same as in the step-down method. Under the step-down method, however, department 1 would now be considered permanently closed and would receive no subsequent allocations from departments 2 and 3.

But, as you can see in figure 134's initial allocation of the accumulated expenses of department 2, department 1 is reopened to receive 10% of department 2 expenses. (Figure 132 indicates that department 2 provides 10% of its services to department 1.) Similarly, department 2 is not closed after the initial allocation of its accumulated expenses but is reopened when the expenses of department 3 are initially allocated.

So, after the initial round of expense allocations for departments 1, 2, and 3, expenses remain in each of these 3 departments. This necessitates a second and final round of expense allocations. These final allocations are made in conformity with the step-down procedure. In other words, once a department's expenses are allocated in the final round, the department is permanently closed.

The results of a double-distribution cost finding will differ somewhat from the results of the step-down method. A comparison is presented in figure 135. It also should be recognized that the double-distribution method, unlike the step-down method, tends to provide fair approximations of the full costs of operating the nonrevenue-producing departments.

Figure 135
Handy Hospital
Comparison of Cost-Finding Results

	Double-Distribution Method	Step-Down Method
Full Costs of Services Provided by:		
Department A	$331,385	$330,115
Department B	337,571	342,719
Department C	211,044	207,166
Totals	$880,000	$880,000

Cost Finding: An Extended Illustration

Now that you have had an opportunity to examine the cost-finding procedure in highly simplified form, let us turn to a more realistic example. The step-down method will be used in this illustration for ease of exposition and also because it is the most widely used method in actual practice. The statistical and accounting data relate to Happy Hamlet Hospital, a hypothetical short-term general hospital of modest size. Because of space and other limitations, certain liberties have been taken with respect to dollar amounts, statistics, and the number of departments involved in the illustration. It also should be understood that differences among hospitals affect the cost-finding procedure and the results it produces. While the illustrated procedure is relevant and generally applicable to all hospitals, the illustration does not include certain of the more troublesome problems which arise in a cost-finding exercise.

WORKSHEET A

Happy Hamlet Hospital's cost finding begins with the placement of a trial balance of expenses and certain revenues on a worksheet (generally referred to as worksheet A) as shown in columns 1–3 of figure 136. Note that the trial balance relates to the 6 months ended June 30, 1978, and includes the following:

1. Departmental cost center expenses
   a. salaries
   b. other expenses
2. Unassigned expenses, classified by major type
3. Certain "other operating" revenues which represent recoveries of specific operating-expense items

Examples of other types of expense recoveries include educational-program tuition fees, telephone revenues, nonpatient room rentals, and sales of scrap. To keep the illustration relatively simple, worksheet A includes only 3 items under expense recoveries (lines 23–25).

Columns 4–7 of worksheet A are used to make various reclassifications and adjustments for cost-finding purposes. The number and types of reclassifications and adjustments depend upon the manner in which direct expenses are accumulated in the accounts and upon the hospital's need for detailed full cost data. In this illustration, we assume that the direct expenses ($245,000) of all nursing units have been recorded by Happy Hamlet Hospital in a single cost center (see account 6021 on line 3). Let us assume, however, that management wishes to obtain from the cost finding the full costs of (a) adult and pediatric nursing units and (b) the newborn nursery. In other words, the single cost center must be reclassified into 2 cost centers. An entry (number 1) therefore is made on the worksheet to reclassify the $245,000 of expense as follows:

Nursing Units—Adult and Pediatric:		
Salaries	$196,000	
Other Expense	22,000	
Newborn Nursery:		
Salaries	24,000	
Other Expense	3,000	
Nursing Units:		
Salaries		$220,000
Other Expense		25,000

This entry eliminates account 6021 from line 3 of the worksheet and establishes 2 new cost centers on lines 29 and 30. Were full cost data required in more detail from the cost finding, additional

Figure 136
Happy Hamlet Hospital
Cost Finding—Worksheet A
Six Months Ended June 30, 1978

Acct. No.		Ledger Balances		
		Salaries	Other	Total
	Nursing services:			
6010	Administrative office	$ 8,000	$ 1,000	$ 9,000
6021	Nursing units	220,000	25,000	245,000
6210	Operating rooms	12,000	6,000	18,000
6230	Emergency rooms	8,000	5,000	13,000
6250	Central supply	10,000	9,000	19,000
	Other professional services:			
7011	Laboratory	20,000	10,000	30,000
7040	Radiology	28,000	12,000	40,000
7070	Pharmacy	14,000	11,000	25,000
7120	Outpatient clinic	9,000	6,000	15,000
7180	Medical records	8,000	4,000	12,000
	General services:			
8050	Dietary	46,000	40,000	86,000
8060	Plant operation and maintenance	25,000	38,000	63,000
8090	Housekeeping	23,000	8,000	31,000
8110	Laundry	17,000	7,000	24,000
8200	Fiscal and administrative services	88,000	12,000	100,000
	Unassigned expenses:			
8510	Depreciation		50,000	50,000
8710	Employee benefits		48,240	48,240
	Expense recoveries:			
5061	Cafeteria sales		(17,000)	(17,000)
5085	Medical record transcript fees		(2,000)	(2,000)
5171	Purchase discounts		(3,000)	(3,000)
	Totals	$536,000	$270,240	$806,240
	Nursing units — adult and pediatric			
	Newborn nursery			
	Totals			

nursing-unit cost centers could easily be established on worksheet A (for example, separate cost centers could be set up for medical and surgical units, pediatric units, psychiatric units, obstetric units, and intensive care units).

As another example, assume that a hospital routinely records the

Adjustments				Adjusted Balances			Worksheet B
Salaries		Other					Line
Add	Deduct	Add	Deduct	Salaries	Other	Total	Number
				$ 8,000	$ 1,000	$ 9,000	8
	(1)220,000		(1) 25,000				
				12,000	6,000	18,000	13
				8,000	5,000	13,000	20
				10,000	9,000	19,000	9
				20,000	10,000	30,000	14
				28,000	12,000	40,000	15
				14,000	11,000	25,000	10
				9,000	6,000	15,000	19
			(2) 2,000	8,000	2,000	10,000	11
				46,000	40,000	86,000	7
				25,000	38,000	63,000	4
				23,000	8,000	31,000	5
				17,000	7,000	24,000	6
			(3) 3,000	88,000	9,000	97,000	3
					50,000	50,000	1
					48,240	48,240	2
					(17,000)	(17,000)	21
			(2) (2,000)				
			(3) (3,000)				
(1)196,000		(1) 22,000		196,000	22,000	218,000	17
(1) 24,000		(1) 3,000		24,000	3,000	27,000	18
$220,000	$220,000	$ 25,000	$ 25,000	$536,000	$270,240	$806,240	

direct expenses of operating an electrocardiology unit in the expense accounts of the laboratory department. This practice may be satisfactory for the purpose of month-to-month expense control but not for the purposes of cost finding. Management may wish to determine the full cost of providing EKG services. If so, a worksheet A reclassification entry is required to remove the direct EKG expenses from the laboratory expenses and establish them in an EKG cost center. The direct expenses associated with the newly created cost centers generally can be estimated from an analysis of payroll and other records.

On the other hand, reclassification entries may be needed to combine 2 or more responsibility accounting cost centers into a single cost center for the purpose of cost finding. Assume, for example, that a hospital operates a school of nursing whose direct expenses are recorded in several cost centers. An entry might be made on the worksheet to combine the direct expenses of these centers into a single cost center for nursing education. This would facilitate the procedure of cost finding.

Entry 2 on worksheet A reduces the direct expenses of the medical records department for the $2,000 of revenues obtained from transcript fees in the medical record. Entry 3 similarly credits fiscal and administrative services for the $3,000 of purchase discounts earned. In some cases, it may be appropriate to offset cafeteria sales to employees and guests against the direct expenses of the dietary department. Happy Hamlet Hospital, however, follows an alternative procedure to be described at a subsequent point.

The adjusted balances, taking into account the reclassifications and adjustments, are extended into columns 8–10 of worksheet A. Column 11 indicates the line numbers of worksheet B (figure 137) to which the adjusted totals shown in column 10 are transferred.

WORKSHEETS B AND B-1

Worksheet B, illustrated in figure 137, begins with the entry of adjusted balances in column 1 (from worksheet A, figure 136). Observe that the sequence in which the cost centers are listed is not the same as the sequence in which they were listed in worksheet A. The cost centers were listed in worksheet A in account-number sequence, the same order in which they appear in the hospital's ledger. In worksheet B, the cost centers are listed in the order in which they will be allocated and closed.

• ***Depreciation***. The allocation of depreciation expense ($50,000) is shown in column 2 of worksheet B. Fiscal and administrative services, for example, received an allocation of $900, plant operation and maintenance was charged with $2,500, and so on. These allocations were determined on the basis of the number of square feet occupied by each department or cost center as indicated in worksheet B-1 (figure 138). Note, in column 1 of worksheet B-1, the listing of square footage (a total of 50,000 square feet) by department or cost center. Since total depreciation expense is $50,000 and there is a total of 50,000 square feet, the *unit cost multiplier* is $1.00 (i.e., $50,000/50,000 square feet). In other words, each department will be allocated $1.00 of depreciation expense for each square foot it occupies. Fiscal and administrative services, for example, uses 900 square feet of space and therefore is charged with $900 of depreciation. A similar computation is made for each department, and the allocations so determined are entered in column 2 of worksheet B. This column then is totaled to be sure that the individual allocations add up to $50,000.

This illustration, of course, makes no distinction between depreciation on the hospital building and depreciation of equipment. When a detailed equipment ledger is maintained, equipment depreciation may be more properly allocated, perhaps on the basis of the investment in equipment by each department. Depreciating the hospital building would be a separate allocation based on square footage. Depreciation on an outlying building which houses boilers or generators, for instance, would be allocated entirely to the plant operation department.

- ***Employee Benefits***. As seen in worksheet B-1, employee benefits are allocated on the basis of departmental payroll dollars as indicated in column 8 of worksheet A. Dividing $48,240 of benefits by $536,000 of payroll dollars provides a unit cost multiplier of 9¢ per dollar of payroll. Or, to put it another way, the amount of employee benefits to be allocated to a department is 9% of the department's gross payroll. The fiscal and administrative services payroll is $88,000, for example, so the allocation for employee benefits is $7,920 (i.e., $88,000 × 9%). The computed allocations then are entered in column 3 of worksheet B. Note that the column adds to the correct total of $48,420.
- ***Fiscal and Administrative Services***. The allocation of fiscal and administrative expenses appears in column 5 of worksheet B. This allocation is based on the accumulated departmental expenses as shown by the subtotals in column 4 of worksheet B. To determine the unit cost multiplier, the subtotals are entered in column 3 of worksheet B-1. The accumulated fiscal and administrative expenses of $105,820 (i.e., $97,000 + $900 of depreciation + $7,920 of employee benefits) divided by the $717,420 of accumulated expenses in all other departments produces a unit cost multiplier of 14.75%. Plant operation and maintenance therefore is charged with $9,993 (i.e., $67,750 × 14.75%) of fiscal and administrative expenses. A similar computation is made for each department, and the results are entered in column 5 of worksheet B.

Fiscal and administrative services, in this illustration, are treated as a single cost center. The results of the cost finding might be considerably more accurate and useful, however, if fiscal and administrative services were broken down into several cost centers, each being allocated on a different basis. On worksheet A, for instance, reclassification entries might be made to create separate cost centers for admitting (to be allocated on the basis of admissions), patient accounting (to be allocated on the basis of patient days), personnel (to be allocated on the basis of number of employees), purchasing (to be allocated on the basis of nonlabor expenses), and so on.

- ***Plant Operation and Maintenance***. The plant operation and maintenance cost center, at this stage of the cost finding, has accumulated expenses of $77,743 which are allocated on the basis of square footage as shown in column 6 of worksheet B. As computed

Figure 137
Happy Hamlet Hospital
Cost-Finding Worksheet B
Six Months Ended June 30, 1978

	(1) Adjusted Balances	(2) Depreciation	(3) Employee Benefits	(4) Subtotals	(5) F & A Services	(6) Plant O & M
Depreciation	$ 50,000	$ 50,000				
Employee benefits	48,240		$ 48,240			
Fiscal and administrative services	97,000	$ 900	$ 7,920	$105,820	$105,820	
Plant operation and maintenance	63,000	2,500	2,250	67,750	$ 9,993	$ 77,743
Housekeeping	31,000	200	2,070	33,270	4,907	$ 334
Laundry	24,000	1,400	1,530	26,930	3,972	2,335
Dietary	86,000	4,200	4,140	94,340	13,915	7,006
Nursing service — adm. office	9,000	200	720	9,920	1,463	334
Central supply	19,000	1,600	900	21,500	3,171	2,669
Pharmacy	25,000	500	1,260	26,760	3,947	834
Medical records	10,000	400	720	11,120	1,640	667
Cost of meals sold						
Operating rooms	18,000	3,000	1,080	22,080	3,257	5,004
Laboratory	30,000	800	1,800	32,600	4,808	1,334
Radiology	40,000	1,400	2,520	43,920	6,478	2,335
Cost of drugs sold						
Nursing units — adult & pediatric	218,000	29,000	17,640	264,640	39,037	48,386
Newborn nursery	27,000	1,400	2,160	30,560	4,508	2,335
Outpatient clinic	15,000	1,500	810	17,310	2,553	2,502
Emergency rooms	13,000	1,000	720	14,720	2,171	1,668
Cafeteria sales	(17,000)			(17,000)		
Totals	$806,240	$ 50,000	$ 48,240	$806,240	$105,820	$ 77,743

in column 4 of worksheet B-1, these allocations were determined by the use of a 1.668 multiplier. The allocation to housekeeping, for example, is $334 (i.e., 200 square feet × 166.8%). Again, where plant operation and maintenance expenses are accumulated in 2 or more cost centers, different allocation bases might be employed. Plant operation, for instance, might be allocated on the basis of a measure of utility usage, whereas plant maintenance expenses might be allocated on the basis of maintenance hours. Since plant operation and maintenance expenses are substantial, this procedure could improve a cost finding markedly.

- ***Housekeeping***. As indicated in column 5 of worksheet B-1,

(7) Hskpg.	(8) Laundry	(9) Dietary	(10) Nursing Adm. Off.	(11) Central Supply	(12) Pharmacy	(13) Medical Records	(14) Subtotals	(15) Net Cost of Meals Sold	(16) Total Costs
$ 38,511									
$ 1,162	$ 34,399								
3,486	$ 200	$118,947							
166	40		$ 11,923						
1,328	6,000		$ 720	$ 35,388					
415	30				$ 31,986				
332	20					$ 13,779			
		$ 27,000					$ 27,000	$ 27,000	
2,490	6,500		896	$ 4,320	$ 2,668		47,215	$ 609	$ 47,824
664	70				552		40,028	516	40,544
1,162	400				644		54,939	709	55,648
					18,400		18,400		18,400
24,069	16,739	91,947	9,211	29,493	7,422	$ 10,610	541,554	6,952	548,506
1,162	2,200		440	405	460	1,102	43,172	557	43,729
1,245	800		304	180	736	1,378	27,008	348	27,356
830	1,400		352	990	1,104	689	23,924	309	24,233
							(17,000)	17,000	
$ 38,511	$ 34,399	$118,947	$ 11,923	$ 35,388	$ 31,986	$ 13,779	$806,240	$ 27,000	$806,240

housekeeping expenses are allocated on the basis of square footage, using a unit cost multiplier of 83¢ per square foot. Hours of housekeeping services also may be an equitable allocation basis. As before, the computed allocations are entered in the appropriate column of worksheet B.

• ***Laundry***. Laundry expenses, as seen in column 6 of worksheet B-1, are allocated on the basis of 10¢ per pound. Laundry might be allocated on the basis of *pieces* of laundry rather than of pounds. Where either pieces or pounds are employed as allocation bases, the number of pieces or pounds may be weighted to take into account that it costs more to process certain laundry items than others.

Figure 138
Happy Hamlet Hospital
Cost-Finding Statistics—Worksheet B-1
Six Months Ended June 30, 1978

	(1) Depreciation	(2) Employee Benefits	(3) F & A Services	(4) Plant O & M
Allocation bases	Square Feet	Payroll Dollars	Accum. Expenses	Square Feet
Fiscal and administrative services	900	$ 88,000		
Plant operation and maintenance	2,500	25,000	$ 67,750	
Housekeeping	200	23,000	33,270	200
Laundry	1,400	17,000	26,930	1,400
Dietary	4,200	46,000	94,340	4,200
Nursing services — administrative office	200	8,000	9,920	200
Central supply	1,600	10,000	21,500	1,600
Pharmacy	500	14,000	26,760	500
Medical records	400	8,000	11,120	400
Cost of meals sold				
Operating rooms	3,000	12,000	22,080	3,000
Laboratory	800	20,000	32,600	800
Radiology	1,400	28,000	43,920	1,400
Cost of drugs sold				
Nursing units — adult and pediatric	29,000	196,000	264,640	29,000
Newborn nursery	1,400	24,000	30,560	1,400
Outpatient clinic	1,500	9,000	17,310	1,500
Emergency room	1,000	8,000	14,720	1,000
Totals	50,000	$536,000	$717,420	46,600
Accumulated expenses per Worksheet B	$ 50,000	$ 48,240	$105,820	$ 77,743
Unit cost multiplier (line 25/line 23)	1.00	.09	.1475	1.668
Worksheet B column number	2	3	5	6

• ***Dietary***. Total dietary expenses (see column 7 of worksheet B-1) are prorated at the rate of $1.50 per meal served. Since 18,000 meals were served by the hospital's cafeteria, $27,000 of dietary expense is allocated to a special cost center (line 12, column 9, of worksheet B) which later will be offset against cafeteria sales

(5)	(6)	(7)	(8)	(9)	(10)	(11)	(12)
Hskpg.	Laundry	Dietary	Nursing Adm. Off.	Central Supply	Pharmacy	Medical Records	Net Cost of Meals Sold
Square Feet	Pounds	Meals Served	Hours	Priced Req.	Priced Req.	Estimated Time	Accum. Expenses
1,400							
4,200	2,000						
200	400						
1,600	60,000		9,000				
500	300						
400	200						
		18,000					
3,000	65,000		11,200	$ 9,600	$ 2,900		$ 47,215
800	700				600		40,028
1,400	4,000				700		54,939
					20,000		
29,000	167,400	61,300	115,137	65,540	8,067	77%	541,554
1,400	22,000		5,500	900	500	8	43,172
1,500	8,000		3,800	400	800	10	27,008
1,000	14,000		4,400	2,200	1,200	5	23,924
46,400	344,000	79,300	149,037	$ 78,640	$ 34,767	100%	$777,840
$ 38,511	$ 34,399	$118,947	$ 11,923	$ 35,388	$ 31,986	$ 13,779	$ 10,000
.83	.10	1.50	.08	.45	.92		.0129
7	8	9	10	11	12	13	15

(worksheet B, column 15). The $91,947 balance of dietary expense is charged to the adult and pediatric nursing units. If the cafeteria is established as a separate cost center by an entry on worksheet A, this likely will improve the cost-finding procedure. In such cases raw food costs may be allocated apart from other dietary expenses.

Figure 139
Happy Hamlet Hospital
Cost Report
Six Months Ended June 30, 1978

Revenue-Cost Centers	(1) Gross Revenues	(2) Costs Direct	(3) Costs Indirect
Operating Rooms	$ 42,909	$ 18,000	$ 29,824
Laboratory	72,346	30,000	10,544
Radiology	95,261	40,000	15,648
Cost of drugs sold	29,408		18,400
Nursing units — adult and pediatric	581,221	218,000	330,506
Newborn nursery	36,382	27,000	16,729
Outpatient clinic	15,290	15,000	12,356
Emergency rooms	21,028	13,000	11,233
Totals	$893,845	$361,000	$445,240
Less deductions from revenues			
Excess of revenues over costs and revenue deductions			

• ***Nursing—Administrative Office***. As may be noted in worksheet B-1, these expenses are allocated on the basis of 8¢ per hour of nursing service worked in cost centers supervised by the nursing service director. The basis for allocation of nursing education expenses generally is hours of assigned student time. It is assumed,

(4)	(5)	(6)	(7)	(8)	(9)
	Units of Service Rendered			Average	
Total	Units	Statistic		Unit Cost	Net
$ 47,824	523	Operations		91.44	$ (4,915)
40,544	11,065	Tests		3.66	31,802
55,648	2,347	Films		23.71	39,613
18,400	7,208	Prescriptions filled		2.55	11,008
548,506	8,244	Patient days		66.53	32,715
43,729	1,077	Newborn days		40.60	(7,347)
27,356	2,180	Visits		12.55	(12,066)
24,233	1,109	Admissions		21.85	(3,205)
$806,240					$ 87,605
					62,569
					$ 25,036

however, that Happy Hamlet Hospital has no school of nursing.

• ***Central Supply***. The expenses of central services and supply are allocated on the basis of 45¢ per dollar of priced requisitions. Other bases of allocation, such as percentage estimates of the time spent in servicing other departments, sometimes may be employed.

Figure 140
Happy Hamlet Hospital
Cost Allocation: Ratio of Costs to Charges Applied to Cost
Six Months Ended June 30, 1978

	Total Costs	Gross Revenues	Cost Converter	Inpatients Revenues	Inpatients Allocated Costs
Department:					
Operating rooms	$ 47,824	$ 42,909	1.114545	$ 42,265	$ 47,106
Laboratory	40,544	72,346	.560418	64,822	36,328
Radiology	55,648	95,261	.584164	70,779	41,346
Cost of drugs sold	18,400	29,408	.625680	24,526	15,346
Nursing units—adult and pediatric	548,506	581,221	.943713	581,221	548,506
Newborn nursery	43,729	36,382	1.201941		
Outpatient clinic	27,356	15,290	1.789143		
Emergency rooms	24,233	21,028	1.152416		
Totals	$806,240	$ 893,845		$ 783,613	$ 688,632

	Gross Revenues	Allocated Costs	Net
Type of Patient:			
Inpatients	$783,613	$ 688,632	$ 94,981
Newborn	38,938	45,198	(6,260)
Outpatients	49,310	47,579	1,731
Emergency	21,984	24,831	(2,847)
Totals	$893,845	$ 806,240	$ 87,605

• ***Pharmacy***. Pharmacy expenses also are allocated on the basis of the dollar value of priced requisitions. As indicated in worksheet B-1, the apportionment is 92¢ per dollar of priced requisitions.

• ***Medical Records***. The cost center for medical records is allocated on the basis of percentage estimates of the time spent in

Newborn		Outpatients		Emergency	
Revenues	Allocated Costs	Revenues	Allocated Costs	Revenues	Allocated Costs
		$ 644	$ 718		
$ 1,266	$ 709	6,258	3,507		
1,143	668	23,339	13,634		
147	92	3,779	2,364	$ 956	$ 598
36,382	43,729				
		15,290	27,356		
				21,028	24,233
$ 38,938	$ 45,198	$ 49,310	$47,579	$ 21,984	$ 24,831

maintaining medical records for the various classifications of patients. These percentages are given in worksheet B-1.

• ***Net Cost of Meals Sold***. Since cafeteria sales were $17,000 and the cost of meals sold was $27,000, the net cost of meals sold is $10,000. As shown in column 12 of worksheet B-1, this $10,000 is allocated on the basis of the accumulated expenses indicated by the subtotals in column 14 of worksheet B. The apportionment uses a unit cost multiplier of .0129. After the computed allocations are entered in column 15 of worksheet B, the worksheet is completed with the computation and entry of total costs in column 16.

COST REPORTS

The results of the cost finding are summarized and reported to the management of Happy Hamlet Hospital in the cost report illustrated in figure 139. The gross revenue data in column 1 are assumed. Column 2 figures are drawn from column 1, lines 18–20, of worksheet B (figure 137); column 4 figures are drawn from column 16 of worksheet B. The indirect costs in column 3 of the cost report may be computed simply by subtracting column 2's figures from column 4's; or the indirect costs of each center may be determined by adding the expense allocations presented in worksheet B.

The units of service rendered by each center are shown in columns 5–7 of the cost report. Column 8 indicates the average cost per unit of service, determined by dividing the total of column 4 by that of column 6. The excess of gross revenues over total costs (or the excess of total costs over gross revenues) is reported in column 9. This tends to indicate the adequacy of the service rates established in each center.

An additional cost report is illustrated in figure 140. This report presents, on lines 16–22, a summary of total costs and gross revenues classified by type of patient: inpatients, newborns, outpatients, and emergency patients. The costs are allocated to these patient groups on the basis of a charge converter or the ratio of costs to charges. This procedure requires an accounting classification of gross revenues by type of patient. Consider, for example, the laboratory department whose total costs are $40,544 and whose gross revenues are $72,346. The cost converter is .560418, computed by dividing $40,544 by $72,346. The revenue for each type of patient is then multiplied by the cost converter to determine the costs to be allocated as follows:

	Gross Revenues	Cost Converter	Cost Allocation
Inpatients	$ 64,822	.560418	$ 36,328
Newborn	1,266	.560418	709
Outpatients	6,258	.560418	3,507
Emergency			
Totals	$ 72,346		$ 40,544

In other words, since laboratory costs are 56.0418% of laboratory revenues, and $64,822 of revenues were derived from services rendered to inpatients, 56.0418% of those revenues (or $36,328) represents the costs allocated to inpatients. The allocations to newborns and outpatients are determined in the same way. (The example assumes that the laboratory provided no services to emergency patients.) This method of allocation is but one of several methods allowed by governmental and other third-party agencies for the purpose of determining reimbursable costs.

QUESTIONS

1. Write a brief definition of *general cost finding*.

2. What are the basic prerequisites for a satisfactory cost-finding procedure?

3. What are the primary purposes of general cost finding?

4. Distinguish briefly between the step-down and the double-distribution methods of cost finding.

5. In what sequence should the expenses of nonrevenue-producing departments be allocated to each other and to the revenue-producing departments in a general cost-finding procedure?

6. Suggest a basis for the allocation of each of the following expenses in a cost finding procedure:

a. Depreciation expense—building
b. Depreciation expense—equipment
c. Employee benefits
d. Insurance

7. Suggest a basis for the allocation of each of the following expenses in a cost finding procedure:

a. Fiscal and administrative services
b. Plant operation and maintenance
c. Housekeeping
d. Laundry
e. Dietary

PROBLEMS

A. Persian Hospital has a single item of unassigned expense, 3 nonrevenue-producing departments (departments 1, 2, and 3), and 3 revenue-producing departments (departments A, B, and C). A trial balance of expenses for the year ended December 31, 1978, is provided below:

Unassigned expense	$ 60,000
Department 1	120,000
Department 2	80,000
Department 3	40,000
Department A	170,000
Department B	240,000
Department C	160,000
	$870,000

The nonrevenue-producing departments rendered services during 1978 to each other and to the revenue-producing departments as indicated below:

Departments Receiving Services:	Departments Rendering Services Dept. 1	Dept. 2	Dept. 3
Dept. 1	---	15%	---
Dept. 2	30%	---	30%
Dept. 3	10	15	---
Dept. A	15	35	25
Dept. B	20	---	45
Dept. C	15	35	---
	100%	100%	100%

Unassigned expenses should be allocated to the nonrevenue-producing and revenue-producing departments on the basis of departmental direct expenses.

Required. Prepare a cost-finding worksheet, using (1) the step-down method and (2) the double-distribution method.

B. Calico Hospital has 2 items of unassigned expense, 4 nonrevenue-producing departments (departments 1, 2, 3, and 4), and 4 revenue-producing departments (departments A, B, C, and D). A trial balance of expenses for the quarter ended December 31, 1978, is provided below:

Unassigned expense (item X)	$ 40,000
Unassigned expense (item Y)	30,000
Department:	
1	100,000
2	80,000
3	50,000
4	30,000
A	150,000
B	220,000
C	110,000
D	90,000
	$900,000

Seventy-five percent of unassigned expense item X is to be allocated to the nonrevenue-producing departments and 25% to the revenue-producing departments, on the basis of departmental direct expenses. Unassigned expense item Y then should be allocated on the basis of accumulated expenses to the nonrevenue-producing and revenue-producing departments. The nonrevenue-producing departments rendered services during 1978 to each other and to the revenue-producing departments as indicated:

Departments Receiving Services:	Departments Rendering Services			
	Dept. 1	Dept. 2	Dept. 3	Dept. 4
Dept. 1	--	10%	15%	--
Dept. 2	20%	--	15	10%
Dept. 3	10	10	--	--
Dept. 4	15	20	10	--
Dept. A	30	--	40	25
Dept. B	10	20	--	--
Dept. C	5	20	--	65
Dept. D	10	20	20	--
	100%	100%	100%	100%

Required. (1) Prepare a cost-finding worksheet under the step-down method. (2) Prepare a cost-finding worksheet under the double-distribution method.

C. Manx Hospital's trial balance of expenses and expense recoveries for the 6 months ended June 30, 1978, is provided below:

	Ledger Balances		
	Salaries	Other	Total
Nursing services			
Administrative office	$ 10,000	$ 3,000	$ 13,000

	Ledger Balances		
	Salaries	Other	Total
Nursing units	200,000	20,000	220,000
Operating rooms	14,000	7,000	21,000
Emergency rooms	6,000	4,000	10,000
Central supply	12,000	10,000	22,000
Other professional services			
Laboratory	23,000	9,000	32,000
Radiology	26,000	11,000	37,000
Pharmacy	15,000	12,000	27,000
Outpatient clinic	8,000	5,000	13,000
Medical records	7,000	3,000	10,000
General services			
Dietary	51,000	44,000	95,000
Plant operation and maintenance	24,000	36,000	60,000
Housekeeping	25,000	9,000	34,000
Laundry	19,000	8,000	27,000
Fiscal and administrative services	79,000	15,000	94,000
Unassigned expenses			
Depreciation		60,000	60,000
Employee benefits		46,000	46.000
Expense recoveries			
Cafeteria sales		(24,000)	(24,000)
Medical record transcript fees		(3,000)	(3,000)
Purchase discounts		(2,000)	(2,000)
Totals	$519,000	$273,000	$792,000

Worksheet A adjustments:

1. The $220,000 of expenses in nursing units is to be reclassified.

	Salaries	Other	Total
Nursing units—adult and pediatric	$171,000	$ 17,000	$188,000
Newborn nursery	29,000	3,000	32,000
Total	$200,000	$ 20,000	$220,000

2. Medical record transcript fees are to be treated as a reduction of the direct expenses of the medical records department.
3. Purchase discounts are to be treated as a reduction of the direct expenses of fiscal and administrative services.

The necessary statistics for a cost-finding procedure are summarized on page 463.

Required. Complete a cost finding for Manx Hospital for the 6 months ended June 30, 1978. This includes worksheets A, B, and B-1, as illustrated on pages 446–453.

D. Tabby Hospital's trial balance of expenses and expense recoveries for the quarter ended March 31, 1978, is provided below:

	Ledger Balances		
	Salaries	Other	Total
Nursing services			
Administrative office	$ 12,000	$ 4,000	$ 16,000
Nursing units	250,000	48,000	298,000
Operating rooms	15,000	8,000	23,000

	Ledger Balances		
	Salaries	Other	Total
Emergency rooms	7,000	4,000	11,000
Central supply	14,000	8,000	22,000
Other professional services			
Laboratory	21,000	9,000	30,000
Radiology	25,000	10,000	35,000
Pharmacy	16,000	11,000	27,000
Outpatient clinic	9,000	5,000	14,000
Medical records	8,000	2,000	10,000
General services			
Dietary	49,000	38,000	87,000
Plant operation and maintenance	23,000	41,000	64,000
Housekeeping	22,000	8,000	30,000
Laundry	20,000	7,000	27,000
Fiscal and administrative services	55,000	16,000	71,000
Unassigned expenses			
Depreciation		51,000	51,000
Insurance on hospital building		12,000	12,000
Employee benefits		48,000	48,000
Expense recoveries			
Cafeteria sales		(26,000)	(26,000)
Telephone service		(3,000)	(3,000)
Purchase discounts		(4,000)	(4,000)
Totals	$546,000	$297,000	$843,000

The $298,000 of expenses accumulated in nursing units is to be reclassified on worksheet A as follows:

	Salaries	Other	Total
Nursing units—adult and pediatric	$218,000	$ 42,000	$260,000
Newborn nursery	32,000	6,000	38,000
Total	$250,000	$ 48,000	$298,000

The necessary statistics for a cost-finding procedure appear on page 464.

Required. Complete a cost finding for Tabby Hospital for the quarter ended March 31, 1978. This includes worksheets A, B, and B-1, as illustrated in the text.

E. Refer to the facts of problem D, and assume the following additional information.

	Gross Revenues	Units of Service	
Operating rooms	$ 48,000	520	Operations
Laboratory	72,000	11,400	Tests
Radiology	96,000	2,400	Films
Cost of drugs sold	30,000	7,200	Prescriptions filled
Nursing units—adult and pediatric	590,000	8,100	Patient days
Newborn nursery	36,000	1,000	Newborn days
Outpatient clinic	17,000	2,200	Visits
Emergency rooms	20,000	1,300	Admissions
Total	$909,000		

Deductions from revenues for the quarter ended March 31, 1978, totaled $62,000.

Manx Hospital
Cost-Finding Statistics

	Square Feet	Pounds of Laundry	Meals Served	Nursing Adm. Hours	Central Supply Priced Req.	Pharmacy Priced Req.	Medical Records
Fiscal and administrative services	900	---					
Plant operation and maintenance	3,500	400					
Housekeeping	300	400					
Laundry	1,600	---					
Dietary	4,400	2,200					
Nursing service — administrative office	200	500					
Central supply	1,800	62,000		9,500			
Pharmacy	600	400					
Medical records	400	300					
Cost of meals sold	---	---	20,000				
Operating rooms	3,000	67,000		11,400	$10,000	$ 3,000	
Laboratory	1,000	800				800	
Radiology	1,400	4,200				1,000	
Cost of drugs sold	---	---				22,000	
Nursing units — adult and pediatric	36,000	168,000	70,000	116,000	68,000	9,000	75%
Newborn nursery	2,400	24,000		6,000	1,000	600	10
Outpatient clinic	1,500	8,800		3,500	500	900	10
Emergency room	1,000	15,000		5,000	2,500	2,700	5
Totals	60,000	354,000	90,000	151,400	$82,000	$40,000	100%

Required. Prepare a cost report similar to that illustrated in figure 139 for Tabby Hospital for the quarter ended March 31, 1978.

Tabby Hospital
Cost-Finding Statistics

	Square Feet	Pounds of Laundry	Meals Served	Nursing Adm. Hours	Central Supply Priced Req.	Pharmacy Priced Req.	Medical Records
Fiscal and administrative services	1,000	100					
Plant operation and maintenance	3,600	500					
Housekeeping	400	500					
Laundry	1,500						
Dietary	4,500	3,000					
Nursing service—administrative office	300	500					
Central supply	1,800	60,000		8,600			
Pharmacy	600	500					
Medical records	400	400					
Cost of meals sold			25,000				
Operating rooms	3,000	62,000		12,000	$12,000	$ 4,000	
Laboratory	1,400	800				800	
Radiology	1,200	4,200				1,000	
Cost of drugs sold						23,000	
Nursing units—adult and pediatric	38,000	168,000	75,000	120,000	66,000	9,000	72%
Newborn nursery	2,800	24,000		6,000	1,000	600	12
Outpatient clinic	1,500	8,800		4,000	500	900	12
Emergency room	1,000	12,700		9,400	5,500	5,700	4
Totals	63,000	346,000	100,000	160,000	$85,000	$45,000	100%

24 Analysis and Interpretation of Financial Statements

The foregoing chapters of this book were concerned primarily with the fundamental mechanics of the accounting process and with the basic accounting concepts underlying the financial statements of the hospital enterprise. Learning effort was directed mainly toward acquiring the abilities to perform accounting operations and to develop financial reports from the information generated by those operations. In this final chapter, attention is directed toward analyzing and interpreting financial statements for the purpose of evaluating the hospital's financial position and operating results.

To introduce the subject of financial analysis and interpretation, let us briefly examine the Handy Hospital financial statements presented in figures 141 and 142. Take a few moments to study these statements, noticing the amounts (in thousands of dollars) reported as revenues, expenses, assets, liabilities, and equity. On the basis of the information provided in these statements, what can you conclude (if anything) concerning Handy Hospital's 1977 operating results and its financial position at December 31, 1977? Are the operating results satisfactory? Is the hospital's financial position strong?

If you were a member of Handy Hospital's top management team, what would be your reaction to the reported 1977 operating results? Are revenues too low? Are expenses too high? Note that the net income for 1977 is $894,000. Is this "good" or "bad"? Is it exciting or disappointing? How can a hospital executive make judgments about the financial impact of operating results for 1977?

Similarly, how would you evaluate the hospital's financial position? The balance sheet, for example, reports $2,450,000 of receivables. Is this amount too large or about "right"? What does it tell you, if anything, about the quality of the hospital's credit and collection efforts? Also reported in the balance sheet are inventories totaling $220,000. What, if anything, does the balance sheet indicate about the quality of inventory management at Handy Hospital? Is the hospital overinvested in this asset, or are the inventories at a dangerously low level? As a final observation, note that the hospital has $3,006,000 of liabilities. Do you regard this as an excessive amount of debt?

Thus, the accounting function does not end with the accumulation of economic data and the communication of that information in financial statements. Once the financial statements are developed, the information they contain should be analyzed and interpreted so as to provide answers to the kinds of questions posed in the above paragraphs. The answers so obtained can be extremely useful to hospital management and external groups in evaluating a hospital's operations and financial status for decision-making purposes. Hospital accountants, either directly or indirectly, are closely involved in the decision-making process by providing relevant information and by assisting in its proper interpretation.

Figure 141
Handy Hospital
Income Statement
Year Ended December 31, 1977

Patient service revenues	$14,517
Less deductions from revenues	1,742
Net patient service revenues	12,775
Other operating revenues	1,225
Total operating revenues	14,000
Less operating expenses:	
Nursing services	4,460
Other professional services	3,361
General services	2,263
Fiscal and administrative services	3,150
Total operating expenses	13,234
Net operating income	766
Add nonoperating revenues	128
Net income for the year	$ 894

BASIC ANALYTICAL TECHNIQUES

In the analysis and interpretation of an item of financial information, one must have a basis of comparison. Consider, for example, the following item from Handy Hospital's December 31, 1977, balance sheet:

Receivables (net)	$2,450

What does this mean? Is the amount too high, too low, or about what it "ought" to be? Standing alone, this bit of information is almost meaningless (except that perhaps we would all agree that $2 million is a large amount). There is no way to evaluate a single figure by itself. It must be compared with, or measured against, something, usually another figure which provides a relevant and useful standard.

It would be helpful, for example, to compare the amount of December 31, 1977, receivables with that of December 31, 1976. Or we could compare the actual amount of receivables at December 31, 1977, with the amount budgeted for that date. Another possibility would be to compare the amount of December 31, 1977, receivables with the amount of total assets at December 31, 1977. And finally, the amount of December 31, 1977, receivables might be compared with net patient service revenues for 1977. Each of these comparisons would be relevant and useful in evaluating the level of receivables at the end of 1977.

Figure 142
Handy Hospital
Balance Sheet
December 31, 1977

Current assets:	
Cash	$ 296
Temporary investments	110
Receivables (net)	2,450
Inventories	220
Prepaid expenses	24
Total current assets	3,100
Long-term investments	430
Plant and equipment (net)	6,370
Total assets	$9,900
Current liabilities:	
Notes payable	$ 50
Accounts payable	366
Accrued expenses payable	651
Other	139
Total current liabilities	1,206
Long-term debt	1,800
Total liabilities	3,006
Unrestricted fund balance	6,894
Total liabilities and fund balance	$9,900

BASIC ANALYTICAL TECHNIQUES

Such comparisons involve the use of 3 basic analytical techniques: (1) horizontal analysis, (2) vertical analysis, and (3) ratio analysis. Let us now illustrate each of these techniques.

HORIZONTAL ANALYSIS

Horizontal analysis consists of the comparison of 2 or more figures across a single line of a financial statement. An example is provided below:

			Increase (Decrease)	
	1977	1976	Amount	Percent
Net patient service revenues	$ 12,775	$ 12,045	$ 730	6.1%

In this analysis, we see that net patient service revenues in 1977 were higher than in 1976. The columns on the right indicate the dollar amount of the increase as well as the percentage increase. The percentage increase (or decrease) is determined by dividing the dollar amount of change by the base-year figure (for 1976 in this example) of $730/$12,045 = 6.1%. Where the base-year figure is zero or a negative value, the dollar change cannot be expressed as a percentage.

Figures 143 and 144 illustrate the horizontal analysis technique applied to Handy Hospital's income statement and balance sheet. In each case, both dollar changes and percentage changes are provided to show the absolute as well as the relative changes. Although not illustrated here, a similar analysis could be made of the hospital's statements of changes in fund balances and statements of changes in financial position. Whatever the statement may be, the purpose of horizontal analysis is to direct the statement reader's attention to those items exhibiting the greatest absolute and relative changes compared to the prior year. Significant changes should be investigated and explained.

Figure 143
Handy Hospital
Comparative Income Statements
Horizontal Analysis
Years Ended December 31, 1977 and 1976

			Increase (Decrease)	
	1977	1976	Amount	Percent
Patient service revenues	$14,517	$13,534	$ 983	7.3%
Less deductions from revenues	1,742	1,489	253	17.0
Net patient service revenues	12,775	12,045	730	6.1
Other operating revenues	1,225	955	270	28.3
Total operating revenues	14,000	13,000	1,000	7.7
Less operating expenses:				
Nursing services	4,460	4,269	191	4.5
Other professional services	3,361	3,167	194	6.1
General services	2,263	1,953	310	15.9
Fiscal and administrative services	3,150	3,129	21	.7
Total operating expenses	13,234	12,518	716	5.7
Net operating income	766	482	284	58.9
Add nonoperating revenues	128	120	8	6.7
Net income for the year	$ 894	$ 602	$ 292	48.5

When more than 2 years are involved in horizontal analysis, trend percentages often are developed. Examine, for example, the illustration in figure 145 of a trend analysis of Handy Hospital's condensed income statements for a 5-year period. In this method of analysis, the figures in the base-year (the earliest year in the comparison) statement are considered to represent 100%. The base year in this example is 1973. The corresponding figures of each succeeding year are expressed as percentages of the base-year figures. The net patient service revenues of 1977 are 165.9% of 1973 net patient service revenues ($12,775/$7,702 = 165.9%). Such percentages can be extremely useful in bringing out unusual relationships and trends which might go unnoticed in an examination of dollar amounts alone. The technique, of course, can also be applied to balance sheets and other financial statements.

Figure 144
Handy Hospital
Comparative Balance Sheets
Horizontal Analysis
December 31, 1977 and 1976

	December 31		Increase (Decrease)	
	1977	1976	Amount	Percent
Current assets:				
Cash	$ 296	$ 230	$ 66	28.7%
Temporary investments	110	80	30	37.5
Receivables (net)	2,450	2,145	305	14.2
Inventories	220	234	(14)	(6.0)
Prepaid expenses	24	11	13	118.2
Total current assets	3,100	2,700	400	14.8
Long-term investments	430	390	40	10.3
Plant and equipment (net)	6,370	6,010	360	6.0
Total assets	$9,900	$9,100	$ 800	8.8
Current liabilities:				
Notes payable	$ 50	$ 200	$ (150)	(75.0)
Accounts payable	366	431	(65)	(15.1)
Accrued expenses payable	651	545	106	19.5
Other	139	124	15	12.1
Total current liabilities	1,206	1,300	(94)	(7.2)
Long-term debt	1,800	1,800	-0-	---
Total liabilities	3,006	3,100	(94)	(3.0)
Unrestricted fund balance	6,894	6,000	894	14.9
Total liabilities and fund balance	$9,900	$9,100	$ 800	8.8

VERTICAL ANALYSIS

Vertical analysis involves the development of component percentages which express the relationships among related data within a particular statement. This procedure also is referred to as *common-size analysis*. Figures 146 and 147 illustrate the application of vertical analysis to Handy Hospital's income statement and balance sheet.

In the vertical analysis of an income statement, total operating revenue usually is selected as the base figure for the computation

Figure 145
Handy Hospital
Trend Analysis of Income Statements
1973–1977

	1977	1976	1975	1974	1973
Amounts					
Patient service revenues	$14,517	$13,534	$11,630	$10,250	$ 8,440
Less deductions from revenues	1,742	1,489	1,245	996	738
Net patient service revenues	12,775	12,045	10,385	9,254	7,702
Other operating revenues	1,225	955	846	782	646
Total operating revenues	14,000	13,000	11,231	10,036	8,348
Less operating expenses:					
Nursing services	4,460	4,269	3,916	3,528	3,084
Other professional services	3,361	3,167	3,074	2,997	2,905
General services	2,263	1,953	1,788	1,433	937
Fiscal and administrative services	3,150	3,129	2,144	1,993	1,265
Total operating expenses	13,234	12,518	10,922	9,951	8,191
Net operating income	766	482	309	85	157
Add nonoperating revenues	128	120	211	70	43
Net income for the year	$ 894	$ 602	$ 520	$ 155	$ 200
Trend Percentages					
Patient service revenues	172.0	160.4	137.8	121.4	100.0
Less deductions from revenues	236.0	201.8	168.7	135.0	100.0
Net patient service revenues	165.9	156.4	134.8	120.2	100.0
Other operating revenues	189.6	147.8	131.0	121.1	100.0
Total operating revenues	167.7	155.7	134.5	120.2	100.0
Less operating expenses:					
Nursing services	144.6	138.4	127.0	114.4	100.0
Other professional services	115.7	109.0	105.8	103.2	100.0
General services	241.5	208.4	190.8	152.9	100.0
Fiscal and administrative services	249.0	247.4	169.5	157.5	100.0
Total operating expenses	161.6	152.8	133.3	121.5	100.0
Net operating income	487.9	307.0	196.8	54.1	100.0
Add nonoperating revenues	297.7	279.1	490.7	162.8	100.0
Net income for the year	447.0	301.0	260.0	77.5	100.0

of component percentages. All other figures (with the following exception noted) in the statement are expressed as percentages of this base figure. In figure 146, for instance, the 1977 base figure is $14,000 of total operating revenues, and each other figure in the 1977 income statement is reported as a percentage of the $14,000 base figure. Similarly, in the 1976 income statement, the $13,000 of total operating revenue serves as the base figure. All figures in the

1976 income statement (with the following exceptions noted) are expressed as a percentage of this $13,000 base figure.

Figure 146
Handy Hospital
Comparative Income Statements
Vertical Analysis
Years Ended December 31, 1977 and 1976

	1977		1976	
	Amount	Percent	Amount	Percent
Patient service revenues	$14,517	100.0%	$13,534	100.0%
Less deductions from revenues	1,742	12.0	1,489	11.0
Net patient service revenues	$12,775	88.0%	$12,045	89.0%
Net patient service revenues (above)	$12,775	91.3%	$12,045	92.7%
Other operating revenues	1,225	8.7	955	7.3
Total operating revenues	14,000	100.0	13,000	100.0
*Less operating expenses:**				
Nursing services	4,460	33.7	4,269	34.1
Other professional services	3,361	25.4	3,167	25.3
General services	2,263	17.1	1,953	15.6
Fiscal and administrative services	3,150	18.3	3,129	21.3
Total operating expenses	13,234	94.5	12,518	96.3
Net operating income	766	5.5	482	3.7
Add nonoperating revenues	128	.9	120	.9
Net income for the year	$ 894	6.4%	$ 602	4.6%

*Natural classification of expenses:				
Salaries and wages	$ 8,364	63.2%	$ 8,024	64.1%
Supplies	1,606	12.1	1,423	11.4
Purchased services	1,945	14.7	1,702	13.6
Depreciation	583	4.4	563	4.5
Interest	138	1.0	120	1.0
Other	598	4.6	686	5.4
Total operating expenses	$13,234	100.0%	$12,518	100.0%

As may be seen at the top of the income statement in figure 146, however, the deductions from patient service revenues generally are expressed as a percentage of gross patient service revenues (rather than of total operating revenues). Otherwise the component percentage would be distorted to the extent of other operating revenues to which the deductions are not related. In other words, while 1977 deductions are 12.4% of total operating revenues ($1,742/$14,000), it means more to say that the deductions are 12% of gross patient service revenues ($1,742/$14,517) or 12¢ of each dollar's worth of services provided to patients.

Notice also in figure 146 that operating expenses are reported both in a functional and in a natural (or object of expenditure) classification. In their external reports particularly, hospitals often present operating expenses in a natural classification because that type of classification signifies more to the general public. The percentages indicated for the natural classification in figure 146 are based upon total operating expenses simply to illustrate the use of an acceptable alternative base figure.

Vertical analysis can be quite useful in appraising the various components of the income statement. In figure 146, for example, we see that nursing service expenses increased from $4,269 in 1976 to $4,460 in 1977. But we also see that nursing service expenses, as a percentage of total operating revenues, decreased from 34.1% in 1976 to 33.7% in 1977. On the other hand, general services expenses increased both absolutely and in relation to total operating revenues. Observations such as these lend perspective to the evaluation of financial statement figures and tend to pinpoint areas for further investigation.

The results of vertical analysis can be viewed in another way. In figure 146, the 1977 operating expenses may be appraised in terms of "cents per dollar of operating revenue." In other words, of each $1.00 of operating revenue, 33.7¢ went for nursing services, 25.4¢ was expended for other professional services, 17.1¢ was employed for general services, and 18.3¢ was taken by fiscal and administrative services. Thus, out of each dollar of 1977 operating revenue, Handy Hospital was able to "bring down" only 5.5¢ into net operating income.

In the Handy Hospital balance sheets illustrated in figure 147, the base figure for asset analysis is total assets, and all other asset figures in the statements are expressed as percentages of total assets. The December 31, 1977, cash balance of $296, for example, is 3.0% of the total asset figure ($296/$9,900). The base figure for the analysis of liabilities and fund balance is their total (the same as total assets), and each component item is converted to a percentage of that base. It can be said, for example, that December 31, 1977, accounts payable are 3.7% of total assets (or of total liabilities and fund balance). This type of analysis is helpful in evaluating the balance sheet in terms of management's allocation of resources and in terms of the sources from which the assets can be financed.

For certain analytical purposes, however, it may be more useful to develop component percentages for current assets, using total current assets as the 100% figure. This is illustrated in figure 148, where it can be seen, for example, that the cash balance is 9.5% of total current assets at December 31, 1977. Similar analyses could be made, of course, of current liabilities or total liabilities.

Regardless of whether horizontal or vertical methods are used for comparing items on the financial statement, these methods merely serve as tools to assist in determining where problems may exist or where further examination of underlying financial data may be desirable. The key question is why certain relationships appear between various figures. Further on in this chapter, techniques for finding the answers to such questions will be described.

Figure 147
Handy Hospital
Comparative Balance Sheets
Vertical Analysis
December 31, 1977 and 1976

	December 31, 1977		December 31, 1976	
	Amount	Percent	Amount	Percent
Current assets:				
Cash	$ 296	3.0%	$ 230	2.5%
Temporary investments	110	1.1	80	.9
Receivables (net)	2,450	24.8	2,145	23.6
Inventories	220	2.2	234	2.6
Prepaid expenses	24	.2	11	.1
Total current assets	3,100	31.3	2,700	29.7
Long-term investments	430	4.3	390	4.3
Plant and equipment (net)	6,370	64.4	6,010	66.0
Total assets	$9,900	100.0%	$9,100	100.0%
Current liabilities:				
Notes payable	$ 50	.5%	$ 200	2.2%
Accounts payable	366	3.7	431	4.7
Accrued expenses payable	651	6.6	545	6.0
Other	139	1.4	124	1.4
Total current liabilities	1,206	12.2	1,300	14.3
Long-term debt	1,800	18.2	1,800	19.8
Total liabilities	3,006	30.4	3,100	34.1
Unrestricted fund balance	6,894	69.6	6,000	65.9
Total liabilites and fund balance	$9,900	100.0%	$9,100	100.0%

RATIO ANALYSIS

A ratio is the quotient which results when one number is divided by another. It is one number expressed in terms of another; it is an expression of the quantitative relationship between the 2 numbers. A ratio may be stated as a common fraction, decimally, or in percentage form. If, for example, we divide Handy Hospital's December 31, 1977, current assets of $3,100 by its December 31, 1977, current liabilities of $1,206, we obtain a ratio known as the *current ratio*. This ratio may be expressed as 3100/1206, as 2.57, or as 257%. It may be said, then, that the current ratio is 257% or 2.57 to 1, or that the hospital has $2.57 of current assets for each dollar of current liabilities.

Ratios are used in financial analysis to expedite comparisons and make relationships more intelligible. Many different ratios can be computed from the data in financial statements. One does not, however, compute all possible ratios. Many, such as the ratio of prepaid expenses to nonoperating revenues, would be totally meaningless for accounting purposes. We must select those ratios which have significance and relevance for the purposes of the analysis. Our discussion here is directed toward the selection, computation, and interpretation of a number of ratios commonly employed in hospital financial analysis.

Figure 148
Handy Hospital
Component Percentage Analysis of Current Assets
December 31, 1977 and 1976

	December 31, 1977		December 31, 1976	
	Amount	Percent	Amount	Percent
Cash	$ 296	9.5%	$ 230	8.5%
Temporary investments	110	3.5	80	3.0
Receivables (net)	2,450	79.0	2,145	79.4
Inventories	220	7.1	234	8.7
Prepaid expenses	24	.9	11	.4
Total current assets	$3,100	100.0%	$2,700	100.0%

ANALYSIS OF OPERATING RESULTS

The management of a hospital is charged with the task of maintaining a satisfactory relationship between revenues and expenses. Opinions differ as to precisely what this relationship should be. Some say that a nonproprietary hospital's financial operating objective should be to break even, that is, to maintain an equality between revenues and expenses. Given the pressures of demand for more and better services, advancing technology, inflation, inadequate reimbursement systems, and other socioeconomic forces, however, others (including this writer) are convinced that a reasonable "profit" objective is both necessary and justifiable. In view of current and emerging conditions in the hospital industry, a "no profit" fiscal objective seems totally unrealistic if the individual hospital is to avoid the erosion of its real capital and its ability to continue to provide the volume and quality of services desired by the community it serves.

EVALUATION OF PROFITABILITY

Since a profit is to be regarded as necessary and desirable for a particular hospital, a judgment must be made as to what that profit should be. A hospital management is likely to have in mind an absolute dollar amount of profit as a financial operating objective. This amount is determined to be the figure required to produce the cash flow needed to meet specific financial requirements such as the payment of bond interest charges, the retirement of long-term debt, the acquisition of new plant assets, the development of new health care programs, and the generation of additional necessary working capital. In addition, a percentage relationship between net operating income and operating revenues or between net operating income and total assets, for example, could be established as a goal or standard against which actual operating results might be measured. For this, the ratios described below are managerially useful.

• ***Operating Income Ratio***. One frequently used measure of profitability is the operating income ratio, sometimes called the *profit margin*. A computation of this ratio for Handy Hospital follows:

	1977	1976
1. Net operating income	$ 766	$ 482
2. Total operating revenues	14,000	13,000
3. Operating income ratio (1 ÷ 2)	5.47%	3.71%

Thus, in terms of the ratio of net operating income to operating revenues, Handy Hospital was more profitable in 1977 than in 1976. In 1977, the hospital was able to earn an operating income that was 5.47% of operating revenues; in 1976, the operating income ratio was only 3.71%. To put it another way, Handy Hospital's 1977 operating income was about 5.5¢ per dollar of operating revenues; the 1976 operating income was only 3.7¢ per dollar of operating revenues. This improved operating performance may be attributable to such factors as an increase in service rates, better management of operating expenses, an increased volume of service, and a more favorable service mix—in other words, relatively greater utilization of those patient services which generate revenues in excess of costs. Whatever the reasons for the improved ratio, they should be identified and evaluated by the hospital's management.

Emphasis sometimes is given to the *operating expense ratio*, the mathematical complement of the operating income ratio. If this operating income ratio is 5.5%, for example, the operating expense ratio must be 94.5%; that is, operating expenses consume 94.5¢ of each dollar of operating revenue. Naturally, the lower the operating expense ratio, the greater the operating income ratio.

• ***Return on Investment***. A weakness of the operating income ratio as a measure of profitability is that it does not take into account the amount of resources invested in the hospital enterprise. Consider, for example, a proprietary hospital having a 1977 operating income of $100,000 and an operating income ratio of 10% which, by most standards, would indicate a high degree of profitability. Suppose, however, that the proprietary hospital's average owner's equity and average total assets were $5 million and $10 million respectively, during 1977. The rate of return (profit) on the owners' investment, then, is only 5% (i.e., $100,000/$5,000,000), and the rate of return on total assets is only 1% (i.e., $100,000/$10,000,000). In most types of business enterprises, such rates of return would be regarded as grossly inadequate to satisfy creditors, pay reasonable dividends to owners, attract new investment capital, obtain new long-term debt funds, or even justify a continuation of the business. Thus, the best and most useful indicator of profitability is the rate of return on the amount of assets invested and employed in a health care institution.

The rates of return on Handy Hospital's average equity and average total assets for 1977 are computed as follows:

	1977
1. Net income for the year	$ 894
2. Average equity ($6,000 + $6,894) / 2	6,447
3. Average total assets ($9,100 + $9,900) / 2	9,500
4. Rate of return on equity (1 ÷ 2)	13.9%
5. Rate of return on total assets (1 ÷ 3)	9.4%

In other words, Handy Hospital earned a 1977 net income that was about 14¢ per dollar of equity and 9.4¢ per dollar of assets. These rates of return probably would be regarded as satisfactory by a majority of profit-seeking businesses.

Although Handy Hospital is a not-for-profit corporation, these ratios are not at all without significance or managerial usefulness. While there are no stockholder-owners interested in cash dividends and appreciation in the value of their stockholdings, Handy Hospital does have owners: the people of the community it serves. These owners presumably *are* interested in the continuation of the hospital as a financially sound and efficient provider of health care services. The hospital's employees are interested in adequate compensation. Banks, hospital bondholders, and other creditors are concerned with the hospital's ability to meet its financial obligations. Management must find the means to finance the acquisition of expensive equipment demanded by an advancing medical technology. If philanthropy and governmental subsidies can be ruled out as important sources of new capital funds, the future of the voluntary not-for-profit hospital is seen to be dependent upon the earning and reinvestment of adequate amounts of profit. It is for this reason that the rate-of-return concept cannot be safely ignored by the management of any hospital enterprise.

• ***Times Interest Earned***. A profitability ratio of particular concern to current and potential investors in hospital bond issues is the *times interest earned* ratio. The computation of the ratio for Handy Hospital is presented below:

	1977	1976
1. Net income for the year*	$ 894	$602
2. Bond interest expense (assumed)	108	108
3. Total (1 + 2)	1,002	710
4. Times interest earned (3 ÷ 2)	9.3	6.6

*Net operating income may be used instead, for a more conservative ratio.

Thus, the hospital earned its bond interest charges 9.3 times in 1977 and 6.6 times in 1976. This is an indicator of the ability of the hospital to pay the annual interest charges on its outstanding bonds. The higher the ratio, the more favorably will investors regard the hospital's bonds as investment opportunities.

INTERNAL ANALYSIS OF REVENUES AND EXPENSES

In addition to the above ratios which may be utilized by groups external to the hospital as well as by management, certain other analytical techniques can be applied by management to evaluate various revenue and expense items. The discussion here will be limited to actual versus budget comparisons and variance analysis.

• ***Analysis of Revenues***. Assume that Handy Hospital's 1977 patient service revenues of $14,517,000 includes $487,275 of daily patient service (routine service) revenues earned in a 20-bed nursing unit referred to as "Three South." The 1977 revenue budget for this unit was $439,600. A management report presented these facts as follows:

	1977		Variance	
	Actual	Budget	Amount	Percent
Daily patient service revenues				
Three South	$487,275	$439,600	$47,675	10.8%

As can be seen, the revenues of this nursing unit were $47,675, or 10.8%, in excess of budgeted revenues. The management question is *why*? What were the factors which caused this favorable revenue variance? How much of the variance is attributable to each factor?

To answer these questions, let us assume that 6,280 patient days of service were budgeted and that actual patient days in this unit were 6,497. Knowledge of the statistical units of service permits the following computation of actual and budgeted average revenue per patient day:

	Actual	Budget
1. Revenues	$487,275	$439,600
2. Patient days	6,497	6,280
3. Average revenue per day (1 ÷ 2)	75	0

Since this nursing unit offers private accommodations only, it is now clear that service rates were increased during the year. So, we become aware that the budget variance is due to 2 factors: (1) an increase in service rates and (2) a higher volume of service than budgeted. The dollar amount of revenues attributable to each of these factors is computed in figure 149. A similar analysis could be made, of course, in a comparison of 1977 actual with 1976 actual.

• ***Analysis of Expenses***. Assume that Handy Hospital's 1977 general services expenses of $2,263,000 include $484,106 of dietary department expense. The 1977 expense budget for the dietary department was $492,750. A management report presented these facts as follows:

	1977		Variance	
	Actual	Budget	Amount	Percent
Operating expenses:				
Dietary department	$484,106	$492,750	$ 8,644	1.75%

Thus, dietary department expenses for 1977 are seen to be $8,644, or 1.75%, less than was budgeted. Why? What were the factors which caused this favorable budget variance? How much of the variance is attributable to each factor?

The statistical unit of service for this department is a served meal. So, let us assume that 328,500 served meals were budgeted and that the actual number of meals served during the year was 336,185. This information permits the following computation of the actual and budgeted average cost per meal served:

	Actual	Budgeted
1. Total expense	$484,106	$492,750
2. Number of meals served	336,185	328,500
3. Average cost per meal served (1 ÷ 2)	$1.44	$1.50

Now we can see that, while the volume of service was 7,685 meals higher than was budgeted (336,185 − 328,500), the average cost per meal was 6¢ less than budgeted ($1.50 − $1.44). The effects of these factors on 1977 dietary department expenses are shown in figure 150. Note that the unfavorable effect of a higher-than-budgeted volume was more than offset by the favorable effect of the lower-than-budgeted cost per meal.

Figure 149
Handy Hospital
Analysis of Budget Variance
Daily Patient Service Revenues—Three South
Year Ended December 31, 1977

Budget Volume Variance:		
Patient days of service		
1977 actual	6,497	
1977 budget	6,280	
Excess of actual days over budgeted days	217	
Budgeted revenue per patient day	× $70	
Budget volume variance (favorable)		$15,190
Budget Rate Variance:		
Average revenue per patient day		
1977 actual	$75	
1977 budget	70	
Excess of actual average revenue over budgeted average revenue	$ 5	
Actual patient days for 1977	× 6,497	
Budget rate variance (favorable)		32,485
Total budget variance (favorable)		$47,675

ANALYSIS OF FINANCIAL POSITION

While operating results and financial strength are treated separately here, both are important considerations, regardless of one's point of view. The information in the balance sheet cannot be ignored when appraising operating results; neither should the income statement be bypassed entirely in evaluating the financial strength of a hospital. Careful attention also should be given the data provided in statements of changes in fund balances and in statements of changes in financial position.

EVALUATION OF CURRENT FINANCIAL POSITION

The current financial strength of a hospital is a matter of great importance not only to its management but also to various external groups. If the hospital is to be able to repay bank loans and meet its short-term obligations to other creditors, it must maintain a sound current financial position. The hospital must have an adequate amount of working capital, it must maintain a satisfactory degree of liquidity, and it must not overinvest in receivables or inventories. Some of the ratios usually applied to obtain insights into the presence or absence of these desired conditions are presented in the following explanation, using the financial statements of Handy Hospital for illustration.

• ***Current Ratio***. One of the most widely used measures of current financial strength is the *current ratio* which indicates the number of dollars of current assets per dollar of current liabilities. It shows the number of times the current assets will "pay off" the current debts of the hospital. The following is a computation of Handy Hospital's current ratio:

	December 31	
	1977	1976
1. Current assets	$3,100	$2,700
2. Current liabilities	1,206	1,300
3. Current ratio (1 ÷ 2)	2.57	2.08

Thus, in terms of the current ratio, Handy Hospital's current debt-paying ability appears somewhat stronger at the end of 1977 than at the end of 1976. There is, however, no one value for the current ratio that is applicable to, or desirable for, all hospitals. What may be an adequate current ratio for one hospital may be dangerously low for another. It also is worth noting that while a particular current ratio may be satisfactory at the end of one year, it may not be satisfactory for the same hospital at the end of the next year.

Figure 150
Handy Hospital
Analysis of Budget Variance
Dietary Department Expenses
Year Ended December 31, 1977

Budget Cost Variance:		
Average cost per meal		
1977 budget	$1.50	
1977 actual	1.44	
Excess of budgeted cost over actual cost	$ .06	
Actual number of meals served	× 336,185	
Budget cost variance (favorable)		$20,171
Budget Volume Variance:		
Number of meals served		
1977 actual	336,185	
1977 budget	328,500	
Excess of actual over budget	7,685	
Budgeted cost per meal served	× $1.50	
Budget volume variance (unfavorable)		(11,527)
Net budget variance (favorable)		$ 8,644

• ***Quick Ratio***. A weakness of the current ratio is that it does not take into account the composition of either current assets or current liabilities. The *quick ratio* (sometimes called the "acid test") is a more valid test of current debt-paying ability than the current ratio in that it gives some consideration to the composition of the hospital's current assets. The computation is as follows:

	December 31	
	1977	1976
1. Cash	$ 296	$ 230
2. Temporary investments	110	80
3. Receivables (net)	2,450	2,145
4. Quick assets (1 + 2 + 3)	2,856	2,455
5. Current liabilities	1,206	1,300
6. Quick ratio (4 ÷ 5)	2.37	1.89

The basic difference between the quick ratio and the current ratio is simply that the computation of the quick ratio excludes inventories and prepaid expense items. An extreme modification of the quick ratio is the division of cash, or the total of cash and temporary investments, by current liabilities.

• ***Current Asset Turnover***. The current asset turnover is said to be an indicator of how "hard" the management of the hospital "works" the current assets, the intensity of current asset utilization. Handy Hospital's turnovers for 1977 and 1976 are computed as follows:

	1977	1976
1. Total operating revenues	$14,000	$13,000
2. Current assets, December 31	3,100	2,700
3. Current asset turnover (1 ÷ 2)	4.52	4.81

Some analysts make the computation using total operating expenses rather than revenues as the numerator; others prefer to use working capital (current assets minus current liabilities) as the denominator (that is, a *working capital turnover*). In any event, a high turnover generally is indicative of efficient and productive employment of current resources.

• ***Analysis of Receivables***. The amount of receivables from patient services in a hospital's balance sheet should not exceed a reasonable proportion of the charges made to patients' accounts during a related period. This relationship may be illuminated by computation of the *accounts receivable turnover*:

	1977	1976
1. Net patient service revenues*	$12,775	$12,045
2. Average receivables (net)**	2,298	1,983
3. Receivables turnover (1 ÷ 2)	5.56	6.07

*Excluding revenues from services rendered on a cash basis and not recorded through accounts receivable.

**January 1 receivables from patients plus December 31 receivables from patients, divided by 2.

This ratio indicates roughly the number of times during the year the receivables from patients were "turned over," or collected. An increase in the turnover generally may be regarded as favorable with respect to the effectiveness of the credit and collection functions.

A more widely used ratio employed by hospitals in the analysis of accounts receivable involves the *number of days' charges uncollected* and in receivables. This ratio is computed for Handy Hospital as follows:

	1977	1976
1. Net patient service revenues	$12,775	$12,045
2. Average daily charges (line 1 divided by 365 days)	35	33
3. Receivables (net), December 31	2,450	2,145
4. Number of days' charges uncollected (3 ÷ 2)	70	65

One may tentatively conclude that, on the average, the quality of receivables management may have declined somewhat between 1976 and 1977. Yet it must be recognized that this ratio is an average; some patients' accounts may be 200 days old while others are only a few days old. It also is extremely informative to compute by major categories of patients and third-party payers, where the information is available, both the receivables turnover and the number of days' charges uncollected.

• ***Analysis of Inventories***. As is true of receivables, a hospital can have an excessive investment in inventories. A reasonable relationship should be maintained between inventories and total current assets. In addition, the relationship between inventories and total cost of supplies used may be computed as an *inventory turnover*:

	1977	1976
1. Total cost of supplies used	$1,606	$1,423
2. Average inventories*	227	209
3. Inventory turnover (1 ÷ 2)	7.07	6.81

*January 1 inventories plus December 31 inventories, divided by 2.

The fact that Handy Hospital "turned over" its inventories a greater number of times in 1977 than in 1976 generally is a favorable indication about the quality of inventory management.

In addition to inventory turnover, the *average number of days' supply* in inventories may be calculated as follows:

	1977	1976
1. Total cost of supplies used	$1,606	$1,423
2. Average daily usage (line 1 divided by 365 days)	4.4	3.9
3. Inventories, December 31	220	234
4. Number of days' supply in inventories (3 ÷ 2)	50	60

In evaluating inventories, it must be understood that a hospital can be understocked as well as overstocked. Either extreme is undesirable. Note also that, where the information is available, both the inventory turnover and the number of days' supply should be computed by major categories of inventory to take properly into account the differing characteristics of various types of supplies.

EVALUATION OF LONG-TERM FINANCIAL POSITION

Many external users of hospital financial statements are interested in the hospital's long-run financial strength as well as in its current financial position. Hospital bondholders and mortgagees, for example, are concerned not only with the ability of the hospital to pay current interest charges but also with the long-run safety of their investments. An intelligent appraisal of a hospital's long-term financial position is also essential to sound long-term financing decisions and long-range planning either on an individual-hospital or area-wide basis. Such an analysis is helpful as well in evaluating the consequences of long-term commitment decisions (bond issues and plant asset acquisitions, for example) which have previously been made and implemented.

In studying a hospital's long-run financial position, an analysis is usually made of (1) changes in the absolute and relative amounts invested by the hospital in the various categories of assets and (2) changes in the absolute and relative amounts of the sources (debt and equity) of its assets. This analysis may take the form of a 5- or 10-year study of the hospital's common-size balance sheets and statements of changes in financial position. Particular attention is given to detecting substantial shifts in the allocation of resources between the current and noncurrent classifications. A study of the hospital's asset structure should also include an examination of assets held in the restricted funds. This is particularly true with respect to the plant replacement and expansion fund, where material amounts might be available for the financing of future construction and equipment needs. Should the hospital have term endowments, their amounts and termination dates should also be considered in evaluating the hospital's long-run financial strength.

An appraisal of a hospital's long-run financial position must necessarily include the detection and investigation of substantial shifts noted in the capital structure, that is, the relative amounts of debt and equity. For this purpose, debt ratios and equity ratios may be computed as shown here:

	December 31	
	1977	1976
1. Total liabilities	$3,006	$3,100
2. Hospital equity	6,894	6,000
3. Total liabilities and equity (assets)	9,900	9,100
4. Debt ratio (1 ÷ 3)	30.4%	34.1%
5. Equity ratio (2 ÷ 3)	69.6%	65.9%

At the end of 1977, we see that 30.4% of Handy Hospital's assets were financed by debt and 69.6% through equity. This position is more conservative (less risky) than that which existed at the end of 1976, when a somewhat greater percentage of the assets was being supplied by creditors.

In some cases, the above ratios are combined into a single *debt/equity ratio*, (i.e., total liabilities divided by total equity). The debt/equity ratio at the end of 1977, for example, is 43.6 (i.e., $3,006/$6,894), meaning that the hospital has about 44¢ of debt for each dollar of equity.

The hospital's asset and capital structure as reflected in its balance sheet should always be viewed in conjunction with its statement of changes in financial position. This latter statement should preferably be presented in comparative form covering several prior periods so that trends in the sources and applications of funds may be clearly discerned. This permits an appraisal of the effectiveness of management's past investing and financing policies in bringing the hospital to its present financial position.

Above all, it must be recognized by all external groups that a successful hospital seldom remains the same. It either changes and grows, or it stagnates and declines. It moves in new directions, developing new programs and services in response to changes in demand and improved technology. This requires adequate financing, satisfactory operating results, and a sound financial position.

QUESTIONS

1. What are "common-size" financial statements?

2. Swellplace Hospital's nursing service expenses were $957,400 in 1978 and $898,300 in 1977. Make a horizontal analysis of these data.

3. What is meant by a vertical analysis of the balance sheet? The income statement?

4. "A hospital with a current ratio of 4 to 1 has greater current financial strength than does a hospital with a current ratio of only 2 to 1." Do you agree? Explain.

5. State how each of the following is computed and explain what might be indicated by the results of the computation:

   a. Operating income ratio
   b. Operating expense ratio
   c. Return on investment
   d. Times interest earned

6. State how each of the following is computed and explain what might be indicated by the results of the computation:

   a. Current ratio
   b. Quick ratio
   c. Current asset turnover

7. State how each of the following is computed and explain what might be indicated by the results of the computation:

   a. Accounts receivable turnover
   b. Number of days' charges uncollected
   c. Ratio of accounts receivable to total current assets

8. State how each of the following is computed and explain what might be indicated by the results of the computation:

   a. Inventory turnover
   b. Average number of days' supply in inventories
   c. Ratio of inventory to total current assets

9. How is the debt/equity ratio computed? Explain what might be indicated by the results of the computation.

10. Goodplace Hospital provides you with the following information:

	Actual	Budget
Daily patient service revenues	$367,500	$360,000
Patient days of service	4,375	4,500

Prepare an analysis of the budget variance in the manner illustrated in figure 149.

11. Warmplace Hospital provides you with the following information:

	Actual	Budget
Laboratory expense	$628,100	$500,000
Number of examinations	114,200	100,000

Prepare an analysis of the budget variance in the manner illustrated in figure 150.

12. Coolplace Hospital has a current ratio of 2 to 1 on June 30, 1978. On July 1, 1978, the hospital obtains a $150,000 short-term loan from a local bank. What is the effect of the loan on the hospital's current ratio, quick ratio, and working capital?

PROBLEMS

A. Realplace Hospital provides you with the following financial statements for 1978 and 1977:

	December 31	
	1978	1977
Cash	$ 240	$ 120
Temporary investments	210	180
Receivables (net)	1,400	1,150
Inventories	300	370
Prepaid expenses	50	80
Total current assets	2,200	1,900
Plant assets (net)	5,800	5,100
Total	$8,000	$7,000
Current liabilities	$ 740	$ 475
Long-term debt	3,530	3,205
Fund balance	3,730	3,320
Total	$8,000	$7,000

	Year Ended 12/31	
	1978	1977
Gross patient service revenues	$6,600	$6,000
Deductions from revenues	790	500
Net patient service revenues	5,810	5,500
Other operating revenues	700	500
Total operating revenues	6,510	6,000
Less operating expenses		
Nursing services	2,100	1,900
Other professional services	1,600	1,500
General services	1,300	1,100
Fiscal and administrative services	1,100	1,400
Total operating expenses	6,100	5,900
Net income for the year	$ 410	$ 100

Operating expenses include the $900 cost of supplies used, $400 of depreciation, and $240 of bond interest expense.

Required. (1) Develop a horizontal analysis of the above statements. (2) Convert the above financial statements to common size. (3) Prepare a ratio analysis of 1978 operating results. (4) Prepare a ratio analysis of December 31, 1978, financial position.

B. Someplace Hospital supplies you with the following information relating to the 1978 operations of its radiology department:

	Actual	Budget
Revenues	$966,400	$930,000
Expenses	393,600	372,000
Number of examinations	60,400	62,000

Required. Prepare an analysis of the budget variances for the radiology department's revenues and expenses for 1978.

C. Wellplace Hospital provides you with the following financial statements for 1978 and 1977:

	December 31 1978	December 31 1977
Cash	$ 268	$ 211
Temporary investments	126	34
Receivables—patients (net)	969	854
Other receivables	42	39
Inventories	296	315
Prepaid expenses	25	29
Total current assets	1,726	1,482
Long-term investments	466	442
Plant assets (net)	8,126	8,185
Other assets	67	88
Total	$10,385	$10,197
Current installments of long-term debt	$ 180	$ 180
Notes payable	125	75
Accounts payable	196	202
Accrued expenses payable	238	217
Payroll taxes withheld	81	63
Advances from third-party payers	75	55
Other	42	29
Total current liabilities	937	821
Long-term debt	1,718	1,865
Fund balance	7,730	7,511
Total	$10,385	$10,197
Patient service revenues	$ 8,830	$ 7,326
Deductions from patient service revenues	1,430	1,465
Net patient service revenues	7,400	5,861
Other operating revenues	505	407
Total operating revenues	7,905	6,268
Less operating expenses		
Nursing services	2,560	2,197
Other professional services	2,050	1,615
General services	1,350	1,033
Fiscal and administrative services	1,925	1,614
Total operating expenses	7,885	6,459
Net operating income (loss)	20	(191)

	1978	1977
Nonoperating revenues	224	176
Net income (loss) for the year	$ 244	$ (15)

The operating expenses include $520 of depreciation, $110 of interest expense, and $790 of supplies used.

Required. (1) Develop a horizontal analysis of the above statements. (2) Convert the above financial statements to common size. (3) Prepare a ratio analysis of 1978 operating results. (4) Prepare a ratio analysis of December 31, 1978, financial position.

D. Softplace Hospital provides you with the following information:

	December 31	
	1978	1977
Cash	$ 50,000	$ 35,000
Temporary investments	80,000	50,000
Receivables (net)	140,000	110,000
Inventories	35,000	28,000
Prepaid expenses	12,000	16,000
Long-term investments	230,000	190,000
Plant assets (net)	420,000	421,000
	$967,000	$850,000
Notes payable	$ 75,000	$ 25,000
Accounts payable	21,000	19,000
Accrued expenses payable	33,000	28,000
Other current liabilities	7,000	22,000
Long-term debt	500,000	450,000
Fund balance	331,000	306,000
	$967,000	$850,000

	Year Ended 12/31	
	1978	1977
Total operating revenues	$840,000	$780,000
Cost of supplies used	210,000	186,000
Depreciation expense	90,000	90,000
Bond interest expense	30,000	27,000
Net patient service revenues	960,000	890,000
Net income	25,000	16,000

Required. (1) Prepare a ratio analysis of operating results for 1978. (2) Prepare a ratio analysis of the hospital's financial position at December 31, 1978.

E. Safeplace Hospital supplies you with the following information relating to the 1978 operations of one of its nursing units:

	Actual	Budget
Revenues	$753,300	$750,000
Expenses	502,200	500,000
Patient days of service	9,300	10,000

Required. Prepare an analysis of the budget variances for revenues and expenses for 1978.

Glossary

This glossary includes selected general accounting terms and certain special terms encountered in hospital financial management. Many of the definitions provided have been adapted from a variety of sources, including the following:

Berman, Howard J., and Weeks, Lewis E. *The Financial Management of Hospitals*. Ann Arbor, Michigan: Health Administration Press, School of Public Health, The University of Michigan, 1974.

Chart of Accounts for Hospitals. Chicago: American Hospital Association, 1976.

Eric L. Kohler. *A Dictionary for Accountants*. Englewood Cliffs, New Jersey: Prentice-Hall, Inc., 1970.

Financial Accounting Standards. Financial Accounting Standards Board, Stamford, Connecticut, 1976.

Hospital Audit Guide. New York: American Institute of Certified Public Accountants, 1972.

Uniform Hospital Definitions. Chicago: American Hospital Association, 1960.

Accelerated depreciation. Depreciation by a method, such as sum-of-years' digits or double-declining balance, which results in the write-off of the cost of a depreciable asset at a more rapid rate than would occur by the straight-line method.

Accounting. The accumulation and communication of historical and projected economic data relating to the financial position of an enterprise and the results of its operations, and the interpretation of the results thereof for purposes of managerial planning and control and for use by decision-making groups external to the enterprise.

Accounting cycle. The procedures involved in maintaining a set of accounting records throughout an accounting period.

Accounting equation. An equation which is both the basic formula for the balance sheet and the foundation of double-entry accounting. Usually written: Assets = Liabilities + Fund Balances.

Accounting period. The period of time covered by an income statement. This period generally is not less than one month nor longer than one year.

Accounting principles. A body of rules, standards, and conventions which determines the manner in which transactions are recorded and in which data are presented in financial statements.

Accounts payable. Liabilities arising from the purchase of goods and services from suppliers on credit.

Accounts receivable. Assets arising from the provision of services or the sale of goods to patients on credit.

Accounts receivable aging schedule. An analysis of accounts receivable according to the length of time the accounts have been outstanding.

Accounts receivable turnover. The amount of charges to patients' accounts, during a given period, divided by the amount of accounts receivable.

Accrual basis of accounting. A method of accounting by which revenues are recognized when earned and expenses when incurred, regardless of the flow of cash.

Accrued expenses. Expenses which have been incurred but not yet paid.

Accrued income. Income which has been earned but not yet received in cash.

Accumulated depreciation. The accumulation to date of depreciation expense—that is, the total portion of the original cost of depreciable assets which already has been allocated to expense in prior and current periods.

Adjusting entry. An entry which is necessary for adjustment of account balances to conform with the accrual basis at the end of the accounting period.

Admission. (1) An inpatient admission is the formal acceptance by a hospital of a patient who is to receive physician's, dentist's, or allied services while lodged in the hospital. (2) An outpatient admission is the formal acceptance by the hospital of a patient who is not to be lodged in the hospital while receiving physician's, dentist's, or allied services at the hospital.

Allowance. The difference between gross revenue from services rendered and amounts received, or to be received, from patients or third-party payers. Allowances are to be distinguished from uncollectible accounts resulting from credit losses.

Allowance for uncollectible accounts. A balance sheet valuation account reflecting the estimated amount of accounts and notes receivable which will prove to be uncollectible by reason of charity care, contractual adjustments, courtesy discounts, and bad debt losses.

Amortization. (1) The systematic allocation of an item to revenue or expense over a number of accounting periods. (2) The repayment of a loan on an installment basis.

Assets. The economic resources of a hospital enterprise which are recognized and measured in conformity with generally accepted accounting principles.

Average daily census. The average number of inpatients maintained in the hospital each day for a given period of time.

Average length of stay. The average number of days of service rendered to each inpatient discharged during a given period.

Bad debt. An account receivable which, although the patient has the ability to pay, is regarded as uncollectible and is charged as a credit loss.

Balance sheet. A statement of financial position showing the hospital's assets, liabilities, and fund balances at a given date.

Board-designated funds. Unrestricted funds set aside by action of the hospital's governing board for specific purposes or projects.

Board-designated investment funds. Unrestricted funds which, at the discretion of the governing board, have been designated for investment to produce income as if they were endowment funds.

Bond. A written promise under seal to pay a sum of money at some definite future time.

Bond discount or premium. The difference between the par or face value of a bond and the amount received (by the issuer) or paid (by the investor) when a bond is issued or purchased.

Bond indenture. The contract between the bondholders and the hospital issuing the bonds.

Bonds sinking fund. A fund in which assets are accumulated in order to liquidate bonds at their maturity date or earlier.

Book value. The amount at which an asset or liability item is carried in accounting records of the hospital.

Budget. A financial plan for future operations.

Capital expenditure. An expenditure chargeable to an asset account when the asset acquired has an estimated life in excess of one year and is not intended for sale in the ordinary course of operations. The opposite of revenue expenditure.

Capital expenditure budgeting. The process of planning and controlling expenditures for property, plant, and equipment items.

Cash basis of accounting. A method of accounting by which revenues are recognized only when cash is received and expenses are recorded only when cash is disbursed.

Cash budget. A projection of cash receipts, disbursements, and balances for a given future period of time.

Cash-flow statement. A statement of actual or projected cash receipts and disbursements for a given period of time.

Chart of accounts. A listing of account titles, with account numbers, indicating the manner in which transaction data are to be classified in the accounting records.

Closing the books. The process of transferring the balances in the revenue and expense accounts, including revenue deductions, to the fund balance account at the end of the fiscal year.

Composite depreciation. Depreciation of a number of similar assets as a group rather than on a unit-by-unit basis.

Compound interest. Interest that is computed on the principal amount invested or borrowed and on any interest earned (on such principal) that has not been paid.

Contingent liabilities. Possible liabilities which may arise upon the happening of some future event which is considered possible but not probable.

Contractual patient. One of a group of patients for whom the hospital has agreed to provide specific inpatient or outpatient facilities and services, payment for which is made to the hospital on the basis of a contract between an outside agency and the hospital.

Control. The process of assuring insofar as possible that the objectives of an organization are realized. Its principal elements are (1) communication of plans, (2) performance appraisal, (3) corrective action, and (4) follow-up.

Control account. A general ledger account, the detail of which is contained in a subsidiary ledger—for accounts receivable, for example.

Controllable cost. In the short run, a cost whose amount is controllable by someone in the organization. It is usually a variable cost.

Controller. The title usually given to the executive responsible for the accounting function in the organization.

Cost. The present value surrendered, or promised to be surrendered in the future, in exchange for goods and services received. Expired costs are expenses; unexpired costs are assets.

Cost basis of accounting. The use of historical, objectively determined cost as the basis of accounting for most assets.

Cost center. An organizational unit whose costs are separately accumulated in the accounts.

Cost control. The attempt to maintain actual costs at, or below, budgeted levels.

Cost finding. The segregation of direct costs by cost centers; the allocation of overhead costs to revenue-producing and other centers by inpatients, outpatients, and other classifications.

Cost or market, lower of. A valuation basis for inventories and temporary investments.

Credit. As a noun, an entry or balance on the right-hand side of an account. As a transitive verb, to make an entry on the right-hand side of an account.

Current assets. Those assets which are cash and will be converted into cash or consumed in the normal operations of the hospital within one year from the balance sheet date.

Current liabilities. Those liabilities which will be discharged with current assets in the normal course of business within one year from the balance sheet date.

Current ratio. The ratio of current assets to current liabilities.

Days' revenue in receivables. The average number of days of billings in accounts receivable which remain uncollected at a given point in time.

Debenture bond. A bond secured, not by specific assets but only by the general credit standing of the issuer.

Debit. As a noun, an entry or balance on the left-hand side of an account. As a transitive verb, to make an entry on the left-hand side of an account.

Deductions from revenues. Revenues uncollectible by reason of charity care, contractual adjustments, courtesy discounts, and bad debts.

Default. Failure to fulfill the requirements of a contract, such as the paying of interest or principal on a debt.

Deferred revenue. Future revenue which has been collected or billed but not yet earned—hence, a liability.

Depreciation expense. That portion of the original cost of a tangible plant asset allocated to a particular accounting period.

Discounting of receivables. A method of short-term financing in which patient receivables are used to secure a loan from a financial institution.

Dishonor. To refuse to honor (pay) a promissory note at maturity.

Donated services. The estimated monetary value of service of personnel who receive no monetary compensation, or partial compensation, for their services. The term is usually applied to services rendered (by members of religious orders, societies, or similar groups) to hospitals operated by, or affiliated with, such organizations.

ECF. Extended care facility—for example, a nursing home.

Endowment funds. Funds with stipulations by the donors that the principal of the funds be maintained inviolate and in perpetuity and that only income from investments of the funds be expended. *See also* Term endowment funds.

Equities. Rights in assets—for example, fund balances.

Expenses. Costs that have been consumed in carrying on some activity and from which no measurable benefit will extend beyond the present. Expenses are expired costs which ordinarily are accompanied by the surrendering of an asset or the incurring of a liability.

FICA. Federal Insurance Contributions Act, commonly known as social security.

FIFO. First-in–first-out method of inventory costing.

Fixed costs. Costs which remain substantially the same in total amount within a given range of production and period of time.

Flexible budget. A budget prepared so that it can be adjusted by interpolation to reflect what expenses should be at any level of activity within a relevant range.

Functional classification. The grouping of expenses according to the operating purposes (patient care, education, research, etc.) for which costs are incurred. Revenues also are classified functionally.

Fund. A self-contained accounting entity set up to account for a specific activity or project.

Fund accounting. A system of accounting in which the hospital's resources, obligations, and fund balances are segregated into logical groups of accounts according to legal restrictions and administrative requirements. Each account group, or fund, constitutes a subordinate accounting entity.

Fund balance. The excess of assets over liabilities (net equity). An excess of liabilities over assets is known as a deficit in fund balance.

Funded debt. Long-term debt.

Funds functioning as endowment. *See* Board-designated investment funds.

Funds held in trust by others. Funds held and administered, at the direction of the donor, by an outside trustee for the benefit of an institution or institutions.

General fund. The name often given to the unrestricted fund.

Governing board. The policy-making body of the hospital. Some of the responsibilities usually attributed to the governing board may be assumed by appropriate committees.

Gross revenues. The value, at the hospital's full established rates, of services rendered and goods sold to patients during a given time period.

HMO. Health Maintenance Organization.

Imprest cash fund. *See* Petty cash fund.

Income statement. A financial statement indicating the results of operations of an enterprise in terms of revenues earned and expenses incurred for a given period of time. Also referred to as an *operating statement*, a *statement of income and expense*, or a *profit-and-loss statement*.

Insolvency. The inability to meet mature obligations.

Interest. A charge for the use of money.

Interim financial statements. Financial statements—for example, monthly balance sheets and income statements—prepared at a date other than the end of the fiscal year.

Internal auditing. The work performed by a hospital's internal auditors.

Internal control. The plan of organization and all the coordinate methods and measures adopted within a hospital to safeguard its assets, check the accuracy and reliability of its accounting data, promote operational efficiency, and encourage adherence to prescribed managerial policies.

Inventory. The aggregate of those items of tangible personal property which (1) are held for sale in the ordinary course of business, (2) are in process of production for sale, or (3) are to be consumed currently in the production of goods or services to be available for sale.

Inventory control. The process of regulating the amount and types of supplies in inventory.

Inventory turnover. Cost of supplies used divided by the average inventory for the period.

Journal. A book of original entry in which transactions are recorded in chronological sequence.

Land improvements. Improvements made to land, including sidewalks, parking lots, driveways, fencing, and shrubbery. Land improvements are depreciable.

Ledger. The group of accounts used in recording the transactions of the hospital. A book of secondary entry.

Liability. The economic obligations of the hospital, as recognized and measured in conformity with generally accepted accounting principles.

LIFO. Last-in–first-out method of inventory costing.

Line of credit. An arrangement whereby a financial institution commits itself to lending up to a specified maximum amount during a specified period.

Liquidity. A hospital's financial position and its ability to meet currently maturing obligations.

Long-term investments. Investments, generally in securities, which the hospital intends to hold for longer than one year from the balance sheet date.

Long-term liabilities. Liabilities which are not payable within one year from the balance sheet (i.e., all liabilities except current ones).

Management. The direction of resources to the attainment of desired objectives through planning and control.

Marketable security. Short-term financial instruments which can be readily purchased or sold without loss in principal.

Matching. An accounting principle which requires the recognition of related revenues and expenses in the same period.

Mortgage. A pledge of designated property as security for a loan—for example, mortgage bonds.

Net assets. The excess of assets over liabilities (i.e., a fund balance).

Net income. The excess of revenues over expenses for a given period of time as presented in the income statements.

Net loss. The excess of expenses over revenues for a given period of time as presented in the income statements.

Net revenues. The excess of gross revenues from patient services over revenue deductions. Also called *net earnings from patient services*.

Net worth. An unsatisfactory term for *net assets* or *fund balance*.

Nonexpendable funds. *See* Endowment funds.

Notes receivable discounted. Notes receivable which have been discounted with recourse at a financial institution.

Objective evidence. A requirement in accounting that all transaction entries be supported, insofar as possible, by properly executed documents.

Object of expenditure classification. A method of classifying expenditures—such as salaries and wages, employee benefits, supplies, and purchased services—according to their natural classification.

Operating ratio. Total operating expenses divided by total operating revenues.

Opportunity cost. The measurable advantage foregone in the past or likely to be sacrificed as a result of a decision involving alternatives.

Organization chart. A diagrammatic illustration of the manner in which a hospital is organized internally.

Overstocked. A condition in which inventory stocks exceed demand.

Patient day. The unit of measure denoting lodging facilities provided and services rendered to one inpatient between the census-taking hour on two successive days.

Percentage of occupancy. The ratio of actual patient days to maximum patient days as determined by bed capacity during any given period of time.

Periodic inventory system. A system of accounting for purchased goods and supplies by which items purchased are charged to expense accounts rather than to inventory.

Permanent funds. *See* Endowment funds.

Perpetual inventory system. A system of accounting for inventories under which a continuous, day-to-day record is kept of inventory levels.

Petty cash fund. A small fund of cash maintained for the purpose of making minor disbursements for which the issuance of a check would be inconvenient or impractical.

Physical inventory. The actual inventory as determined by physical count, usually at the end of a reporting period.

Planning. The process of establishing programs for the achievement of objectives.

Plant. Physical properties used for hospital purposes (i.e., land, land improvements, buildings, and equipment). The term does not include real estate or properties of restricted or unrestricted funds not used for hospital operations.

Plant replacement and expansion funds. Funds donated for renewal or replacement of the hospital plant.

Pooled investments. Assets of two or more funds consolidated for investment purposes.

Position control plan. A management tool for controlling the number of employees on the hospital payroll and for assuring the utilization of each employee to the point of maximum effectiveness.

Posting. The process of transferring the information in the journals to the ledger.

Preferred stock. A type of stock which has preference over common stock with respect to dividends, or to assets in case of liquidation, or both.

Prepaid expense. An expense-type outlay which benefits (is applicable to) subsequent accounting periods and therefore is an asset.

Prepaid income. *See* Deferred revenue.

Present value. The value today of a future receipt or payment, or successive receipts or payments, discounted at the appropriate discount rate.

Profit-and-loss statement. A less than satisfactory term for *income statement*.

PSRO. Professional Standards Review Organization.

Purchase order. A business document used in purchasing.

Qualified audit report. An audit report which includes one or more qualifications or exceptions.

Quantity discount. A reduction in unit purchase cost received by those who purchase supplies in a quantity in excess of a set amount.

Quick assets. Cash, temporary investments, and receivables.

Quick ratio. The ratio of quick assets to current liabilities.

Ratio. The quotient which results when one number is divided by another.

Receiving report. A business document in which a record is made of incoming quantities of supplies.

Record date. The date on which a list of stockholders is prepared to determine those who are entitled to receive a declared dividend.

Referred outpatient. One who is admitted exclusively to a special diagnostic or therapeutic facility or service of the hospital for diagnosis or treatment on an ambulatory basis.

Refunding. The process of replacing one debt with another, usually having a lower interest cost.

Registered bond. A type of bond whose principal, and usually whose interest, is payable only to the owner as recorded by the issuer.

Relative value units. Index numbers assigned to various procedures based on the relative amounts of labor, supplies, and capital required to perform the procedure.

Reserve. A term generally undesirable in accounting usage but sometimes employed in *reserve for bad debts* and *reserve for depreciation*.

Responsibility accounting. A system of accounting which accumulates and communicates historical and projected monetary and statistical data relating to revenues and controllable expenses classified according to the organizational units which produce the revenues and are responsible for incurring the expenses.

Restricted funds. Funds restricted by donors for specific purposes. The term refers to specific-purpose and endowment funds.

Retirement of indebtedness funds. Funds required by external sources to be used to meet debt service charges and the retirement of indebtedness on plant assets. The term *sinking funds* is sometimes used to describe these funds.

Revenue. Income which results from the sale of goods and the rendering of services and is measured by the charge made to patients, clients, or tenants for goods and services furnished to them. Revenue also includes gains from the sale or exchange of assets, interest, and dividends earned on investments and unrestricted donations of resources to the hospital.

Revenue expenditure. An expenditure charged against operations.

Salvage value. The estimated amount for which a plant asset can be sold at the end of its useful life. Also called *scrap value*.

Self-responsible patient. A patient who pays either all or part of his hospital bill from his own resources, as opposed to one which a third party pays.

Semivariable costs. Costs which are partly variable and partly fixed in behavior, in response to changes in volume.

Sinking fund. *See* Retirement of indebtedness funds.

Specific-identification method. A system of inventory costing. Also applied in the determination of the costs of securities sold.

Specific-purpose fund. Funds restricted by donors for a specific purpose or project. Board-designated funds do not constitute specific-purpose funds.

Statement of changes in financial position. A financial statement which summarizes the movement of funds (working capital) within a hospital for a given period of time.

Statement of changes in fund balances. A financial statement setting forth the changes that have occurred in the amount of the fund balances during a given period of time.

Stock dividend. A dividend paid in the form of additional shares of stock.

Stockout. A condition in which demand exists for inventory items currently not available.

Straight-line method. A method of depreciation. Also a method of amortizing bond premium and discount.

Subsidiary ledger. A group of accounts which is contained in a separate ledger and which supports a single account (a control account) in the general ledger.

SYD. Sum-of-years'-digits method of depreciation.

Tangible asset. An asset—such as equipment—having physical existence.

Temporary fund. Name formerly given to *specific-purpose fund.*

Temporary investments. Investments, generally in marketable securities, which a hospital does not intend to hold for more than one year from the balance sheet date.

Term endowment funds. Donated funds which by the terms of the agreement become available either for any legitimate purpose designated by the governing board or for a specific purpose, designated by the donor, upon the happening of an event, or upon the passage of a stated period of time.

Term loan. A loan, generally obtained from a bank or insurance company, with a maturity period of more than one year. Term loans are generally amortized.

Trade credit. Debt arising from transactions in which supplies and services are purchased on credit from suppliers.

Trial balance. A list of the accounts in a ledger, with their balances, at a given date.

Unamortized bond discount (or premium). That portion of bond discount (or premium) that has not yet been amortized.

Unemployment taxes. Taxes levied by federal and state governments to finance payments to the unemployed.

Unexpended plant funds. *See* Plant replacement and expansion funds.

Unexpired cost. An asset. *See* Cost.

Unrestricted funds. Funds which bear no external restrictions as to use or purpose (i.e., funds which can be used for any legitimate purpose designated by the governing board, as distinguished from funds restricted externally for specific operating purposes, for plant replacement and expansion, and for endowment).

Useful life. An estimate made of the number of years an item of plant equipment will be used by a hospital.

Variable cost. A cost which varies directly in total with changes in the level of activity.

Voucher system. A system for the processing and control of cash disbursements.

Weighted-average costing. A method of determining the cost of supplies used and the valuation of inventory.

Working capital. Generally, the excess of current assets over current liabilities. Sometimes called *net working capital*.

Worksheet. A device used in accounting to facilitate the preparation of financial statements.

Yield. The actual rate of return on an investment, as opposed to the nominal rate of return.

Index